Dietary fibre perspectives — 1
reviews and bibliography

Edited by Anthony R. Leeds
Bibliographical editor Alison Avenell

Foreword by D. P. Burkitt

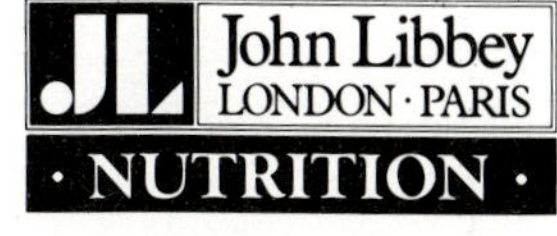

British Library Cataloguing in Publication Data:

Dietary fibre perspectives: reviews and bibliography 1.

1. Fiber in human nutrition—Bibliography
1. Leeds, Anthony. R   2. Avenell, Alison
016.6132'8   Z6663.N9

ISBN 0 86196 052 1

First published in 1985 by
John Libbey and Company Limited
80/84 Bondway, London SW8 1SF, England
(01) 582 5266

© 1985. Copyright. All rights reserved.

Unauthorised duplication contravenes applicable laws.

Typeset by Activity Limited, Salisbury, Wiltshire
Printed by Whitstable Litho Limited, Whitstable, Kent
Bound by Biddles Limited, Guildford, Surrey

Foreword

D. P. Burkitt

Nothing more dramatically illustrates the phenomenal growth of interest in dietary fibre which has been witnessed during the last 15 years than the explosive increase in scientific publications on the subject. Within a decade the annual rate of publications on the subject rose a remarkable 40-fold. A valuable contribution of this book is likely to be the carefully documented and chronologically arranged lists of references to scientific papers dealing with the nature and properties of fibre that appeared in numerous journals between the 16th century and the end of 1982.

This rapidly expanding field of medical and nutritional science more than justifies the production of what may for some appear just another book about which so much has already been written. The crucial importance of this work is that it consists largely of reviews and these are virtually essential for those who want to keep abreast of developments in this rapidly expanding field. The very fact that studies in dietary fibre have implications in almost every department, not only of human medicine and nutrition but also in veterinary practice, results in publications on the subject in so many journals dealing with varied disciplines that it is difficult for any individual to keep abreast of what is going on in the overall field.

Both the reviewers and their subjects have been well chosen. The function and properties of fibre in the large gut (Chapter 1) have from the outset assumed paramount importance and diseases of this organ are prominent amongst those recognized as characteristic of modern Western culture. Although fibre's relationship to lipid metabolism (Chapter 2) is less clear than is its effects on bowel content and behaviour its potential role is immeasurable in view of the overwhelming importance of cardiovascular disease to morbidity and mortality in more economically developed communities.

Since the management of diabetes and obesity has already been revolutionized through increased understanding of the role of fibre in the pathogenesis of these disorders, all doctors and nutritionists must want to know the progress already made and the direction in which mounting evidence is leading. Associated with the challenge of diabetes and obesity is the additional possibility of a role for dietary fibre in the treatment of gallstones (Chapters 3, 4, 5 and 6).

The change of direction witnessed in the introduction of diets rich in starch and fibre for diabetes and the allowance of liberal starch foods to the obese are comparable to the complete reversal of diets prescribed for diverticular disease of the colon. The clarification of misconceptions regarding the effects of fibre on mineral status (Chapter 7) is urgently necessary and relationships between fibre and food products (Chapter 8) brings studies that might appear of only theoretical interest down to practical fundamentals of eating practically.

There are many diseases characteristic of modern Western culture that can be reduced if, and only if, causative environmental factors can be identified and reduced. McKeown has recently expressed the opinion that this realization is comparable in magnitude to the realization in the 19th Century that the same applied to infective diseases and observations that dramatically reduced infections as killing diseases. Since it is now generally believed that diets with inadequate fibre are a major factor determining the emergence of Western diseases, the importance of a better and wider understanding of fibre could scarcely be exaggerated.

Contents

The Authors and Editors

Alison AVENELL
St Bartholomew's Hospital Medical College, West Smithfield, London EC1, England

D. P. BURKITT FRS
The Old House, Bussage, Near Stroud, Gloucestershire, England

P. R. ELLIS
Department of Food and Nutritional Sciences, Queen Elizabeth College (University of London), Campden Hill Road, London W8 7AH, England

Barbara F. HARLAND
Department of Human Nutrition and Food, School of Ecology, Howard University, Washington DC 20059, United States of America

Kenneth W. HEATON
Department of Medicine, Bristol University Medical School, British Royal Infirmary, Marlborough Street, Bristol, BS2 8HW, England

Patricia A. JUDD
Department of Food and Nutritional Sciences, Queen Elizabeth College (University of London), Campden Hill Road, London W8 7AH, England

Marcin KROTKIEWSKI
Department of Rehabilitation Medicine, Sahlgren's Hospital, University of Göteborg, S–413 45, Göteborg, Sweden

Anthony R. LEEDS
Department of Food and Nutritional Sciences, Queen Elizabeth College (University of London), Campden Hill Road, London W8 7AH, England

C. LEITZMANN
Institut für Ernährungswissenschaft der Justus-Liebig Universität, D–6 300 Giessen, Federal Republic of Germany

Eugene R. MORRIS
Research Chemist, United States Department of Agriculture, Agricultural Research Service, Human Nutrition Research Center, Beltsville, MD 20705, United States of America

David B. PETERSON
MRC Training Fellow in Nutrition, Diabetes Research Laboratories, University of Oxford, Radcliffe Infirmary, Woodstock Road, Oxford OX2 6HE, England

G. ROTH
Institut für Ernährungswissenschaft der Justus-Liebig Universität, D–6 300 Giessen, Federal Republic of Germany

Kjeld RYTTIG
Medical Department, Farma Food A/S, Copenhagen, Denmark

Ulf SMITH
Department of Medicine II, Sahlgren's Hospital, University of Göteborg, S–413 45 Göteborg, Sweden

Hugh C. TROWELL
Windhover, Woodgreen, Near Fordingbridge, Hants SP6 2AZ, England

A. Stewart TRUSWELL
Department of Nutrition, University of Sydney, Sydney, NSW 2006, Australia

Introduction

Fibre perspectives has been designed and produced as a starting point for those with an interest in dietary fibre and as a desk-top handbook for checking literature sources for those with a long-standing interest. It arises out of the evident usefulness to my own students of Hugh Trowell's bibliography produced in 1978. Initially we produced annual bibliographies, published separately in the Journal of Plant Foods, in each case delaying preparation until at least 18 month after the end of the year in question in order to produce a complete rather than partial bibliography. In all cases the bulk of the work was done by Alison Avenell, while Hugh Trowell and I made observations at various stages. By 1983 it seemed reasonable to reprint all of the bibliographies, with corrections and addenda, as the separate items might not be widely available. In order to broaden the scope of the work I invited colleagues and fellow scientists to contribute short review essays, limited in total number in order to restrict the size of the book, thus keeping the final cost down and giving *Fibre perspectives* a better chance of wider availability.

Great care has been taken to correct the bibliographies, but inevitably mistakes will still be present. If readers feel inclined to help I would appreciate being told of errors as those would then be corrected in the next edition.

The method of use of the bibliography is probably clear with little explanation. The grey bars on the right lateral edges of the relevant pages mark the start of the subject indexes (bars on the upper half of the page) and the start of the author indexes (bars on the lower half of the page). Having extracted references for the period up to the end of 1982, you need then run your computer search only for the years 1983 to the present time.

There is an Index to the reviews at the back of the book, prepared with help from my wife, Jacqueline – thus we take responsibility for any errors and inadequacies. Many individuals have helped bring this work to publication – I am grateful to all of them, named and unnamed.

The initial excitement, perhaps over-excitement, with the topic of dietary fibre has now disappeared and we are at the stage where many individuals are carrying out sound, steady work. Since the subject is young, and the experimental procedures sometimes quite difficult it will take another decade or so of work before we really feel confident about the role of fibre in the widely differing areas of health where its involvement has been suggested.

If this publication causes a slight acceleration in the rate of accumulation of knowledge about fibre I shall be content.

Kings College London
4 July 1985

Anthony R. Leeds

The editors and publishers gratefully acknowledge the generous support given by the Kellogg Company of Great Britain Ltd to sustain the original publication of Dr Hugh C. Trowell's 'Dietary fibre in human nutrition: a bibliography'. We thank the Kellogg Company of Great Britain for permisson to include it here — as pages 107-167.

1
Fibre and the large gut

G. Roth and C. Leitzmann

Introduction

Of the numerous effects ascribed to dietary fibre in human nutrition, none are as obvious as those on the large gut. Almost every measurable incident which occurs in the large bowel is affected by fibre. This applies among others to faecal bulk and constituents; transit time, stool frequency and colonic motility; microflora and associated fibre digestibility, production of gas and short-chain fatty acids; various diseases.

Effect of fibre on faecal bulk and constituents

The effects of fibre on bowel habits are well known, ie shortened transit time, altered colonic metabolism and increased faecal output. Recent studies have led to additional interpretations of the role of fibre in the colon (Cummings, 1982), focusing on the large variation of fibre from different plant foods and its different reactions in individuals despite similar fibre intakes. Comparisons of *in-vitro* and *in-vivo* effects of different sources of fibre showed an inverse relation between water-holding capacity and stool weight; bran and bagasse produced the largest increase whereas pectin led to virtually no change in stool weight (Stephen & Cummings, 1979). The inadequacy of *in-vitro* measurements of water-holding capacity for predicting water contents of stools was shown by different preparations of soya pulp or fibre, with very high water-holding capacities *in vitro*, which had no effect on the mean percentage water content of the faeces (Schweitzer, 1983).

The ability of certain foods to increase stool weight decreases in the following order: carrots, cabbage, sugar beet pulp, peas and wheat bran (Eastwood, 1978). The water-holding capacities of cell wall preparations from potato, banana and bran are about 2–3 g water/g, while fibre from cucumber, carrot, and lettuce holds 20–24 g water/g (Cummings, 1982). The ingestion of 20 g fibre in the form of bran, cabbage, apple and guar gum increased stool weight by 127, 59, 40 and 20 per cent respectively. The pentose fraction of the noncellulosic polysaccharides of fibre is most closely related to changes in stool weight; the greater the amount of pentose, the greater the increase in faecal weight (Cummings *et al.*, 1978; Selvendran, 1984).

The pentose hypothesis cannot be used as the only explanation for differences in stool weight, however, since identical intakes of pentose in fibre fed at different particle sizes lead to different stool weights. Coarse rather than fine bran was most effective in promoting bulkier stools of high moisture content (Heller *et al.*, 1980; Wrick *et al.*, 1983). Potatoes, turnips, cauliflower, and rhubarb did not increase stool weights in contrast to bran, carrots, oranges, apples, potatoes, Brussels sprouts and spring cabbage (Eastwood, 1978, Eastwood *et al.*, 1983). Fibre of sufficiently large particle size ensures an intact cell wall structure and sufficient lignification to resist extensive fermentation of cell wall constituents. This is most effective in promoting bulkier stools of high moisture; it also ensures more frequent defecation (Wrick *et al.*, 1983).

Since faecal output varies considerably from one person to another, variables other than diet alone must determine stool production (Schweizer *et al.*, 1983). Water-holding capacity is altered rapidly by bacterial fermentation, which depends on the digestibility of the fibre and individual intestinal transit time, those with the slowest transit time having the lowest stool weights (Cummings *et al.*, 1978). The age of subjects showed no effect on transit time, faecal constituents and stool weight; however, faecal output is associated with an increase in faecal constituents (Eastwood *et al.*, 1982).

Bacteria are made up of about 80 per cent water and play an important role in the water-holding capacity of the gut (Stephen & Cummings, 1980). The dry matter in stools consists of minerals, fats, carbohydrates and nitrogen-containing compounds; the amount of carbohydrates depends on the transit time (Wiggins, 1983). On a control diet faecal solids were made up of 55 per cent bacteria, 17 per cent undigested fibre and 24 per cent water-soluble material. Digestible fibre causes an increase in faecal weight by stimulating bacterial growth. For example, cabbage — which is almost completely digested — produces a smaller increase in fibre excretion, but a greater increase in bacterial solids, than bran. The increase in bacterial solids almost completely explains the increase in faecal weight. Both stool output and intestinal transit time have been reported as significantly correlated with faecal bacterial mass ($r = 0.84$ and -0.80 respectively) (Stephen & Cummings, 1980).

Since stool weight also correlates with protein intake, it has been suggested that undigested protein should be considered part of the fibre composite (Nutrition Reviews, 1984; Saunders & Betschart, 1980). With cabbage fibre there was an increase of 63 per cent in the nitrogen excretion of the bacterial fraction, whereas with wheat fibre it increased only by 34 per cent; no nitrogen was detected from faeces during a fibre-free diet (Brauer, Slavin & Marlett, 1981).

Faecal substrate concentrations differ with the type of fibre. Lignin or lignin-rich fibre, such as the sequestering agent bagasse, increases the daily faecal loss of acid steroids and fatty acids while having no effect on neutral substances. Since bagasse causes an increase in faecal bulk, the faecal concentration of bile acids was similar to control values, while neutral steroids were diluted (Baird *et al.*, 1977; Story, Kritchevsky & Eastwood, 1979).

Gel-forming fibres, such as pectin or guar, are able to 'trap' substrates and therefore increase the faecal loss of acid steroids, neutral steroids, fat and amino acids such as tryptophan. Since the increase in faecal bulk is smaller than the increase in faecal loss of steroids, there is an increase in faecal concentration of both acid and neutral steroids (Hill, 1982*a*). Totally fermentable, non-gel-forming fibre, such as lactulose or mannitol, do not increase faecal loss of steroids or fat. However, they are potent faecal bulking agents and thus cause a nonspecific reduction of the faecal concentration of acid steroids, fats and neutral steroids (Hill, 1982*a*).

4

Cereal fibre causes no additional loss of faecal steroids so that their concentration is reduced in proportion to the increase in stool bulk (Hill, 1982*a*; Stephen & Cummings, 1980). These findings apply particularly to wheat bran, whereas oatmeal behaves differently having a greater effect on faecal bile acid loss (Kay, 1981).

Consumption of 15–30 g fibre, as an addition to the amount present in the usual diet, is probably sufficient to achieve the desired effects on faecal bulk and stool softness (Dwyer *et al.*, 1979). The minimal faecal weight to ensure transit times of 2 days or less is about 120 g/day (Spiller *et al.*, 1982).

Effect of fibre on transit time, stool frequency and colonic motility

Qualitative changes in bowel function related to fibre are, among others: softer stools, decreased intestinal transit time (ITT), and greater frequency of bowel movements (Connell, 1978; Devroede, 1978; Smith, 1982; Wienbeck and Erckenbrecht, 1982).

Measurements of intestinal transit time

Modern measurements of ITT use radio opaque markers that can be counted in the stool by X-rays. The original method defined ITT as the time taken for at least 80 per cent of the markers to be excreted (Hinton, Lennard-Jones & Young, 1969). Other methods use dyes such as carmine, ball bearings and gravel, radioactive chromic oxide, radio pills or chromium sesquioxide (Connell, 1981; Mathers & Blake, 1983; Van Soest, Uden & Wrick, 1983). Time between ingestion and the excretion of a nonabsorbable dye is perhaps the easiest method to assess gut transit, although faecal concentration cannot be easily determined, and dyes may not be visible in faecal samples from constipated subjects (Marlett, Slavin & Brauer, 1981). The simple measurement of ITT using foods with intense colours (blueberries, beets) remains a reliable standby (Roth & Leitzmann, 1983).

Because of the variability of the radio opaque method as used in single studies, Cummings, Jenkins & Wiggin (1976) introduced the measurement of 'mean transit time' (MTT) by giving a small dose of marker to subjects with each meal continuously over a period of weeks; the range of MTT in their studies was from 20 to 145 h. With a typical South Indian diet including 30–40 g fibre/d MTT was lower (33 ± 9 h) than on those reported in Western countries (Shetty & Kurpad, 1983).

Marlett *et al.* (1981) did not agree that MTT is a more reproducible method than ITT. Their results suggested that the variation observed with ITT (method of Hinton *et al.*, 1969) is a genuine biological variation in colonic function and that the more complicated measurement of MTT does little to reduce this variation (Marlett *et al.*, 1981; Wyman *et al.*, 1976).

Factors that influence intestinal transit time

Several factors influence ITT: the act of defecation, suppression of the urge to defecate, sudden emotional stress, exercise and — probably the most important — the diet itself. Foods that contain specific cathartics such as prunes or rhubarb have an obvious effect. The fibre content of food seems to be the most important variable in decreasing ITT, but the effect of fibre on faecal weight is even more obvious

5

(Connell, 1981). No significant effect on ITT of dietary protein level (Cummings *et al.*, 1979*a*), or of phases of the menstrual cycle, was noticed (Wyman *et al.*, 1976).

The results after ingestion of different fibres on ITT showed that foods can be ranked in descending order as follows: bran, mango, carrot, apple, lettuce, winter cabbage, peas, cauliflower, banana, potato and turnip (Mitchell & Eastwood, 1976). Although increasing the fibre content of the diet usually decreased ITT, no effect was observed when cellulose or Solka Floc (a refined cellulose product extracted from woodpulp) was ingested (Slavin & Marlett, 1980) while Solka Floc with a pectin supplement lowered ITT (Spiller *et al.*, 1980). The failure of cellulose to decrease ITT significantly in healthy women indirectly supports the suggestion that physiological amounts of fibre alter ITT only when it is very short or very long (Marlett *et al.*, 1981).

It is assumed that ITT is the result rather than the cause of colonic events. However, there is also some evidence that ITT itself influences events in the large gut and that it may not be the effect of a particular diet or environmental factor. That ITT is an independent factor modifying colonic function can be demonstrated by changing ITT. By slowing ITT pharmacologically stool weight was decreased, and conversely, by speeding it up, stool weight was increased (Stephen & Cummings, 1980). Faster transit is thus associated with the incomplete metabolism of fibre and ITT determines how an individual will respond to identical amounts of fibre.

Stool composition and frequency
Fibre's effects on stool composition and stool frequency do not parallel effects of ITT, ie stool water content is neither a function of ITT nor of fibre level, but of the fibre source. A delayed ITT does not necessarily cause hard dry stools, as can be seen with vegetable fibre which induce a sufficiently large microbial mass that has a high water content (Wrick, 1983). If colonic transit is influenced by fibre without a change in stool frequency, but correlates well with stool weight, this may imply that the size of the bowel and the length of segment emptied at defecation are factors involved. Frequency of bowel contraction is greater on the left side of the large gut than on the right side, thereby creating conditions of storage within the right colon (Devroede, 1978).

Apparent digestibility of fibre
Fibre from mixed diets, bran, pectin and guar are substantially digested during passage through the gut. The site of digestion by bacteria is considered to be the right colon (Cummings & Stephen, 1980). Many of the effects of fibre in the colon relate to the fact that it is extensively broken down in this part of the gut. Since this fibre breakdown is an anaerobic process, it should be called fermentation. The degree of digestion depends on the constituents and amount of fibre, ITT, particle size, the extent and kind of processing before ingestion, and the degree of lignification (Cummings, 1984; Slavin, Brauer & Marlett, 1981).

The different methods employed to determine the amount of fibre being digested give different results. The 'Neutral detergent fibre' method (NDF) of Van Soest — used by Dintzis *et al.* (1979); Farrell, Girle & Arthur (1978), Fetzer, Kies & Fox

6

(1979) and Holloway, Tasman Jones & Lee (1978) — does not remove starch from foodstuffs, and therefore, the amount of undigested nitrogen in faecal NDF is a possible source of error in digestibility measurements (Marlett & Lee, 1980; Nutrition Reviews, 1984). Slavin & coworkers (1981) determined the mean apparent NDF digestibility after correcting for protein contamination, as well as removing residual starch in NDF food residues by an alpha-amylase treatment of the NDF residue. Hemicellulose was calculated as NDF minus directly measured cellulose including lignin.

In most of the published studies only short-term digestibilty of fibre was assessed, without the time needed to adapt to a particular fibre intake. One month was regarded as an adequate time period for subjects to adapt to a particular fibre intake in order to examine changes in fibre digestibilty (Slavin et al., 1981). In a low cellulose diet containing fruits, vegetables (Prynne & Southgate, 1979) and refined grains more than half of the fibre was degraded, while the apparent digestibility of refined cellulose was minimal. Highly crystalline celluloses were much less susceptible to enzymatic breakdown than the cellulose present in fruit and vegetable cell walls (Cummings, 1982). Studies with ruminants indicated that cellulose digestion may proceed for up to 48 h, supporting a similar concept for man (Cummings et al., 1979b).

Digestion of water-insoluble fibre was about 80 per cent when a low fibre diet was consumed (Farrell et al., 1978; Holloway et al., 1978) but decreased when bran or cellulose supplements were added (Farrell et al., 1978; Slavin et al., 1981). Pectin was completely fermented in the gut by all subjects (Cummings et al., 1979b).

There was no relationship between fibre digestibility and ITT with pectin (Cummings et al., 1979b), but when more than 50 per cent of fibre was digested on a low cellulose diet, digestibility and ITT were related (Slavin et al., 1981). Apparent digestibility of fibre was found to be related also to fibre particle size (Dintzis et al., 1979; Heller et al., 1980). Reduction in particle size increased the digestibility of cellulose and hemicellulose, indicating a greater digestibility of the finely ground than of the coarse bran (Ehle, Robertson & Van Soest, 1982; Heller et al., 1980).

In contrast to polysaccharide fibres, the breakdown of lignin is an aerobic process which, contrary to expectation, does occur in the anaerobic regions of the large gut. The more lignified a cell wall or plant structure (wheat bran), the less liable it is to fermentation in the gut. Lignin inhibits the fermentation of the polysaccharide fibres to a certain extent (Cummings, 1982; Dwyer et al., 1979).

The three main end-products of fermentation are short-chain fatty acids, various gases and energy (Cummings, 1982). These products may be absorbed, may alter the chemical environment of the colon, or may exert a specific physiological action, ie promote peristalsis (Eastwood & Kay, 1979).

Effect of fibre on the microflora of the large gut
Efforts to identify and quantify the microflora of the intestine have been complicated by the difficulties associated with maintaining strictly anaerobic conditions during the aquisition of samples and their culturing. Many researchers have cultured faecal samples, assuming that this material is representative of the colonic contents. But the number of microbes in the intra-abdominal colon (10^9/g) are less than in faeces (10^{11}/g) (Fleming & Calloway, 1983). From faecal studies it

appears that the five major genera of the colon are *Bacteroides, Eubacteria, Bifidobacteria, Peptostreptococci* and *Fusobacteria* (Salyers, 1979). Of these, the *Bacteroides* are thought to account for about one-third of the total organisms.

Bacteroides are strict anaerobes capable of fermenting complex carbohydrates including starch, cellulose, xylans, pectins, galactomannans and mucins or glycoproteins (Bryant, 1978; Decker & Palmer, 1981). It has been suggested that gastrointestinal movements and secretions, such as mucins and bile acids, are able to control the activity of *Bacteroides* and that anger/stress situations can influence their dominance in relationship to the total microflora (Fleming & Calloway, 1983; Moore, Cato & Holdeman, 1978). *Bacteroides*, which produce hydrogen, formate, acetate, propionate, butyrate, succinate and lactate, are involved in bile acid transformation and able to form the potential carcinogen indole from tryptophan.

To simplify the metabolic activities of intestinal flora, bacteria are divided into three major groups (Smith & Bryant, 1979): the first group consists mainly of fermentative bacteria, converting complex carbohydrates to short-chain fatty acids (SCFA) and carbon dioxide hydrogen, and hydrolysing proteins and lipids to similar products plus branched-chain and aromatic amino acids. The second group comprises obligate hydrogen-forming acetogenic aromatic bacteria which ferment fatty acids and many of the aromatic compounds to hydrogen, acetate and carbon dioxide. The third group consists of methanogenic bacteria that cleave acetate to methane and carbon dioxide and reduce carbon dioxide to methane using electrons derived from oxidation of hydrogen. Products from one group can obviously be utilised as substrates by another group.

Effects of fibre on bacterial metabolism can be discussed under three headings: (a) the effect of fibre on substrate concentration (see 'Effect of fibre on faecal bulk and constituents' at the beginning of this chapter); (b) the influence of fibre on intestinal physiology and consequently on bacterial enzyme activity, and, (c) the effect of the products of fibre metabolism on bacterial enzyme action (Hill, 1982*a*; Van Soest, 1984).

The suggestion that fibre may modify bacterial enzyme activity by modifying the composition of the flora itself was investigated by measuring the activity of 'sentinel enzymes' like β-glucoronidase or azoreductase; reports of sentinel enzyme activity changes have come mainly from animal studies. In human studies faeces showed a large day-to-day variation in enzyme activity but little evidence of any effect of diet (Hill, 1982*a*).

Short-term changes in the diet have produced no recognisable change in the faecal bacterial flora. Only studies of populations from different countries, consuming widely different diets, looked likely to reveal differences in faecal flora. As most of the activity of the intestinal flora is carried out in the right colon, nutrition is more likely to have an effect on this part. The value of measurements of faecal flora has been questioned because a number of studies showed that big changes in the physiology of the right colon revealed only small differences in faecal physiology (Hill, 1982*b*).

Faecal flora remain largely constant even with added fibre. Although the daily faecal mass is doubled, bacterial content per gram of faeces remains unchanged. Thus the total number of bacteria excreted daily per gram of human faeces is directly related to fibre intake (Bornside, 1978). The constancy of faecal microflora can be disrupted by oral administration of certain antibiotics, but afterwards faecal flora returns to its original level within a few days (Bornside, 1978).

A decrease of intestinal flora occurs on starvation, but the small amount of faeces that is produced monthly is qualitatively and quantitatively similar (Finegold & Sutter, 1978). Therefore, it seems very likely that utilization of mucins and endogenous substances is responsible for the stability of the flora (Salyers, 1979). Although species composition of the colonic microflora is not significantly affected by diet (Ruckdeschel, 1980) changes in diet may produce changes in the metabolic activities of the flora by inducing enzymes. This may be achieved by monitoring the response of intestinal flora to changes in diet using enzyme assays (Salyers, 1979).

Since bacteria grow preferentially on solid surfaces, rather than freely suspended in fluids, there are high concentrations of both substrates and bacterial enzymes at the matrix surface of fibre. The effect of this increase in surface area of the colonic contents on bacterial enzyme activity has not been studied, but would undoubtedly yield interesting results (Hill, 1982*a*).

In general, bacterial metabolism is affected by the concentration of steroids in the bile, the flow rate of bile, the ITT, and the site and rate of absorption (Bokkenheuser *et al.*, 1978). Bacterial enzymes metabolizing steroids tend to have pH optima close to 7; in particular, the 7-alpha-dehydroxylase that produces lithocholic acid from chenodeoxycholic acid and deoxycholic acid from cholic acid has greatly reduced activity at acid pH. Lactulose might greatly reduce the extent of bile acid metabolism to the dehydroxylated products (Thornton & Heaton, 1980).

ITT has generally been assumed to be the major factor in determining the extent to which a substrate is metabolized by bacterial enzymes. But this does not hold true for the extent of reduction of cholesterol, bran, fibrogel, pectin and guar (Hill, 1982*b*). Since metabolism of cholesterol to coprostanol by bacteria is facile, while lactulose, pectin and guar are readily metabolized to fatty acids and carbon dioxide, bacteria have little effect on the proportion of cholesterol undergoing reduction in the colon (Hill, 1982*b*). In contrast a correlation was shown between ITT and the amount of urinary volatile phenol produced by bacterial metabolism of tyrosine (Cummings *et al.*, 1979*a*).

Adsorption of bacteria to fibre may prevent or alter bacterial metabolism of the latter. Fermentation by bacteria alters chemically active groups on the fibre molecule and modifies physical structure, thus altering important physiological effects (Eastwood & Kay, 1979).

Gases produced by the microflora of the large gut
Gases produced by organisms may diffuse into the blood for expiration in breath, or may be expelled through the rectum as flatus. Thus, breath gas composition can be used as an indicator of intestinal gas composition (Fleming & Calloway, 1983; Wolever *et al.*, 1983). Breath hydrogen concentrations have been reported as elevated following consumption of soybeans, California small white beans, lima beans and mung beans (Fleming & Calloway, 1983). The gas producing oligosaccharides (raffinose and stachyose) are constituents of legume seeds (Tadesse & Eastwood, 1978), some cereal brans (Bond & Levitt, 1978) and some

purified food fibres including pectin (Marthinsen & Fleming, 1982). Oat bran or oat gum did not increase breath hydrogen excretion (Marthinsen & Fleming, 1982).

The volume and composition of flatus are also influenced by the diet. The former depends on many factors including anxiety and stress. The composition of flatus is determined by endogenous secretions, the microbial population and the substrates available for fermentation (Fleming & Calloway, 1983). Generally, hydrogen production increases on high-fibre diets ; xylan and pectin ingestion results in a higher flatus volume of hydrogen and carbon dioxide. The period of microbial and enzymatic adaption seems to be 3–5 days, because relatively constant levels of gas excretion were obtained thereafter (Marthinsen & Fleming, 1982).

Short-chain fatty acids produced by the microflora

Short-chain fatty acids (SCFA) were believed to increase stool weight because of possible poor absorption from the colon and water retention by osmosis. However, recent work has shown that SCFA are absorbed from the human colon, as they are in all animals, its rate of absorption being dependent on their concentration (Ruppin *et al.*, 1980). SCFA may exert effects perhaps by stimulating mucus secretion or by affecting colonic motility (Cummings & Stephen, 1980). They are absorbed with an attendant stimulation of the absorption of salt (net Na^+) and water (Cummings, 1981) and by accumulating bicarbonate ions (McNeil *et al.*, 1978; Ruppin *et al.*, 1980). These bicarbonate ions are considered responsible for maintaining a relatively constant pH within the lumenal contents, even when large quantities of SCFA are being produced.

Different results were obtained with lactulose, where the local concentration of SCFA is sufficient to cause a fall in the pH to about 4.8 in the caecum and ascending colon. This can be used for preventing ammonia intoxification as the acid pH would provide a gradient against which ammonia (NH_4^+) could not be absorbed (Hill, 1982*a*). Since no increased faecal concentration of ammonia occurred, it was suggested that products of lactulose metabolism are utilized in the synthesis of new bacterial mass (Stephen & Cummings, 1980).

Although some of the absorbed SCFA appears in the blood and is metabolized as an energy source (Smith & Bryant, 1979), it appears that a large proportion of these SCFA is metabolized by the gut epithelium and does not appear in the blood (Fleming & Rodriguez, 1983). If SCFA are absorbed and are used as energy by the host, the extent to which these fibres can supply energy via their fermentation can be calculated. When excretion is directly proportional to the lumenal concentration of SCFA, it can be assumed that excretion is a relative indicator of absorption (Fleming & Rodriguez, 1983). Following absorption into the mucosal cell, SCFA particular butyrate provide an important source of energy for the colonic mucosa. Acetate and propionate are transported directly to the liver, where they are available for energy metabolism in the usual way (Roediger, 1980; 1982).

It is tempting to conclude that the substrate fermented to yield SCFA is the fibre component of the diet, if this is the only dietary ingredient being changed. However, interactions among dietary components must be considered, because

10

the presence of fibre may reduce the digestibility of an otherwise completely digestible component (Fleming & Rodriguez, 1983; McNeil, 1984).

Diseases of the large gut associated with lack of fibre

The fibre hypothesis formulated by Burkitt and coworkers (see Introductory chapter) draws particularly upon epidemiological data on the association of the lack of fibre in the diet of populations in industrialised countries and Western diseases of the large gut. There has been a dramatic increase in these diseases parallel with a reduction of fibre in the human diet. Some of these diseases can easily be treated, or are completely healed, given an adequate consumption of fibre; others are only difficult to reverse. Since most of these diseases take many years to develop the literature mainly comprises reports of retrospective epidemiological studies. A summary follows of the recent findings for common diseases of the large gut associated with a lack of fibre in the diet.

Constipation

Constipation due to lack of fibre in food is one of the commonest gastroenterological symptoms. It can be defined as the infrequent passage of small hard stools, passed with difficulty and sometimes accompanied by a feeling of incomplete emptying of the rectum (Brodribb, 1983). Most feeding studies suggest that for every gram of extra cereal fibre consumed, mean wet weight of stool increases from 3–9 g (Brodribb, 1983). In a carefully controlled study the mean increase in stool weight was 4.1 g/g of added fibre for coarse wheat bran (resistant to fermentation), as compared to 1.9 g/g when fruit and vegetables (highly fermentable) were used (Stasse-Wolthuis *et al.*, 1980). Cooked wheat bran had a reduced stool-bulking capacity, probably due to structural alterations leading to greater bacterial degradation (Wyman *et al.*, 1976). It has been reported that frequency, stool consistency, abdominal pain and signs of venous stasis improved after treatment for 4 weeks with ispaghula husk (Borgia *et al.*, 1983). Increasing wheat bran intake for 6 months in persons with diverticular disease improved both excessive frequency and infrequency of defecation (Brodribb, 1983).

Infants between the ages of 6 and 16 months suffering from constipation show normal bowel movements after a month of a diet containing bran. At the same time a decrease in blood levels of calcium, phosphate, and trace elements occurred, indicating that bran should be used in infancy with extreme caution (Zoppi *et al.*, 1982). Little doubt exists that lack of fibre, inactivity and old age exacerbate the problem of constipation. Patients with simple constipation, ie without associated disease, often have excessive segmenting movements of the colon, which restrict the passage of stool, or appear to have reduced peristaltic movements. The mechanisms that control this smooth muscle activity are not yet well understood (Lancaster-Smith & Williams, 1982).

Depending on individual physio-anatomical differences, it appears that 150 to 300 g/d of faeces are needed to prevent constipation; very little decrease in ITT is found after the 300 g/d faecal weight level is reached (Spiller; 1982*a*).

Diverticular disease

Diverticular disease (DD) is characterized by constipation or diarrhoea,

11

flatulence, abdominal pain, colicky pain, mucus and blood in the stools, and tenesmus. The physiological basis of the formation of diverticula is a rise in pressure in a given segment of the colon, predominantly the sigmoid, favoured by the gastrocolic reflex (Almy & Howell, 1980; Heinkel, 1983).

DD has been linked with low fibre intake in developed Western countries, and conversely, low prevalence of DD among vegetarians in developed countries has been attributed to their high intake of fibre, particularly of cereal origin (Gear *et al.*, 1979; Hasik *et al.*, 1982). The changes of fibre intake since 1945 in the Japanese diet resemble the pattern of the rapid decline that took place in the United States during the period of the 1930s to the 1950s. Although the prevalence of DD is still relatively low in Japan, it shows signs of a sudden steep rise, mainly because of a decline in consumption of fibre from cereals. In Japanese diverticula are predominantly (75 per cent) located in the ascending or right colon, while among Westerners they are found overwhelmingly along the left side of the colon, suggesting a genetic factor (Ohi *et al.*, 1983).

Fibre reduces intracolonic pressure and spasm. These features are important in treating DD, in which the colon tends to become narrow with increased spasm. Although there is still some controversy due to deficiencies in methodology, about whether fibre reduces these symptoms, evidence has been reported that 60 per cent of all symptoms were abolished and a further 28 per cent relieved after 6 months on a high fibre diet (Brodribb, 1983).

Cereal fibre is poorly digested by colonic bacteria, has maximal effect in increasing stool weight and reducing ITT, is empirically used in the treatment of symptomatic DD and may be most effective in protection against DD (Ohi *et al.*, 1983). Coarse wheat bran (15–30 g/d) reduces both pressure and symptoms. Fine or processed bran is less effective (Smith, Drummond & Eastwood, 1981). Thus coarse wheat bran may be the therapy of choice in uncomplicated DD (Kay, 1982). Diets rich in coarse wheat bran, apples, oranges and currants have been recommended (Eastwood, 1978; Hyland & Taylor, 1980), while others have concluded that dietary measures are probably harmless and may do some good (Connell, 1978; Mendeloff, 1978). Significant differences in objective measurements, such as increased stool weight and increased stool frequency, were achieved in 59 patients consuming bran crispbread of ispaghula husk for 4 months; however, it was not possible to demonstrate an improvement in the whole spectrum of symptoms of DD (Ornstein, 1981, Ornstein *et al.*, 1981).

Irritable bowel syndrome

Irritable Bowel Syndrome (IBS) affects the entire gastrointestinal tract and is probably a result of an inappropriate reaction of the gastrointestinal muscles to stress and to physical factors in the gut, of which deficiency of fibre is only one component (Eastwood & Passmore, 1983). A bacterial rather than an immunological mechanism has been suggested as underlining IBS (Bayliss *et al.*, 1984) and motility disturbances, psychiatric disorders and dietary deficiencies have been discussed as causes (Floch, 1981). Although a subjective improvement and a reduction in colonic motor activity in subjects treated with wheat bran has been reported (Manning *et al.*, 1977), others failed to document an ameliorative effect (Hill, 1983; Soltoft *et al.*, 1976). Bran may be particularly serviceable among soothing substances which can be administered to counter the peristaltic reflex after eating which triggers the occurrence of the painful symptoms of IBS. Since the main causes of IBS are of a psychological nature, the problem does not lie only in the gut. Nevertheless early therapy, including proper dietary intake with plenty of fibre to relax the colon, is called for, if muscle hypertrophy and spasm are to be avoided (Heinkel, 1983). Fibre alone should not be the therapeutic agent, since studies showed that a combination of a tranquilliser, antispasmodic, and bulking agent such as ispaghula husk, were more effective in treating IBS than any single agent or pair of agents (Ritchie & Truelove, 1979; Fielding, 1982).

Inflammatory bowel disease
The term inflammatory bowel disease is widely used to describe two diseases of unknown aetiology, namely ulcerative colitis and Crohn's disease (Heaton, 1981). Fibre appears to have no specific therapeutic value in ulcerative colitis, but it may reduce recurrence in Crohn's disease (Heaton, Thornton & Emmett, 1979*b*). Elemental diets with low fibre content are recommended in both diseases, to calm down the colon segment (Kasper, 1982; Levin, 1982), and to minimize the amount of ileostomy fluid (Hori, Hudson & Hill, 1983). There is some evidence that if there is a stricture ie in Crohn's disease, a high fibre diet may be contraindicated (Eastwood & Passmore, 1983).

Refined sugar intake was higher in Crohn's disease patients before they became ill than in matched controls (Heaton, 1981; Heaton *et al.*, 1979*a,b*; Kasper & Sommer, 1979; Martini & Brandes, 1976; Miller, 1982; Miller *et al.*, 1976; Thornton, Emmett & Heaton, 1979). This raises the possibility that refined carbohydrates promote the development of the disease but this need not necessarily be linked to a reduced fibre intake. Heaton (1981) showed that although neither cereal fibre nor cooked vegetable fibre intake were markedly different, there was a marked lack in the intake of raw fruit and vegetable fibre in Crohn's disease patients. When a diet providing 33 g fibre/d was given to these patients, even if they had strictures, the results of this full-fibre diet were beneficial and not detrimental (Heaton, 1981).

Bile acids have been linked with Crohn's disease but were not found to be involved in the inflammatory process (Kurtz *et al.*, 1981). A positive correlation found in England between eating cornflakes and Crohn's disease (James, 1977) was not confirmed by others (Mayberry, Rhodes & Newcombe, 1980; Thornton *et al.*, 1979). A fibre-rich, unrefined carbohydrate diet (Heaton *et al.*, 1979; 1981), as well as a low carbohydrate diet excluding refined sugar (Brandes & Lorenz-Meyer, 1981; Kasper, 1982), appears to have a favourable effect on the course of Crohn's disease. A large double–blind trial is in progress to resolve this apparent contradiction (Hill, 1983).

Cancer
Epidemiological and laboratory evidence suggests that a high intake of total fat increases susceptibility to cancer, including colon cancer. Fruits and vegetables, especially cruciferous vegetables (such as cabbage, broccoli, Brussels sprouts, cauliflower) appear to be associated with a decrease in the incidence of cancer (Palmer & Bakshi, 1983). It was shown that ovolactovegetarians and strict vegetarians had lower levels of faecal mutagens than nonvegetarians (Kuhnlein *et*

al., 1981). Besides fibre these vegetables contain potential protective compounds such as isothiocyanates, flavones, indoles, protease inhibitors, β-sitosterol and naturally occurring phenols (Palmer & Bakshi, 1983).

The incidence of colon cancer in Denmark and New York is higher than in England, although the per capita fat intake of these three populations is similar and a higher intake of dietary fibre is not observed in England. However, higher intake of fibre-containing foods appears to be the dietary factor associated with low risk of colon cancer in populations such as that of Finland (Reddy *et al.*, 1978).

There are several postulated mechanisms whereby fibre may protect against large-bowel cancer. Increasing the bulk of faeces by fibre dilutes potentially noxious substances in the bowel. Increasing fibre intake has been shown to decrease ITT which is closely related to the effect that a particular fibre exerts on faecal output (Cummings & Branch, 1982). Slower transit allows more time for gut bacteria to degrade intraluminal components, to produce carcinogens and to enable such carcinogens to act (Reddy, 1982). The stimulation of microbial growth, which is seen when fibre is fed, or when ITT is speeded up, has a number of important implications (Cummings & Branch, 1982). The adsorption by fibre of harmful substances such as bile acids could be important, as could alterations of colonic pH towards the acid side by the production of SCFA due to bacterial digestion of fibre (Spiller & Freeman, 1981).

It is very difficult to generalize about the diluting effect of fibre since most studies are carried out with faeces, which may not reflect changes in the caecum and right colon. The protective role of fibre can, therefore, be assessed only indirectly. There are some types of fibre that may cause a fall in the concentration of substances in faeces, such as carcinogens, bile acids, SCFA and ammonia (Cummings & Branch, 1982). It was shown that faecal bile acid concentrations were increased both in subjects with carcinoma of the colon and in populations with an increased risk of large-bowel cancer (Hill *et al.*, 1975; Reddy, 1982). Concentrations of bile acids greater than 6 mg/g faecal solids signify an increased risk. Low fibre diets allow greater conversion of bile salts to potential carcinogens, and thus bile acids in high-incidence countries are much more degraded (Bornside, 1978).

Adding wheat fibre to the diet decreased the concentration of faecal bile acids and neutral steroids because of the bulking effect of fibre, whereas the addition of pectin to the diet increased the faecal steroid and bile acid output (Kay, 1981). It is apparent that the faecal excretion of bile acids varies with the type and amount of fibre (Reddy, 1982). To date, however, no active carcinogen derived from bile acids has been isolated from human faeces and, therefore, the effect of bile acids on bowel formation of tumours of the bowel is not fully resolved (Palmer & Bakshi, 1983).

The relation between fibre consumption and carcinogens has been studied in experimental animals using 3-methyl-4-aminobiphenyl, 3-methyl-2-naphthylamine, cycasin and methylazoxymethanol and their derivates such as azoxymethane and 1,2-dimethylhydrazine, methylnitrosourea or N-methyl-N'-nitro-N-nitrosoguanidine and 3-methylcholanthrene. The data have been reviewed by Reddy (1982).

Some correlation data supported the hypothesis that fibre itself protects against large bowel cancer (MacLennan *et al.*, 1978). Other results suggested an inverse

14

correlation of the pentosan content and mortality from colon cancer (Bingham *et al.*, 1979). Bran and cellulose was found to protect against 1,2-dimethylhydrazine-induced (DMH) tumours (Freeman, Spiller & Kim, 1980; Trudel, Senterman & Brown, 1983), but not against tumours induced by azoxymethane of N-nitroso-N-methylurea (Watanabe *et al.*, 1978).

At colonic pH, a greater percentage of DMH was bound by wheat bran than by citrus pulp or pectin. Therefore, it is possible that certain fibres bind carcinogens at colonic pH, thus making it unavailable for contact with the colonic mucosa. Soluble fibres such as pectin do not bind DMH, but may modify the metabolism of carcinogens in the liver and/or in the colonic mucosa (Smith-Barbaro *et al.*, 1981). Chemicals formed during the cooking of meat, for example the mutagen 2-amino-3-methylimidazo (4,5-*f*)-quinoline (IQ), were found to be bound to fibre. At pH 6.5 corn bran, wheat bran and alfalfa meals were able to bind approximately 50 per cent of the available IQ after incubation for 1 hour. The optimal binding occurred between pH 4–6, overlapping the pH range in the human gastrointestinal tract; binding was probably due to a cation-exchange mechanism. It is likely that the extent of IQ binding to fibre *in vivo* will be highly individual and dependent on the number of saccharolytic bacteria in the gut (Barnes, Maiello & Weisburger, 1983).

The major anions in the stool are SCFA, which remained unchanged when wheat fibre was added to the diet. Since concentrations of SCFA depend not only on their production, but also on their absorption in the colon, production rates and absorption of SCFA from the colon may be important in tumourigenesis, butyrate possibly having antitumour properties by lowering the concentration of free ammonia (Cummings & Branch, 1982). Ammonia is also a product of bacteria and has been linked to colonic tumour formation (Visek, 1978). Data show a decrease in faecal dialysate ammonia, in association with a decrease in ITT, in subjects given fibre from carrot, cabbage, apple, bran and guar (Cummings *et al.*, 1979*b*). The concentration of ammonia in faecal dialysate is dependent on production from urea and from protein by bacteria, absorption across the mucosa and incorporation into bacterial protein. It is probably the latter pathway that leads to an overall fall in ammonia, since fibre is known to stimulate microbial cell growth in the colon (Cummings & Branch, 1982; Stephen & Cummings, 1980; Wrong & Vince, 1984).

The metabolic activity of the gut microflora may be modified by dietary components eg microbial reduction by metronidazole is increased by pectin supplementation and decreased by carrageenan. Dietary pectin significantly increased the rate of reduction of p-nitrobenzoic acid and metronidazole in rats by increasing β-glucuronidase activity (Bauer *et al.*, 1979; Ross & Leklem, 1981; Wise, Marlett & Rowland, 1982). In contrast, carrageenan greatly decreased the activity of the microflora towards these substrates, but it was impossible to determine whether this effect was substrate-specific. This suggests that carrageenan decreases the toxicity of those nitrocompounds which depend on microbial nitroreduction for their toxic effects (Rowland *et al.*, 1983).

Faecal β-glucuronidase and mucinase are important enzymes of the colonic microflora which degrade protective mucins in the colon of rats and humans. Elevated levels were found to be associated with diets high in animal protein and fat, factors associated with increased risk of colon cancer. The enzyme β-glucuronidase is of interest because it hydrolizes biliary glucuronides when they reach the colon and mucinase is responsible for degrading the protective mucins of the colon. Fibre caused lower specific activities and less total output of these enzymes than did the fibre-free diet. This supports the hypothesis that fibre (guar, pectin, carrageenan) may reduce colon carcinogenesis by decreasing β-glucuronidase levels. Total daily output of mucinase was highest in rats fed fibre-free diets or cellulose and lower in rats fed more readily fermentable fibre such as pectin, guar or carrageenan (Shiau & Chang, 1983).

Other large-gut-associated diseases
A soft, formed stool, which can be passed easily without straining, usually produces an improvement in the symptoms resulting from haemorrhoids, anal fissures and perianal haematoma. These disorders are often precipitated by a period of constipation and thus a high fibre intake might be useful (Brodribb, 1983; Burkitt, 1981).

Straining by raising intra-abdominal pressures, has been postulated to be the major cause of hiatus hernia. The transmission of these pressures to the major veins draining the legs has been incriminated as an important cause of varicose veins. Consequently, fibre by removing the necessity to strain at stool may be considered protective against these diseases (Burkitt, 1981).

A comparison of food diaries from patients with acute appendicitis and control patients showed a significant difference in fibre intake. Results support the hypothesis that diet, in particular a lack of fibre, may be a determining factor in the pathogenesis of acute appendicitis (Arnbjörnsson, 1983; Burkitt, 1981).

Concluding remarks
Although a growing number of increasingly sophisticated experiments in the last few years have furthered our understanding of the interaction between fibre and the large gut, many questions remain and new ones have been added. Fibre and the large gut are highly complex structures, both of which are not fully understood in detail. However, despite the multi-faceted interactions most data so far support the simple dietary fibre hypothesis as put forward by Burkitt and Trowell about 15 years ago. Some of the recurring questions in the literature concentrate on the validity of employing isolated fibres, the use of data from animal experiments, analytical problems, individual variabilities in humans and a recommendation for the proper daily intake of fibre. These and other important points of discussion are reflected in recent publications.

The question arises, how useful are results if highly purified fibres such as pectin and cellulose are used in animal studies — should natural high-fibre products such as wheat bran, carrot powder and other nonpurified sources be employed instead?

Both approaches are probably important, but effects of highly purified fibre polymers must not be extrapolated to natural products and foods. On the other hand, there is a great problem in human studies due to the absence of agreement as to the way fibre analysis of foods should be presented and which method of analysis should be used. This lack of sufficient published data makes the task of the epidemiologist a difficult and often impossible one (Spiller, 1982*b*).

16

The effect a particular fibre has on colonic function depends on its digestibility and, thus, its physical and chemical composition. How these factors control digestion by the microflora has yet to be established in humans. The differing response of individuals to the same fibre source may relate to the characteristics of their colonic bacteria (Cummings & Stephen, 1980). The extreme variability of the anatomy and physiology of the alimentary tract in different mammalian species requires that these mechanisms be studied in humans (Wiggins, 1983).

Looking at total fibre intake, not only a quantitative decrease but also a qualitative change has occurred during the last 100 years. The decreased intake of cellulose- and lignin-rich foods such as cereals parallels an increased intake of pectin-containing fruits. Since fibres from cereals are regarded as more important because of their special physical properties, an increased consumption of fruit may not compensate for the decreased intake of cereal fibre. We have therefore recommended that fibre intake should be double its present level (20–25 g/d) and that the greater part of this should come from cereals (Leitzmann, 1983).

References

Almy T. P., Howell D. A. (1980): Diverticular disease of the colon. *New Engl. J. Med.* **302**, 324–331.

Arnbjörnsson E. (1983): Acute appendicitis and dietary fiber. *Arch. Surg.* **118**, 868–870.

Baird I. M., Walters R. L., Davies P. S., Hill M. J., Drasar B. S., Southgate D. A. T. (1977): The effects of two dietary fiber supplements on gastrointestinal transit, stool weight, and frequency, and bacterial flora, and fecal bile acids in normal subjects. *Metabol.* **26**, 117–127.

Barnes W. S., Maiello J., Weisburger J. H. (1983): In vitro binding of the food mutagen 2-amino-3-methylimidazo (4,5-*f*)-quinoline to dietary fibres. *J. Nat. Cancer Inst.* **70**, 757–760.

Bauer H. G., Asp N., Oste R., Dahlquist A., Fredlund P. (1979): Effect of dietary fibre on the induction of colorectal tumors and fecal β-glucuronidase activity in the rat. *Cancer Res.* **39**, 3752–3756.

Bayliss C. E., Houston A. P., Jones V. A., Hishon S., Hunter J. O. (1984): Microbiological studies on food intolerance. *Proc. Nutr. Soc.* **43**, 16A.

Bingham S., Williams D. R., Cole T. J., James W. P. T. (1979): Dietary fibre and regional large-bowel cancer mortality in Britain. *Br. J. Cancer* **40**, 456–463.

Bokkenheuser V. D., Winter J., Kelly W. G. (1978): Metabolism of biliary steroids in human fecal flora. *Am. J. Clin. Nutr.* **31**, S221–S226.

Bond J. H., Levitt M. D. (1978): Effect of dietary fiber on intestinal gas production and small bowel transit time in man. *Am. J. Clin. Nutr.* **31**, S169–S174.

Borgia M., Sepe N., Brancato V., Costa G., Simone P., Borgia R., Lugli R. (1983): Treatment of chronic constipation by a bulk-forming laxative (Fibrolax^R). *J. Int. Med. Res.* **11**, 124–127.

Bornside G. H. (1978): Stability of human fecal flora. *Am. J. Clin. Nutr.* **31**, S141–S144.

Brandes J. W., Lorenz-Meyer H. (1981): Zuckerfreie Diät: Eine neue Perspektive zur Behandlung des Morbus Crohn? *Z. Gastroenterol.* **19**, 1–4.

Brauer P. M., Slavin J. L., Marlett J.A. (1981): Apparent digestibility of neutral detergent fiber in elderly and young adults. *Am. J. Clin. Nutr.* **34**, 1061–1070.

Brodribb A. J. M. (1983): Dietary fibre as a tool of the clinician. In *Dietary Fiber*, ed G. G. Birch, K. J. Parker, pp. 195–204. London and New York; Applied Science Publishers.

Bryant M. P. (1978): Cellulose digesting bacteria from human faeces. *Am. J. Clin. Nutr.* **31**, S113–S115.

Burkitt D. (1981): Diet and disease. *Irish Med. J.* **74**, 36–38.

Connell A. M. (1978): The effects of dietary fiber on gastrointestinal motor function. *Am. J. Clin. Nutr.* **31**, S152–S156.

Connell A. M. (1981): Dietary fiber. In *Physiology of the gastrointestinal tract*, ed L. R. Johnson, Vol. 2, pp. 1291–1299. New York: Raven Press.

Cummings J. H., Jenkins D. J. A., Wiggins H. S. (1976): Measurement of the mean transit time of dietary residue through the human gut. *Gut* **17**, 210–218.

Cummings J. H., Southgate D. A. T., Branch W. J., Houston H., Jenkins D. J. A., James W. P. T. (1978): Colonic response to dietary fiber from carrot, cabbage, apple, bran, and guar gum. *Lancet* **1**, 5–9.

Cummings J. H., Hill M. J., Jivraj T., Heaston H., Branch W. J., Jenkins D. J. A. (1979a): The effect of meat protein and dietary fiber on colonic functions and metabolism. I. Changes in bowel habit, bile acid excretion, and calcium adsorption. *Am. J. Clin. Nutr.* **32**, 2086–2093.

Cummings J. H., Southgate D. A. T., Branch W. J., Wiggins H. S., Houston H., Jenkins D. J. A., Jivraj T., Hill M. J. (1979b): The digestion of pectin in the human gut and its effect on calcium absorption and large bowel function. *Br. J. Nutr.* **41**, 477–485.

Cummings J. H., Stephen A. M. (1980): The role of dietary fibre in the human colon. *Can. Med. Ass. J.* **123**, 1109–1114.

Cummings J. H. (1981): Short chain fatty acids in the human colon. *Gut* **22**, 763–779.

Cummings J. H. (1982): Consequences of the metabolism of fiber in the human large intestine. In *Dietary fiber in health and disease* ed G. V. Vahouny, D. Kritchevsky, pp. 9–22. New York and London: Plenum Press.

Cummings J. H., Branch W. J. (1982): Postulated mechanisms whereby fiber may protect against large bowel cancer. In *Dietary fiber in health and disease*, ed G. V. Vahouny, D. Kritchevsky, pp. 313–325. New York and London. Plenum Press.

Cummings J. H. (1984): Microbial digestion of complex carbohydrates in man. *Proc. Nutr. Soc.* **43**, 35–44.

Dekker J., Palmer J. K. (1981): Enzymatic degradation of the plant cell wall by a bacteroides of human fecal origin. *J. Agric. Fd Chem.* **29**, 480–484.

Devroede G. (1978): Dietary fiber, bowel habits, and colonic function. *Am. J. Clin. Nutr.* **31**, S157–S160.

Dintzis F. R., Legg L. M., Deatherage W. L., Baker F. L., Inglett G. E., Jacob R. A., Reck S. J., Munoz J. M., Klevay L. M., Sandstead H. H., Shuey W. C. (1979): Human gastrointestinal action on wheat, corn, and soy hull bran — preliminary findings. *Cereal Chem.* **56**, 123–127.

Dwyer J. T., Goldin B., Gorbach S., Patterson J. (1979): Dietary fiber supplements in the therapy of gastrointestinal disorders. In *Drug therapy reviews*, ed R. R. Miller, D. J. Greenblatt, Vol. 2, pp. 394–427. Amsterdam: Elsevier/North-Holland, Biomedical Press.

Eastwood M. A. (1978): *Fiber in the gastrointestinal tract. Am. J. Clin. Nutr.* **31**, S30–S32.

Eastwood M. A., Kay R. M. (1979): An hypothesis for the action of dietary fiber along the gastrointestinal tract. *Am. J. Clin. Nutr.* **32**, 364–367.

Eastwood, M. A., Baird, J. D., Brydon, W. G., Smith, J. H., Helliwell, S., Pritchard J. L. (1982): Dietary fiber and colon function in a population aged 18–80 years. In *Dietary fiber in health and disease*, ed. G. V. Vahouny, D. Kritchevksy, pp 23–34. New York and London: Plenum Press.

Eastwood, M. A., Passmore, R. (1983): Dietary fibre. *Lancet* **2**, 202–206.

Eastwood, M. A., Robertson, J. A., Brydon, W. G., MacDonald, D. (1983): Measurement of water-holding properties of fibre and their faecal bulking ability in man. *Br. J. Nutr.* **50**, 539–547.

Ehle, F. R., Robertson, J. B., Van Soest, P. J. (1982): Influence of dietary fibres on fermentation in the human large intestine *J. Nutr.* **112**, 158–166.

Farrell, D. J., Girle, L., Arthur, J. (1978): Effects of dietary fiber on the apparent digestibility of major food components and on blood lipids in men. *Aust. J. Exp. Biol. Med. Sci.* **56**, 469–479.

Fetzer, S. G., Kies, C., Fox, H. M. (1979): Gastric disappearance of dietary fiber by adolescent boys. *Cereal Chem.* **56**, 34–37.

Fielding, J. F. (1982): Domperidone treatment in the irritable bowel syndrome. *Dig.* **23**, 125–127.

Finegold, S. M., Sutter, V. L. (1978): Fecal flora in different populations, with special reference to diet. *Am. J. Clin. Nutr.* **31**, S116–S122.

Fleming, S. E., Calloway, D. H. (1983): Determination of intestinal gas excretion. In *Dietary Fibre*, ed G. G. Birch, K. J., Parker, pp. 221–254. London and New York: Applied Science Publishers.

Fleming, S. E., Rodriguez, M. A. (1983): Influence of dietary fiber on fecal excretion of volatile fatty acids by human adults. *J. Nutr.* **113**, 1613–1625.

Floch, M. H. (1981): *Nutrition and diet therapy in Gastrointestinal disease*, New York and London: Plenum.

Freeman, H. J., Spiller, G. A., Kim, Y. S. (1980): A double-blind study on the effects of differing purified cellulose and pectin fiber diets on 1,2-dimethyl-hydrazine-induced rat colonic neoplasia. *Cancer Res.* **40**, 2661–2665.

Gear, J. S. S., Ware, A., Fursdon, P., Mann, J. I., Nolan, D. J., Brodribb, A. J. M., Vessey, M. P. (1979): Symptomless diverticular disease and intake of dietary fibre. *Lancet* **1**, 511–514.

Hasik, J., Hryniewiecki, L., Klincewicz, H., Gadzinowska, A. (1982): Feeding habits in patients with ulcerative colitis and colon diverticulitis. In *Colon and nutrition*, ed. H. Kasper, H. Goebell, pp. 153–157. Falk Symposium No. 32. Lancaster: MTP.

Heaton, K. W., Thornton, J. R., Emmett, P. M. (1979a): Dietary factors in Crohn's disease. *Z. Gastroenterol.* **17**, S140–S144.

Heaton, K. W., Thornton, J. R., Emmett, P. M. (1979b): Treatment of Crohn's disease with an unrefined carbohydrate, fibre-rich diet. *Br. Med. J.* **2**, 764–766.

Heaton, K. W. (1981): What is the place of refined carbohydrate and dietary fiber in inflammatory bowel disease? In *Dietary fibre: progress towards the future*, ed. I. M. Baird, M. H. Ornstein, pp. 59–64. Manchester, England.

Heinkel, K. (1983): Therapy of irritable colon and diverticular disease. In *Current therapy of gastrointestinal disorders*, ed. G. Dobrilla, C. Liguory, G. Misiewicz, pp. 117–121. New York: Raven Press.

Heller, S. N., Hackler, L. R., Rivers, J. M., Van Soest, P. J., Roe, D. A., Lewis, B. A., Robertson, J. (1980): Dietary fiber: the effect of particle size of wheat bran on colonic function in young men. *Am. J. Clin. Nutr.* **33**, 1734–1744.

Hill, M. J., Drasar, B. S., Williams, R. E. O., Meade, T. W., Cox, A. G., Simpson, J. E. P., Morson, B. C. (1975): Fecal bile acids and clostridia in patients with cancer of the large bowel. *Lancet* **1**, 535–538.

Hill, M. J. (1982a): Colonic bacterial activity: effect of fiber on substrate concentration and on enzyme action. In *Dietary fiber in health and disease*, ed. G. V. Vahouny, D. Kritchevsky, pp. 35–52. New York and London: Plenum Press.

Hill, M. J. (1982b): Influence of nutrition on the intestinal flora. In *Colon and nutrition*, ed. H. Kasper, H. Goebell, pp. 37–44. Falk Symposium No. 32. Lancaster: MTP.

Hill, M. J. (1983): Bacteria, dietary fiber and chronic intestinal disease. In *Dietary fibre*, ed. G. G. Birch, K. J. Parker, pp. 255–273. London and New York: Applied Science Publishers.

Hinton, J. M., Lennard-Jones, J. E., Young, A. C. (1969): A new method for studying gut transit-times using radio-opaque markers. *Gut* **10**, 842–847.

Holloway, W. D., Tasman-Jones, C., Lee, S. P. (1978): Digestion of certain fractions of dietary fiber in humans. *Am. J. Clin. Nutr.* **31**, 927–930.

Hori, S., Hudson, M., Hill, M. J. (1983): Microbiological and oligosaccharide content of ileostomy fluid in subjects taking an unrefined and a refined carbohydrate diet. *Proc. Nutr. Soc.* **42**, 109A.

Hyland, J. M. P., Taylor, I. (1980): Doses of a high fibre diet prevent the complications of diverticular disease? *Br. J. Surg.* **67**, 77–79.

James, A. (1977): Breakfast and Crohn's disease. *Br. Med. J.* **1**, 943–945.

Kasper, H., Sommer, H. (1979): Dietary fiber and nutrient intake in Crohn's disease. *Am. J. Clin. Nutr.* **32**, 1898–1901.

Kasper, H. (1982): Ballaststoff-reiche und ballaststoff-freie Diät. Anwendung bei gastroenterologischen Erkrankungen. *Münch. Med. Wschr.* **124**, 1108.

Kay, R. M., (1981): Effects of diet on the fecal excretion and bacterial modification of acidic and neutral steroids, and implications for colon carcinogenesis. *Cancer Res.* **41**, 3774–3777.

Kay, R. M. (1982): Dietary fiber. *J. Lip. Res.* **23**, 221–242.

Kuhnlein, U., Bergstrom, D., Kuhnlein, H. (1981): Mutagens in feces from vegetarians and non-vegetarians. *Mutat. Res.* **85**, 1–12.

Kurtz, W., Leuschner, U., Strohm, W. D., Kon, H. (1981): Ileal and colonic mucosal bile acids in Crohn's disease and colonic carcinoma. Int. Symp. on Inflammatory Bowel Disease, Jerusalem Israel (abstract).

Lancaster-Smith, M., Williams, K. G. D. (1982): Constipation and other problems with defecation. In *Problems in gastroenterology*, pp. 97–101. Basel: Karger.

Leitzmann, C. (1983): Ballaststoffe — Definition, Zusammensetzung, Eigenschaften und Verzehr in der Bundesrepublik. *Münch. Med. Wschr.* **125**, 398–402.

Levin, B. (1982): Nutritional assessment and intervention in inflammatory bowel disease: an overview of recent studies. In *Colon and nutrition*, ed. H. Kasper, H., Goebell, pp. 259–265. Falk Symposium No. 32. Lancaster: MTP.

MacLennan, R., Jensen, O. M., Mosbech, J., Vuori, H. (1978): Diet, transit time, stool weight, and colon cancer in two Scandinavian populations. *Am. J. Clin. Nutr.* **31**, S239–S242.

Manning, A. P., Heaton, K. W., Harvey, R. F., Uglow, P. (1977): Wheat fibre and the irritable bowel syndrome. *Lancet* **2**, 417–418.

Marlett, J. A., Lee, S. C. (1980): Dietary fiber, lignocellulose and hemicellulose contents of selected foods determined by modified and unmodified Van Soest procedures. *J. Fd Sci.* **45**, 1688–1693.

Marlett, J. A., Slavin, J. L., Brauer, P. M. (1981): Comparison of dye and pellet gastrointestinal transit time during controlled diets differing in protein and fiber levels. *Dig. Dis. Sci.* **26**, 208–213.

Martini, G. A., Brandes, J. W. (1976): Increased consumption of refined carbohydrates in patients with Crohn's disease. *Klin. Wschr.* **54**, 367–371.

Marthinsen, D., Fleming, S. E. (1982): Excretion of breath and flatus gases by humans consuming high-fiber diets. *J. Nutr.* **112**, 1133–1143.

Mathers, J. C., Blake, J. S. (1983): Transit time through the human gut of markers taken at different times of the day. *Proc. Nutr. Soc.* **42**, 111A.

Mayberry, J. F., Rhodes, J., Newcombe, R. G. (1980): Increased sugar consumption in Crohn's disease. *Dig.* **20**, 323–326.

McNeil, N. I., Cummings, J. H., James, W. P. (1978): Short chain fatty acid absorption by the human large intestine. *Gut* **19**, 819–822.

McNeil, N. I. (1984): The contribution of the large intestine to energy supplies in man. *Am. J. Clin. Nutr.* **39**, 338–342.

Mendeloff, A. I. (1978): Fiber and gastrointestinal tract. Summary and recommendations. *Am. J. Clin. Nutr.* **31**, S145–S147.

Miller, B., Fervers, F., Rohbeck, R., Strohmeyer, G. (1976): Zuckerkonsum bei Patienten mit Morbus Crohn. *Verh. Dt. Ges. Inn. Med.* **82**, 922–924.

Miller, B. (1982): Crohn's disease and nutrition — aetiological aspects. In *Colon and nutrition*, ed H. Kasper, H., Goebell, pp. 251–256. Falk Symposium No. 32. Lancaster: MTP.

Mitchell, W. D., Eastwood, M. A. (1976): Dietary fiber and colonic function. In *Fiber in human nutrition*, ed G. A. Spiller, R. J., Amen, pp. 192–206. New York: Plenum Press.

Moore, W. E. C., Cato, E. P., Holdeman, L. V. (1978): Some current concepts in intestinal bacteriology. *Am. J. Clin. Nutr.* **31**, S33–S42.

Nutrition Reviews (1984): The effect of fiber on protein digestibility. *Nutr. Rev.* **42**, 23–24.

Ohi, G., Minowa, K., Oyama, T., Nagahashi, M., Yamazaki, N., Yamamoto, S., Nagasako, K., Hayakawa, K., Kimura, K., Mori, B. (1983): Changes in dietary intake among Japanese in the 20th century: a relationship to the prevalence of diverticular disease. *Am. J. Clin. Nutr.* **38**, 115–121.

Ornstein, M. H., Littlewood, E. R., Baird, I. M., Fowler, J., North, W. R. S., Cox, A. G. (1981): Are fibre supplements really necessary in diverticular disease of the colon? A controlled clinical trial. *Br. Med. J.* **282**, 1353–1356.

Ornstein, M. H. (1981): Diverticular disease of the colon — what is the real use of dietary fibre? In *Dietary fibre — progress towards the future*, ed I. M., Baird, M. H., Ornstein, pp. 71–76. Manchester, England.

Palmer, S., Bakshi, K. (1983): Diet, nutrition and cancer: interim dietary guidelines. *J. Nat. Cancer Inst.* **70**, 1151–1170.

Prynne, C. J., Southgate, D. A. T. (1979): The effects of a supplement of dietary fiber on fecal excretion by human subjects. *Br. J. Nutr.* **41**, 495–503.

Reddy, B. S., Hedges, A. R., Laakso, K., Wynder, E. L. (1978): Metabolic epidemiology of large bowel cancer: fecal bulk and constituents of high-risk North American and low-risk Finnish population *Cancer* **42**, 2832–2838.

Reddy, B. S. (1982): Dietary fiber and colon carcinogenesis, a critical review. In *Dietary fiber in health and disease*, ed G. V. Vahouny, D. Kritchevsky, pp. 265–312. New York and London: Plenum Press.

Ritchie, J. A., Truelove, S. C. (1979): Treatment of irritable bowel syndrome with lorazepam, hyoscine butyl-bromide, and ispaghula husk. *Br. Med. J.* **1**, 376–378.

Roediger, W. E. W. (1980): The colonic epithelium in ulcerative colitis: an energy-deficiency disease? *Lancet* **2**, 712–715.

Roediger, W. E. W. (1982): The effect of bacterial metabolites on nutrition and function of the colonic mucosa. Symbiosis between man and bacteria. In *Colon and nutrition*, ed H. Kasper, H., Goebell, pp. 11–24. Falk Symposium No. 32. Lancaster: MTP.

Ross, J. K., Leklem, J. E. (1981): The effect of dietary citrus pectin on the excretion of human fecal neutral and acid steroids and the activity of 7α-dehydroxylase and β-glucuronidase. *Am. J. Clin. Nutr.* **34**, 2068–2077.

Roth, G., Leitzmann, C. (1983). The longterm influence of cereal products containing different levels and kinds of dietary fibers on digestion and metabolism of healthy adults Fourth Europ. Nutr. Conf. (Amsterdam), Paper WO-4, p. 133.

Rowland, I. R., Marlett, A. K., Wise, A., Bailey, E. (1983): Effect of dietary carrageenan and pectin on the reduction of nitro-compounds by the rat caecal microflora. *Xenobiotica* **13**, 251–256.

Ruckdeschel, G. (1980): Darmflora und Elementardiät. *Akt. Ern. Med.* **5**(2), 81–88.

Ruppin, J., Bar-Meir, S., Soergel, K. H., Wood, C. M., Schmitt, M. C. (1980): Absorption of short-chain fatty acids by the colon. *Gastroenterol.* **78**, 1500–1507.

Salyers, A. A. (1979): Energy sources of major intestinal fermentative anaerobes. *Am. J. Clin. Nutr.* **32**, 158–163.

Salyers, A. A., Palmer, J. K., Balascio, J. (1979): Digestion of plant cell wall polysaccharides by bacteria from the human colon. In *Dietary fibers: chemistry and nutrition*, ed G. E. Inglett, S. I., Falkehag, pp. 193–201. New York: Academic Press.

Saunders, R. M., Betschart, A. A. (1980): The significance of protein as a component of dietary fiber. *Am. J. Clin. Nutr.* **33**, 960–961.

Schweizer, T. F., Bekhechi, A. R., Koellreutter, B., Reimann, S., Pometta, D., Bron, B. A. (1983): Metabolic effects of dietary fiber from dehulled soybeans in humans. *Am. J. Clin. Nutr.* **38**, 1–11.

Selvendran, R. R. (1984): The plant cell wall as a source of dietary fiber: chemistry and structure. *Am. J. Clin. Nutr.* **39**, 320–337.

Shetty, P. S., Kurpad, A. (1983): Intestinal transit times and faecal weights of South Indian subjects. *Proc. Nutr. Soc.* **42**, 110A.

Shiau, S-Y., Chang, G. W. (1983): Effects of dietary fiber on fecal mucinase and β-glucuronidase activity in rats. *J. Nutr.* **113**, 138–144.

Slavin, J. L., Marlett, J. A. (1980): Apparent cellulose digestibility in human subjects consuming low and high cellulose diets. *Fed. Proc.* **39**(3), 1.

Slavin, J. L., Brauer, P. M., Marlett, J. A. (1981): Neutral detergent fibre, hemicellulose and cellulose digestibility in human subjects. *J. Nutr.* **111**, 287–297.

Smith, A. N., Drummond, E., Eastwood, M. A. (1981): The effect of coarse and fine Canadian Red Spring wheat and French soft wheat bran on colonic motility in patients with diverticular disease. *Am. J. Clin. Nutr.* **34**, 2460–2463.

Smith. A. N. (1982): Effects on fibre on colonic function and motility. In *Colon and nutrition*, ed H. Kasper, H. Goebell, pp. 181–187. Falk Symposium No. 32. Lancaster: MTP.

Smith, C. J., Bryant, M. P. (1979): Introduction to metabolic activities of intestinal bacteria. *Am. J. Clin. Nutr.* **32**, 149–157.

Smith-Barbaro, P., Hansen, D., Reddy, B. (1981): Carcinogen binding to various types of dietary fiber. *J. Natl. Cancer Inst.* **67**(2), 495–497.

Soltoft, J. E., Gudmand-Hoyer, E., Krag, B., Kristensen, E., Wulff, H. R. (1976): A double blind trial of the effect of wheat bran on symptoms of irritable bowel syndrome. *Lancet* **1**, 270–272.

Spiller, G. A., Chernoff, M. C., Hill, R. A., Gates, J. E., Nassar, J. J., Shipley, E. A. (1980): Effect of purified cellulose, pectin, and a low-residue diet on fecal volatile fatty acids, transit time, and fecal weight in humans. *Am. J. Clin. Nutr.* **33**, 754–759.

Spiller, G. A., Freeman, H. J., (1981): Recent advances in dietary fiber and colorectal diseases. *Am. J. Clin. Nutr.* **34**, 1145–1152.

Spiller, G. A. (1982a): Nutritional factors in the aetiology and treatment of constipation. In *Colon and nutrition*, ed H. Kasper, H. Goebell, pp. 189–192. Falk Symposium No. 32. Lancaster: MTP.

Spiller, G. A. (1982b): Colon cancer and dietary fiber, an overview. In *Dietary fiber in health and disease*, ed G. V. Vahouny, D. Kritchevsky, pp. 237–238. New York and London: Plenum Press.

Spiller, G. A., Wong, L. G., Whittam, J. H., Scala, J. (1982): Correlation of gastrointestinal transit time to fecal weight in adult humans at two levels of fiber intake. *Nutr. Rep. Int.* **25**, 23–30.

Stasse-Wolthuis, M., Albers, H. F. F., van Jeveren, J. G. C., de Jong, J. W., Hautvast, J. G. A. J., Hermus, R. J. J., Katan, M. B., Brydon, W. G., Eastwood, M. A. (1980): Influence of dietary fiber from vegetables and fruits, bran or citrus pectin on serum lipids, fecal lipids, and colonic function. *Am. J. Clin. Nutr.* **33**, 1745–1756.

Stephen, A. M., Cummings, J. H. (1979): Water-holding by dietary fibre in vitro and its relationship to faecal output in man. *Gut* **20**, 722–729.

Stephen, A. M., Cummings, J. H. (1980): Mechanism of action of dietary fibre in the human colon. *Nature* **284**, 283–284.

Story, J. A., Kritchevsky, D., Eastwood, M. A. (1979): Dietary Fiber — bile acid interactions. In *Dietary fibers: chemistry and nutrition*, ed G. E. Inglett, S. I. Falkehag, pp. 49–55. New York: Academic Press.

Tadesse, K., Eastwood, M. A. (1978): Metabolism of dietary fiber components in man assessed by breath hydrogen and methane. *Br. J. Nutr.* **40**, 393–396.

Thornton, J. R., Emmett, P. M., Heaton, K. W. (1979): Diet and Crohn's disease: characteristics of the pre-illness diet. *Br. Med. J.* **2**, 762–764.

Thornton, J. R., Heaton, K. W. (1980): Lactulose and bile: evidence linking colonic bacteria and cholesterol gallstones. *Gut* **21**, 906–908.

Trudel, J. L., Senterman, M. K., Brown, R. A. (1983): The fat/fiber antagonism in experimental colon carcinogenesis. *Surgery* **94**, 691–696.

Van Soest, P. J., Uden, P., Wrick, K. L. (1983): Critique and evaluation of markers for use in humans and farm and laboratory animals. *Nutr. Rep. Int.* **27**, 17–28.

Van Soest, P. J. (1984): Some physical characteristics of dietary fibres and their influence on the microbial ecology of the human colon. *Proc. Nutr. Soc.* **43**, 25–33.

Visek, W. J. (1978): Diet and cell growth modulation by ammonia. *Am. J. Clin. Nutr.* **31**, S216–S220.

Watanabe, K., Reddy, B. S., Wong, C. Q., Weisburger, J. H. (1978): Effects of dietary undegraded carrageenan on colon carcinogenesis in F 344 rats treated with azoxymethane or methylnitrosourea. *Cancer Res.* **38**, 4427–4430.

Wienbeck, M., Erckenbrecht, J. (1982): Motility of the colon and its function. In *Colon and nutrition*, ed H. Kasper, H. Goebell, pp. 105–113. Falk Symposium No. 32. Lancaster: MTP.

Wiggins, H. S. (1983): Gastroenterological functions of dietary fibers. In *Dietary Fibre*, ed G. G. Birch, K. J. Parker, pp. 205–220. London and New York: Applied Science Publishers.

Wise, A., Marlett, A. K., Rowland, I. R. (1982): Dietary fibre, bacterial metabolism and toxicity of nitrate in the rat. *Xenobiotica* **12**, 111–118.

Wolever, M. S., Thorne, M-J., Thompson, L. U., Cohen, Z., Jenkins, D. J. A. (1984): Digestibility of carbohydrate from bread and lentils using a breath hydrogen technique and a human ileostomy model. *Proc. Nutr. Soc.* **43**, 15A.

Wrick, K. L., Robertson, J. B., Van Soest, P. J., Lewis, B. A., Rivers, J. M., Roe, D. A., Hackler, L. R. (1983): The influence of dietary fiber source on human intestinal transit and stool output. *J. Nutr.* **113**, 1464–1479.

Wrong, O. M., Vince, A. (1984): Urea and ammonia metabolism in the human large intestine. *Proc. Nutr. Soc.* **43**, 77–86.

Wyman, J. B., Heaton, K. W., Manning, A. P., Wicks, A. C. B. (1976): The effect on intestinal transit time and the faeces of raw and cooked bean in different doses. *Am. J. Clin. Nutr.* **29**, 1474–1479.

Zoppi, G., Gobio-Casali, L., Deganello, A., Astolfi, R., Saccomani, F., Cecchettin, M. (1982): Potential complications in the use of wheat bran for constipation in infancy. *J. Ped. Gastroenterol. Nutr.* **1**, 91–95.

2
Dietary fibre and blood lipids in man

Patricia A. Judd and A. Stewart Truswell

Introduction

It is now 30 years since Walker & Arvidsson first put forward the hypothesis that the low blood cholesterol levels of South African Bantu prisoners might be due, in part, to their high intakes of dietary fibre (Walker & Arvidsson, 1965).

The idea was further advanced by Trowell, Burkitt and others, as the 'dietary-fibre hypothesis' developed, and attention was drawn to the rarity of ischaemic heart disease (IHD) and gallstones in certain African populations consuming traditional diets, high in complex carbohydrate and fibre (Trowell, 1972; Burkitt, 1973; Trowell, Painter & Burkitt, 1974). Evidence of similar patterns of high fibre intake and low IHD incidence was also apparent in Northern India (Malhotra, 1967). In Westernised populations, observation of those consuming vegetarian diets (Barrow *et al.*, 1961; Burr *et al.*, 1981; Hardinge *et al.*, 1958; Phillips *et al.*, 1978; Sacks *et al.*, 1975) or diets high in fruits, vegetables and legumes (Keys, Fidanza & Keys, 1955) also seemed to indicate low concentrations of plasma cholesterol or delayed onset of IHD.

The apparent negative association between dietary fibre intakes and IHD cannot be taken as a causal link. IHD is a multifactorial condition and many other aspects of diet and lifestyle may differ in the populations cited. However, the effect of dietary fibre on plasma lipids has proved a fertile area for study and in the last 10–15 years there have been a large number of short-term experiments in man and laboratory animals.

A picture is beginning to emerge of the effect of dietary fibre and fibre components on plasma lipids. Some types of dietary fibre have repeatedly been shown to lower cholesterol, some have not and others remain to be fully tested. In many experiments larger amounts of dietary fibre have been consumed than may appear practical on a daily basis and the question may be asked as to whether lowering plasma chloesterol levels by such means is beneficial. Although high plasma cholesterol levels have been accepted as an independent risk factor for IHD (Department of Health and Social Security, 1974; Royal College of Physicians, 1976), it has proved difficult to show that lowering these reduced morbidity or mortality from the disease. However, the recently reported results from the Lipid Research Clinic's coronary prevention trial (Anon, 1984*a,b*) have shown that reduction of total and LDL cholesterol was associated with a significant reduction in the risk of coronary heart disease (deaths and non-fatal infarcts) by 19 per cent after 7 years. The reduction in cholesterol levels was achieved by a combination of a diet, in which the polyunsaturated:saturated fat ratio was increased from 0.48 to 0.67 over the 7 years, and cholestyramine, a bile acid sequestrant. It is suggested by Oliver (1984) that the men were well-motivated to continue this regimen as they were part of an 'at-risk' population, being between 35 and 55 years of age and categorised as having type II hypercholesterolaemia (mean plasma cholesterol levels 7.6 mmol/litre), but this does not detract from the effectiveness of the trial.

Two other observations show the size of the possible protective effect of dietary fibre. About 0.52 mmol/l (20 mg/dl) of the difference in mean plasma cholesterol levels of men in Naples (170 mg/dl) and in Minnesota (233 mg/dl) (Keys et al., 1955) could not be explained by their pattern of fatty acid and cholesterol intake (Keys, Anderson & Grande, 1965). Keys, Anderson & Grande (1960) suggested that much of this could be explained by the higher consumption of fibre from fruit, vegetables and legumes in the Mediterranean diets.

In a comparison of three lipid-lowering diets of different types, that rich in fruit or vegetable fibre, as well as being a modified fat diet, lowered plasma cholesterol by 0.45 mmol/l more than the low fibre diet with fat similarly modified (Lewis et al., 1981).

The difference between the present mean plasma cholesterol level in middle-aged US men (5.44 mmol/l or 210 mg/dl) and the 'feasible mean' (4.92 mmol/l or 190 mg/dl) recommended as a medium-term objective by a World Health Organisation Expert Committee (1982) is 0.52 mmol/litre (20 mg/dl). There are considerable differences in mortality or incidence of IHD between communities whose mean (age-standardised) plasma chloesterol levels differ by only 0.52 mmol/l and the regression equation from the Seven Country Study predicts an increase of nearly 50 per cent of coronary deaths when the community mean cholesterol level rises from 5.18 to 5.70 mmol/l (Blackburn, 1980).

These observations suggest that a hypocholesterolaemic effect of dietary fibre could be useful in the general population and in those with hypercholesterolaemia.

The cholesterol-lowering effect of dietary fibre

Concentrated sources of dietary fibre
Much of the initial interest in dietary fibre was centred around wheat-bran as a source of fibre and many of the early experiments investigating lipid-lowering effects used this. Twenty-three reports of studies using wheat fibre have been summarised elsewhere (Kay & Truswell, 1980) and nine others noted since then (Angelico et al., 1979; Avgerinos, Fuchs & Flock, 1977; van Dokken, 1978; Flanagan et al., 1980; Liebman et al., 1983; Lindegärde & Larsson 1984; Salvioli, Salati & Lugli, 1980; Stasse-Wolthuis et al., 1979; Stasse-Wolthuis et al., 1980). Mean plasma total cholesterol was reduced in only eight reports, in the rest plasma cholesterol either rose (in two cases significantly) or remained unchanged.

The studies using wheat fibre illustrate some of the problems of experiments intended to look at the effect of a treatment on blood lipids. The studies above all had different protocols and used different sources of wheat fibre; of the eight studies which demonstrated a cholesterol-lowering effect one noted a significant result using bran (Avgerinos et al., 1977), another reported a reduction in cholesterol with hard red spring wheat bran but not with ordinary soft white wheat bran (Munoz et

24

al., 1979*a*). Several other investigations used only one-way designs, ie control periods followed by test periods, and few plasma cholesterol measurements (Farrell, Girle & Arthur, 1978; Letchford *et al.*, 1978; Mathur, Singh & Chadda, 1977; Persson *et al.*, 1975; van Berge-Henegouwen, 1979). All the subjects were outpatients and in some cases ate ad-lib (van Berge-Henegouwen, 1979; Mathur *et al.*, 1977) thus clouding any effect of dietary fibre with other possible dietary changes.

In contrast the majority of the articles reporting no change in plasma cholesterol are studies with control-test-control (Kay & Truswell, 1977*a*) or crossover design (Liebman *et al.*, 1983), or parallel control groups (Stasse-Wolthuis *et al.*, 1980; Heaton, Manning & Hartog, 1976) or a long trial (Heaton *et al.*, 1976; Tarpila, Miettinen & Metsaranto, 1978; Brodribb & Humphreys, 1976); in some studies all food was provided for the subjects in a metabolic unit (Kay & Truswell, 1977; Raymond *et al.*, 1977; Jenkins, Hill & Cummings, 1975). In nearly all these negative reports frequent estimations were made of plasma cholesterol levels.

It appears that, in studies where plasma cholesterol was reduced, changes in laboratory standardisation or seasonal variation may not have been allowed for. In such studies it is essential to: (i) ensure that the dietary period is of adequate length and allow time for adjustment to the basal diet, (ii) have a control period at each end of the treatment period, or a parallel-running control, (iii) repeat measurements for each period and, ideally, (iv) analyse samples as a research procedure with different dates in the same batch and the analyst unaware of the treatment.

Other cereal brans or similar 'particulate' fibre concentrates have been examined with mixed results. Maize bran did not lower cholesterol levels (Munoz *et al.*, 1979*a*) and cellulose has similarly not lowered cholesterol levels in human experiments (Behall, Lee & Moser, 1984; Eastwood *et al.*, 1973; Kaur, Bhat & Godara, 1981; Keys, Grande & Anderson, 1961; Prather, 1964; Stanley *et al.*, 1972) except when given to children in very large doses (100 g/day) (Shurpalekar *et al.*, 1971).

Oat bran, however, has been reported to lower plasma cholesterol (Anderson & Chen, 1979; Chen *et al.*, 1981; Kirby *et al.*, 1981; Kretsch, Crawford & Calloway, 1979) but differs from the other brans in that it contains a soluble β-glycan as part of the non-cellulosic polysaccharide fraction and is partly mucillaginous (Preece & Hobkirk, 1953).

Fibre-rich foods
Different legumes have been reported to lower plasma cholesterol in several controlled trials; 100 g/day of brown beans (*Phaseolus vulgaris*) lowered plasma cholesterol by 12 mg/dl (Luyken *et al.*, 1962); a mixture of 115 g brown beans, lima beans (*Phaseolus lunatus*) and split peas (*Pisum sativum*) was effective in middle-aged men (Grande, Anderson & Keys, 1965) and Bengal gram (*Cicer arietinum*) substituted for wheat flour over a period of 20 weeks caused a slow fall in cholesterol levels (Mathur, Khan & Sharma, 1968). Freeze-dried peas (30 g/day) have been reported to lower plasma cholesterol by 15 mg/dl in a study in Ireland (Gormley *et al.*, 1979). Other workers have failed to confirm these observations, albeit in a short-term study (Grande *et al.*, 1974).

Soybeans have been the subject of much recent research, with the emphasis mainly on a postulated cholesterol-lowering effect of vegetable protein. Sirtori and co-workers (1979) reported striking reductions in plasma cholesterol levels when 60–90 g/day of a soyabean isolate, or 60–120 g/day of a soy protein concentrate, replaced most of the animal protein in the diets of patients with type-II hypercholesterolaemia (Sirtori *et al.*, 1979; Descovich *et al.*, 1980). These products contain around 20 per cent carbohydrate, mostly 'unavailable', which may have accounted for some of the effect (Helms, 1977). van Raaij *et al.* (1981) were unable to confirm the effect in normolipidaemic subjects and in a further study (van Raaij *et al.*, 1982) comparing soy isolate (80 per cent protein) with soy concentrate (57 per cent protein) in middle-aged volunteers found a small effect only for the isolate, both in lowering plasma low density lipoprotein (LDL) cholesterol and raising high density lipoprotein (HDL) cholesterol. This suggests that any effect of soya is not due to its dietary fibre content and is further reiterated by two recently reported studies in which concentrated dietary fibre or polysaccharide from dehulled soya beans failed to lower serum cholesterol levels. In the first of these, purified soya fibre fed to six healthy volunteers for 3 weeks resulted in an increase in low density liproprotein cholesterol of 19 per cent (Schweizer *et al.*, 1983) and in the second 25 g of soy polysaccharide taken by 14 young men resulted in unchanged serum lipid levels (Tsai *et al.*, 1983). It should be noted, however, that the subjects' mean serum cholesterol levels in both studies were initially low (4.01 and 4.94 mmol/l respectively) and Sirtori has suggested that soya protein products are only effective in hypercholesterolaemic subjects (Sirtori, Descovich & Noseda, 1980). Soya bean hulls, as distinct from polysaccharides from the cotyledon, have been shown to reduce cholesterol by 14 per cent in healthy men (Munoz *et al.*, 1979*a*) but these are not normally eaten.

Other foods which have been suggested to have hypocholesterolaemic effects include rolled oats (de Groot, Luyken & Pikaar, 1963; Luyken *et al.*, 1965), carrots, (Robertson, *et al.*, 1979) and apples (Canella, Golinelli & Melli, 1962; Gormley *et al.*, 1977). Other studies have not confirmed the hypocholesterolaemic effects of the fibre of rolled oats or carrots (Jenkins *et al.*, 1979). Rolled oats contain more fat than other cereals (7–10 per cent of dry weight; Morrison *et al.*, 1975) and this is predominantly unsaturated. When 125 g/day of rolled oats was given to healthy subjects in place of wheat and corn products and the fat in the oats was compensated for, seven out of ten subjects showed a fall in cholesterol levels. The mean fall was only 8 per cent, however, and not significant (Judd & Truswell, 1981).

Diets where mixed vegetables and/or fruits have been used to increase fibre in the diet have also been investigated with similarly mixed results. Stasse-Wolthuis *et al.* (1980) gave a mixture of fruits and vegetables known to be relatively high in pectins and demonstrated small reductions in cholesterol levels. Keys & co-workers (1960) also demonstrated lower cholesterol levels in their subjects when 17 per cent of energy was replaced by fresh fruit, vegetables and legumes or 500 kcal of mixed vegetables were given. Lower cholesterol levels have also been demonstrated when diets high in legumes, fruit and vegetables have been given as part of the treatment of diabetic patients (Anderson, 1982) but these studies are complicated by concomitant changes in the diet and other workers have not shown lower plasma cholesterol levels (Behall, Kelsay & Prather, 1978).

Viscous polysaccharides and other fibre components
The use of purified fibre components, which can be added to defined diets, reduces

the problems associated with using foodstuffs as it becomes possible, theoretically,, to maintain intakes of fat and other nutrients. From this type of experiment evidence for the mechanisms of action of hypocholesterolaemic fibres is suggested and has been studied extensively in animals.

It is now well accepted that viscous polysaccharides such as pectin and guar gum are hypocholesterolaemic agents. Table 1 summarises the reports in the literature for pectin. The fall in cholesterol levels was significant in at least ten reports involving normolipidaemic and hyperlipidaemic subjects; and in those studies where no effect was seen, either no details of the experiment were given (Fahrenbach et al., 1965), or a small dose (6 g/day) was given (Delbarre, Fondier & de Gery, 1977). A dose response can be seen (Kay & Truswell, 1977b) which appears to be linear up to about 15 g/day but that may flatten above this. For guar gum, the doses given have been between 15 and 36 g/day, but effects have been reported with as little as 6 g/day (Fahrenbach et al., 1965). The effect has been seen in normolipidaemic subjects (Fahrenbach et al., 1965; Jenkins et al., 1975) and in patients with hyperlipidaemia (Jenkins et al., 1979, 1980; Miettinen 1983; Tuomilheto et al., 1981). Two recent reports of the additive effect of guar gum in patients with familial hypercholesterolaemia already being treated by the lipid-lowering drugs cholestryamine (Schwandt et al., 1982) and bezafibrate (Wirth et al., 1982) also illustrate its potential usefulness. HDL cholesterol levels have been reported unchanged in studies with guar gum (Jenkins et al., 1980b) as with pectins (Table 1) and although less work has been done on the mechanism of the hypocholesterolaemic effect of this gum, it is highly viscous in aqueous solution and has been shown to increase faecal bile acid excretion in at least one study (Jenkins et al., 1976).

Other viscous polysaccharides also appear to be effective hypocholesterolaemic agents. Psyllium seed gum (composed mainly of arabinose and galacturonic acid units) at 24 g/day lowered cholesterol in normal subjects by 16 per cent (Kies & Fox, 1977), confirming an early report in two subjects only (Forman et al., 1968). Gum acacia, 15 g/day for 4 weeks, has recently been reported to cause a 10 per cent reduction in plasma cholesterol in five hyperlipidaemic subjects. Locust bean gum has been found effective in normal men (Behall et al., 1984) and hyperlipidaemic adults and children (Hanson et al., 1983). Behall et al. (1984) also reported that carboxymethylcellulose gum and gum karaya also had a hypocholesterolaemic effect after 4 weeks of supplementing the subjects diets at a dose of 0.75 g gum/100 kcal.

Effect of fibre on lipoprotein fractions
Most earlier work concentrated on total cholesterol in plasma, but evidence is now appearing for selective changes in lipoprotein fractions. Usually it is the cholesterol in the low density lipoprotein (LDL) fraction which is reduced, as with oat bran (Kirby et al., 1981), rolled oats (Judd & Truswell, 1982; Schwandt et al., 1982) and locust bean or other gums (Hanson et al., 1982); Behall et al., 1984). Combined treatments such as soya bean and pectin (Schwandt, Richter & Weisweiler, 1981), cholestyramine and guar, or bezafibrate and guar, show similar effects (Schwandt et al., 1982; Wirth et al., 1982).

Table 1. *Effects of pectin on plasma and faecal lipids in man*

Author	Pectin: type, amount	Duration	Experimental conditions	Plasma lipids %			Faecal lipid excretion		
				Total chol	HDL chol	TG	Total fat	Neutral steroids	Bile acid
Delbarre *et al.* (1977)	6 g low methoxyl or 6 g high methoxyl	6 weeks	10 hyperlipidaemic subjects	0	XR	XR	————	XR*	————
Durrington *et al.* (1976)	12 g citrus NF* (in orange juice)	3 weeks	12 healthy young men	−8	XR	XR	————	XR	————
Farenbach *et al.* (1965)	6–12 g (pre-swelled)	7–9 weeks	23 mental patients	−6	XR	XR	————	XR	————
Fisher *et al.* (1965)			? hypercholesterolaemic diet	−18	?	?	————	?	————
Jenkins *et al.* (1975, 1976)	36 g NF + orange juice	2 weeks	7 healthy young men	−12	XR	XR	+43	−	+34
Judd & Truswell (1982)	15 g NF (jelly) 15 g low methoxyl	3 weeks 3 weeks	10 healthy young adults, 5m, 5f 10 healthy young adults, 5m, 5f	−18 −16	0 0	0 0	———— ————	XR XR	———— ————
Kay & Truswell (1977*a*)	15 g NF (jelly)	3 weeks	9 healthy volunteers	−13	XR	0	+44	+17	+35
Keys *et al.* (1961)	15 g NF (biscuit)	3 weeks	24 subjects	−5	XR	XR	————	XR	————
Langley & Thye (1977)	10 g	4 weeks	11 subjects	sig fall ?%	XR	sig fall ?%	————	XR	————
Lopez *et al.* (1968)	20–23 g NF	5 weeks	3 subjects	−13	XR	XR	All increased		?%
Miettinen & Tarpila (1977)	40–50 g NF as jam	2 weeks	9 subjects, 7 hyperlipidaemic	−15	XR	0	XR	+57	+58
Palmer & Dixon (1968)	10 g NF in capsules	4 weeks	16 healthy young men	−6	XR	XR	————	XR	————
Schwandt *et al.* (1982)	12 g apple	8 weeks	6 hyperlipidaemic patients on cholestyramine	−19	LDL −35	0	————	XR	————
Stasse-Wolthuis *et al.* (1980)	9 g NF	5 weeks	15 healthy adults, 10 m, 5 f	−10	0	XR	+75	+25	+50

*NF = National Formulary; XR = Not reported (— XR — denotes values not reported)

Generally, high density lipoprotein (HDL) cholesterol levels remain unchanged, thus increasing the ratio of HDL:LDL cholesterol, a desirable effect as higher HDL levels are associated with reduced risk of atherosclerotic heart disease (Castelle *et al.*, 1977; Lewis *et al.*, 1974). Some studies have reported increased levels of HDL cholesterol, not necessarily accompanied by a decrease in total cholesterol. Thus, guar gum (Jenkins *et al.*, 1980*a*), wheat bran under various conditions (McDougall *et al.*, 1978; Salvioli *et al.*, 1980; Tarpila, Miettinen & Metsaranta, 1978), mixed fibres (Tarpila & Miettinen, 1980) and psyllium colloid (Tarpila & Miettinen, 1977), have all been reported as increasing this lipid fraction, but negative effects have also been summarised by Miettinen (1983).

Plasma triglyceride levels
Plasma triglyceride levels have been unchanged in most reports of the hypolipidaemic effects of dietary fibre, although there have been some reports of reductions in plasma triglyceride levels, usually in hyperlipidaemic or diabetic patients. In each case the fibre has been from leguminous seeds and there have been other changes in diet which might contribute to the hypotriglyceridaemic effect (Anderson & Ward, 1979; Jenkins *et al.*, 1983; Rivellese *et al.*, 1980).

Interest has been shown recently, however, in the possibility that fat absorption may be modified by dietary fibre or its components and post-prandial rises in plasma triglyceride levels have been studied in a few experiments. Anderson & Chen (1979) first observed a reduction of post-prandial triglyceride levels in diabetic patients fed high carbohydrate, high fibre diets and suggested that these diets may attenuate the post-prandial rise in chylomicrons. Irie, Hara & Goto (1982) have confirmed the observations in ten subjects (one with hypertriglyceridaemia), studied for 6 hours after a meal containing two egg yolks and 1½ cups of ice cream, with and without guar gum. Plasma triglyceride levels were found to be reduced at 2 and 4 hours after the guar-gum-containing meals, but were higher at 6 hours.

Gatti *et al.* (1984) have recently reported similar suppression of the expected rise in plasma triglyceride levels after meals containing guar-enriched pasta products, and we have also demonstrated a delay in the rise of plasma triglycerides on feeding a test breakfast with guar gum to six healthy young men compared to the same meal without gum (Schnell & Judd, unpublished results) (Figure). We have demonstrated similar effects when rats (Schnell, Pacy & Judd, 1984) were fed guar gum in a test meal and triglyceride rise and chylomicron composition measured at intervals for 3 hours. The rise in triglycerides was delayed by guar gum and the size distribution of the chylomicrons suggested that they were being synthesised in the distal small intestine as well as the proximal part (Wu *et al.*, 1975). If viscous polysaccharides alter the site of absorption and hence the composition of chylomicron particles in man this may also change their subsequent utilisation. This may also be affected by a slower, steadier rate of delivery of triglycerides to peripheral tissues. Viscous polysaccharides are known to reduce post-prandial glucose and insulin responses to carbohydrate feeding and the latter may also result in slower clearance of triglyceride (Anderson & Chen, 1979). Jenkins (1977) suggested that guar and pectin promote greater absorption of fat via the lymphatic route and this may also alter subsequent metabolism. More work on the effects of

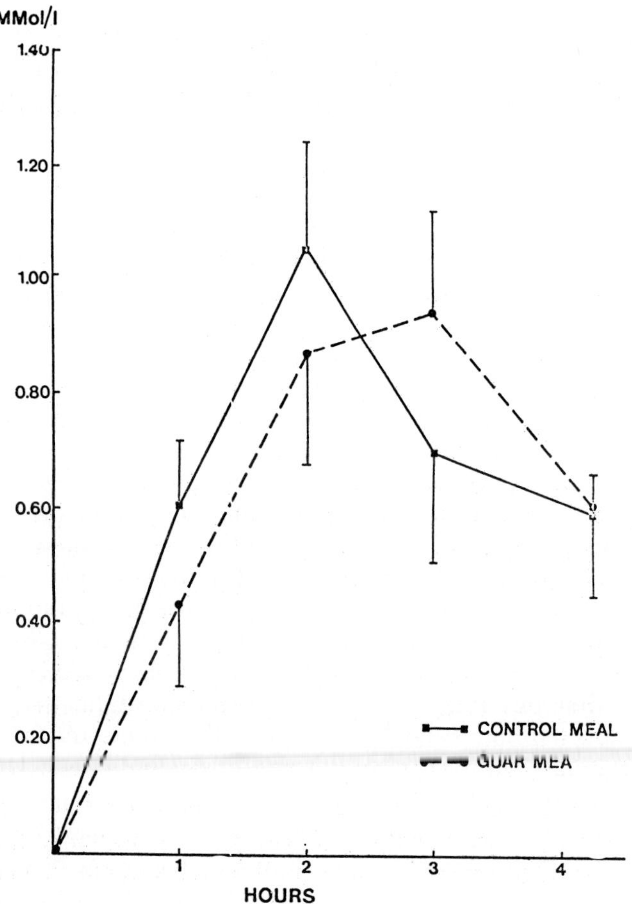

Figure. *Post-prandial chylomicron triglycerides (mean of 6 subjects) after a breakfast containing 50 per cent of energy as fat, with or without 7.5 g guar gum (mean and s.e.m.).*

different types of dietary fibre and fibre-containing diets on lipid absorption would be useful.

Mechanisms of the lipid-lowering effects of dietary fibre

Clarification of our understanding of the mechanisms of the cholesterol-lowering effect of dietary fibres and fibre components has come largely from animal studies where observations may be made on the distribution throughout the body of cholesterol as well as of plasma lipids. Several mechanisms have been suggested for the effect, as outlined in Table 2. Each of these proposed mechanisms has been studied in some detail and there have been recent authoritative reviews on several of them, including intestinal absorption of lipids (Vahouney, 1982), bile salt metabolism (Kay & Truswell, 1980; Miettinen, 1983; Story & Thomas, 1982), and lipoprotein metabolism (Story & Kelly, 1982). Only a brief outline will therefore be given here.

30

Table 2. *Suggested mechanisms for the hypocholesterolaemic effects of dietary fibre.*

1 Reduction of fat and energy intake
2 Reduction of cholesterol and fat
  absorption
3 Changes in endocrine response

4 Effects of colonic metabolites
5 Increased bile acid excretion

Reduction in fat and energy intake

In many studies on the hypocholesterolaemic effects of fibre, difficulties in interpretation have arisen due to concomitant changes in diet. Foods which are concentrated sources of fibre are often low in fat and bulky and may therefore displace other fat and energy containing foods in the diet. Kay, Sabry & Czisma (1980) have reported an inverse correlation between percentage of energy from fat and dietary fibre intake in a normal population. Reduction in saturated fat intake will itself have hypocholesterolaemic effects.

Changes in energy intake resulting in weight loss may also have hypolipidaemic effects, especially in hypertriglyceridaemic subjects, and evidence is accumulating to show that dietary fibre reduces the availability of energy supplying nutrients (Farrell *et al.*, 1978; Judd, 1982; Kay & Truswell, 1977*a*; Kelsay *et al.*, 1981; Southgate & Durnin, 1970). The differences in daily faecal energy are small (Southgate suggested between 20 and 95 kcal/day and our results showed an increase of 179 kcal/day when mean fibre intake increased from 27 g/day to 45) but their cumulative effect may be important (Southgate & Durnin, 1970, Judd, 1982).

Reduction in fat and cholesterol absorption

Reduction in fat absorption, as demonstrated by increased faecal fat excretion, has been described with viscous polysaccharides such as guar and pectin and with other types of fibre. The quantities are usually small and may depend on the form of fat in the diet. Levine & Silvis (1980) recently demonstrated that when fat was in the form of peanuts, increasing the fibre content of the diet had no effect on faecal fat excretion, but when 20 g of crude fibre was added to a diet containing peanut oil faecal fat increased significantly. A study of the effects of pectin on small intestinal absorption in patients with ileostomies has confirmed that it reduces absorption in the small intestine. The ileostomy contents of fat were markedly higher during the pectin period than before and after (Sandberg *et al.*, 1983).

The possible changes in rate and site of absorption of fat have been outlined above and the effects on absorption of cholesterol discussed in detail by Vahouney (1982). Cholesterol absorption (expressed as increases in faecal neutral steroids) has been shown to be decreased in man, but is usually not so pronounced as the changes in bile acid excretion.

Changes in endocrine responses

High fibre, high carbohydrate diets (Anderson & Chen, 1979) and viscous polysaccharides have been shown to modify glucose absorption and result in lower insulin responses as discussed in Chapter 4 of this volume. As insulin has been shown to increase cholesterol synthesis (Bhathena, Avigan & Schreiner, 1974) it may be significant that the viscous polysaccharides which markedly alter insulin responses also appear to have the greatest effect on plasma cholesterol levels.

Changes in gut hormones may contribute to the lower insulin levels when viscous polysaccharides are fed. Gastric inhibitory polypeptide (GIP) and gut glucagon-like immunoreactivity (GLI) are able to stimulate insulin release (Marks & Turner, 1977) and feeding either guar gum (Morgan *et al.*, 1979) or pectin (Jenkins *et al.*, 1980*a*) resulted in lower levels of GIP under various conditions. Other hormones affecting lipoprotein metabolism such as glucagon have also shown altered blood levels when high levels of fibre are fed (Miranda & Horwitz, 1978; Munoz, Sandstead & Jacob, 1979*b*).

Effects of colonic metabolites
Fermentation of fibre in the large gut may result in alteration in colonic flora, changes in bile acid metabolites and production of varying amounts of short chain fatty acids (SCFA). In rats the cholesterol-lowering effect of pectin was not suppressed by antibiotics (Leveille & Sauberlich, 1966; Rosenberg & Anderson, 1982; Wells & Ershoff, 1961) suggesting that fermentation in the large gut is not an important factor in its hypocholesterolaemic effect. Anderson & Chen (1979), however, proposed that SCFA metabolites produced by fermentation of fibre might alter hepatic fatty acid and triglyceride metabolism. Recent work from their laboratory has demonstrated changes in glucose metabolism in isolated rat hepatocytes exposed to acetate, proprionate or oleate (Anderson & Bridges, 1982). Investigations of the contribution of colonic fermentation products to metabolism is currently in the early stages and may prove to be significant.

Increased bile acid excretion
In studies of the hypocholesterolaemic effects of pectins, where bile acid excretion has been measured these metabolites have usually been shown to be increased (see Table 1). Other viscous polysaccharides have been shown to increase bile acid excretion at the same time as decreasing plasma cholesterol levels, eg psyllium colloid (Forman *et al.*, 1968; Stanley *et al.*, 1972), guar gum (Jenkins *et al.*, 1977; Miettinen, 1980). Cellulose (Shurpalekar *et al.*, 1971; Stanley *et al.*, 1972), bagasse (Walters *et al.*, 1975) and in some circumstances wheat fibre and mixed wheat fibres have also shown increased bile acid excretion, but this is not always so and sometimes has not been accompanied by reductions in plasma cholesterol levels. Kay & Truswell (1980) and Miettinen (1983) have summarised the effects of dietary fibre on faecal bile acid excretion.
It is not yet clear how the loss in faecal bile acid is achieved. Binding of bile acids *in vitro* has been studied by various workers and found to be dependent on various chemical and physical characteristics of the fibres and bile salts used (Eastwood & Hamilton, 1968; Eastwood & Mowbray, 1976; Kay *et al.*, 1979).
Fibres or fibre components known to be hypocholesterolaemic, such as oat fractions (Chenoweth & Benninck, 1976) and lignin (Eastwood & Girdwood, 1968; Judd, Kay & Truswell, 1976; Kay *et al.*, 1979; Thiffault, Belanger & Pauliot, 1970), have been shown to bind bile acids; but this has also been demonstrated with other fibres which do not appear to be hypocholesterolaemic, eg fibre-enriched wheat bran (Flóren & Nilsson, 1982; Lindgärde & Larrsson, 1984).
Binding has been attributed to chemical effects such as hydrophobic bonding, but it is thought that physical effects such as sequestration of bile acids within a

32

complex 'gel-matrix' may be more important for viscous polysaccharides (Eastwood, 1978). Although it has proved difficult to demonstrate bile acid binding *in vitro* for these types of fibre, recent studies with equilibrium dialysis techniques and NMR appear to confirm this (Pfeffer *et al.*, 1981); the workers suggested that interactions between pectin and bile salts were due to viscosity effects and that approximately 20 mg of bile acid was bound by each gram of pectin. The authors pointed out that this was similar to the increase in faecal bile acids in Kay & Truswell's subjects (1977*a*).

Changes in viscosity of the gut contents have been observed in rats fed guar gum by Blackburn & Johnson (1981), and in our studies examination of gut contents showed definite differences in consistency and an obvious 'gel' in pectin fed rats compared to controls (Judd & Truswell, 1985) that could effect fat and cholesterol absorption, as well as sequestering bile salts.

Increased loss of bile acids in the faeces is thought to result in reduction in plasma cholesterol levels due to increased synthesis of bile acids from cholesterol in the liver. Some evidence for this is provided by the observation of increased plasma concentrations of methyl sterols in humans (Miettinin & Tarpila, 1977), and by a study showing increased conversion of acetate[1-^{14}C] to cholesterol in rats (Mokady, 1974) when viscous types of fibre are fed.

Conclusions

The cholesterol-lowering effect of certain types of dietary fibre and fibre-containing foods is now well established. Further research on the mechanisms of the effect on fat and cholesterol absorption is required, but currently it would appear that diets high in fibre-containing foods – such as fruits vegetables and legumes – may be of benefit to the general population, irrespective of whether the effects are due to replacement of saturated fat and sugar in the diet or to modifications in rate of absorption. Such observations may enable 'prudent' diets to be designed (Lewis *et al.*, 1981).

Viscous polysaccharides, which have more profound lipid-lowering effects, may be of particular use to hyperlipidaemic subjects. The usefulness of these supplements was thought to be limited in the past due to their low palatability and the high dose required (approximately 15 g/day). However, new food products containing these gums are being produced and tested (Burley *et al.*, 1984; Judd *et al.*, 1983; Schwandt *et al.*, 1981) and may enable a variety of products to be used to supply the required dose.

References

Avgerinos, G. C., Fuchs, H. M., Floch, M. H. (1977): Increased cholesterol and bile acid excretion during a high fiber diet. *Gastroenterology* **72**, 1026, Abstract.

Barrow, J. G., Quinlain, C. B., Edmando, R. E. (1961): Prevalence of atherosclerotic complications in Trappist and Benedictine monks. *Circulation* **24**, 881, Abstract.

Behall, K. M., Kelsay, J. L., Prather, E. S. (1978): Effect of fibre from fruits and vegetables on serum levels of triglycerides, free fatty acids, cholesterol, glucose, lactate, insulin, growth hormone, cortisol and phosphorus of human subjects. *Fed. Proc.* **37**, 543, Abstract.

Behall, K. M., Lee, K. H., Moser, P. B. (1984): Blood lipids and lipoproteins in adult men fed four refined fibres. *Am. J. Clin. Nutr.* **39**, 209–214.

van Berge-Henegouwen, G. P., Huybregts, A. W., van de Werf, S., Demacker, P. Schade, R. W. (1979): Effect of a standardized wheat bran preparation on serum lipids in young healthy males. *Am. J. Clin. Nutr.* **32**, 794–798.

Bhathena, S. J., Avignon, J. Schreiner, M. E. (1974): Effect of insulin on sterol and fatty acid synthesis and hydroxymethylglutaryl coA reductase activity in mammalian cells grown in culture. *Proc. Natl. Acad. Sci.* **71**, 2174–2178.

Blackburn, H. (1980): Diet-lipid-atherosclerosis relationship: epidemiological evidence and public health implications. In *Atherosclerosis V.* Proceedings of the Fifth International Symposium, ed A. M. Gotto, L. C. Smith, B. Allen. pp. 220–234. New York: Springer-Verlag.

Blackburn, N. A. Johnson, I. (1981): The effect of guar gum on the viscosity of the gastrointestinal contents and on glucose uptake from the perfused jejunum in the rat. *Br. J. Nutr.* **46**, 239–246.

Brodribb, A. J. M., Humphreys, D. M. (1976): Diverticular disease. Three studies. *Br. Med. J.* **1**, 424–430.

Burkitt, D. P. (1973): Some disease characteristics of modern Western civilisations. *Br. Med. J.* **1**, 274–278.

Burley, V., Leeds, A. R., Ellis, P. R., Peterson, D. B. (1985): Wholemeal guar bread: acceptability and efficacy combined. A study of blood glucose, plasma insulin and palatability in normal subjects. *Proc. Nutr. Soc.* **43**, 48A.

Burr, M. L., Bates, C. J., Fehily, A. M., St Leger, A. S. (1981): Plasma cholesterol and blood pressure in vegetarians. *J. Hum. Nutr.* **35**, 437–441.

Canella, C., Golinelli, G., Melli, A. (1962): Influenza sui valori colesterolemici della polpa de mela aggiunta all normale alimentazione. *Archispedale S. Anna de Ferrara* **15**, 803–814.

Castelle, W. B., Doyle, J. T., Gordon, T., Hames, C. G., Hjortland, M. C., Hulley, S. B., Kagan, A., Zekel, W. J. (1977): HDL cholesterol and other lipids in coronary heart disease: the cooperative lipoprotein phenotyping study. *Circulation* **55**, 767–772.

Chen, W. J. L., Anderson, J. W., Gould, M. R. (1981): Cholesterol-lowering effects of oat bran and oat gum. *Fed. Proc.* **40**, 852, Abstract.

Chenoweth, W. L., Benninck, H. R. (1976): Hypocholesterolaemic effect of oat fibre. *Fed. Proc.* **35**, 495 (A1598).

Delbarre, F. J., Fondier, J., De Gery, A. (1977): Lack of effect of two pectins on idiopathic or gout-associated hyperdyslipidemic hypercholesterolemia. *Am. J. Clin. Nutr.* **30**, 463–464.

Department of Health and Social Security (1974): *Diet and coronary heart disease.* Rep. Hlth Soc. Subj. No. 7 London: HMSO.

Descovich, G. C., 14 others, and Sirtori, C. R. (1980): Multicentre study of soybean protein diet for outpatient hypercholesterolaemic patients. *Lancet* **2**, 709–712.

van Dokkum, W. (1978): Zemelen in brood: verteerbaarheid en invloed op het defectatiepatroon, de mineralen-balans en de serum-lipidconcentraties bij de mens. *Voedingsmiddelentechnologie* **11**, 18.

Durrington, P. N., Manning, J. P., Bolton, C. H., Hartog, M. (1976): Effect of pectin on serum lipids and lipoproteins, whole gut transit time and stool weight *Lancet* **2**, 394–396.

Eastwood, M. A. (1978): Vegetable fibre: its physical properties. *Proc. Nutr. Soc.* **32**, 137–144.

Eastwood, M. A., Girdwood, R. H. (1968): Lignin – a bile salt sequestering agent. *Lancet* **2**, 1170–1172.

Eastwood, M. A., Hamilton, D. (1968): Studies on the absorption of bile salts to non-absorbed components of the diet. *Biochem. Biophys. Acta* **152**, 165–173.

Eastwood, M., Mowbray, L. (1976): The binding of components of mixed micelles to dietary fibre. *Am. J. Clin. Nutr.* **29**, 1461–1467.

Eastwood, M. A., Kirkpatrick, J. R., Mitchell, W. D., Bone, A., Hamilton, T. (1973): Effects of dietary supplements of wheat bran and cellulose on faeces and bowel function. *Br. Med. J.* **4**, 392–394.

Fahrenbach, M. H., Riccardi, B. A., Saunders, J. C., Lourie, N., Heider, J. C. (1965): Comparative effects of guar gum and pectin on human serum cholesterol levels. *Circulation, Suppl.* II to Vols **31** and **32**, 11.

Farrell, D. J., Girle, L., Arthur, J. (1978): Effects of dietary fibre on the apparent digestibility of major food components and on blood lipids in man. *Austr. J. Exp. Biol. Med. Sci.* **56**, 469–479.

Fisher, H., Griminger, P., Sostman, E. R., Brush, M. K. (1965): Dietary pectin and plasma cholesterol. *J. Nutr.* **86**, 113.

34

Flanagan, M., Little, C., Milliken, J., Wright, E., McGill, A. R., Weir, D. G., O'Moore, R. R. (1980): The effects of diet on high density lipoprotein. *J. Hum. Nutr.* **34**, 43–45.

Florén, C. H., Nilsson, Å. (1982): Binding of bile salts to fibre-enriched wheat bran. *Hum. Nutr. Clin. Nutr.* **36C**, 381–390.

Forman, D. T., Garvin, J. E., Forestner, J. E., Taylor, C. B. (1968): Increased excretion of faecal bile acids by an oral hydrophilic colloid. *Proc. Soc. Exp. Biol. Med.* **127**, 1060–1063.

Gatti, E., Catenazzo, G., Camisasca, E., Tori, A. (1984): Effects of guar-enriched pasta in the treatment of diabetes mellitus and hyperlipidaemia. *Ann. Nutr. Metab.* **28**, 1–10.

Gormley, T. R., Kevany, J., Egan, J. P., McFarlane, R. (1977): Effect of apples on serum cholesterol levels in humans. *Irish J. Fd Sci. Tech.* **1**, 117–128.

Gormley, T. R., Kevany, J., O'Donnel, B., McFarlane, R. (1979): Effect of peas on serum cholesterol levels in humans. *Irish J. Fd. Sci. Tech.* **3**, 101–109.

Grande, R., Anderson, J. T., Keys, A. (1965): Effect of carbohydrates of leguminous seeds, wheat and potatoes on serum cholesterol concentration in man. *J. Nutr.* **86**, 313–317.

Grande, F., Anderson, J. T., Keys, A. (1974): Sucrose and various carbohydrate-containing foods and serum lipids in man. *Am. J. Clin. Nutr.* **27**, 1043–1051.

de Groot, A. P., Luyken, R., Pikaar, N. A. (1963): Cholesterol-lowering effect of rolled oats. *Lancet* **2**, 304.

Hardinge, M. G., Chambers, A. C., Crooks, H., Stare, F. J. (1958): Nutritional studies of vegetarians. III Dietary levels of fiber. *Am. J. Clin. Nutr.* **6**, 523–525.

Heaton, K. W., Manning, A. P., Hartog, M. (1976): Lack of effect on blood lipid and calcium concentrations of young men on changing from white to wholemeal bread. *Br. J. Nutr.* **35**, 55–60.

Helms, P. (1977): Soybean-protein diet and plasma-cholesterol. *Lancet* **1**, 805.

Hopson, J. J. (1967): Studies on the effect of dietary pectin on plasma and fecal lipids. M.Sc. thesis, University of Iowa. [Quoted by Chenoweth, W. L. and Leveille, G. A.: Metabolism and physiological effects of food pectins. In *Physiological effects of food carbohydrates*, ed. A. Jeanes J. Hodge, pp. 312–324].

Irie, N., Hara, T., Goto, Y. (1982): The effects of guar gum on post-prandial chylomicronaemia. *Nutr. Rep. Int.* **26**, 207–214.

Jenkins, D. J. A., Hill, M. S., Cummings, J. H. (1975): Effect of wheat fiber on blood lipids, fecal steroid excretion and serum iron. *Am. J. Clin. Nutr.* **28**, 1408–1411.

Jenkins, D. J. A., Leeds, A. R., Newton, C., Cummings, J. H. (1975): Effect of pectin, guar gum and wheat fibre on serum cholesterol. *Lancet* **1**, 1116–1117.

Jenkins, D. J. A., Leeds, A. R., Gassull, M. A., Houston, H., Goff, D. V., Hill, M. J. (1976): The cholesterol lowering effect of guar and pectin. *Clin. Sci. Mol. Med.* **51**, 8.

Jenkins, D. J. A. (1977): Action of dietary fibre in lowering fasting serum cholesterol and reducing post-prandial glycaemia. In *International conference on atherosclerosis*, Milan, 1977, ed L. A. Carlson, R. Paolotti, G. Weber, p. 173. New York: Raven Press.

Jenkins, D. J. A., Leeds, A. R., Slavin, B., Mann, J., Jepson, E. M. (1979): Dietary fiber and blood lipids: reduction of serum cholesterol in Type II hyperlipidaemia by guar gum. *Am. J. Clin. Nutr.* **32**, 16–18.

Jenkins, D. J. A., Reynolds, D., Leeds, A. R., Waller, A. L., Cummings, J. H. (1979): Hypocholesterolemic action of dietary fibre unrelated to fecal bulking effect. *Am. J. Clin. Nutr.* **32**, 2430–2435.

Jenkins, D. J. A., Bloom, S. R., Albequerque, R. H., Leeds, A. R., Sarson, D. L., Metz, G. L., Alberti, K. G. M. M. (1980a): Pectin and complications of gastric surgery: normalisation of post-prandial glucose and endocrine responses. *Gut* **21**, 574–579.

Jenkins, D. J. A., Reynolds, D., Slavin, B., Leeds, A. R., Jenkins, A. K., Jepson, E. M. (1980b): Dietary fiber and blood lipids: treatment of hypercholesterolaemia with guar crispbread. *Am. J. Clin. Nutr.* **33**, 575–581.

Jenkins, D. J. A., Wong, G. S., Patten, R., Bird, J., Hall, M., Buckley, G. C., McGuire, V., Reichart, R., Little, J. A. (1983): Leguminous seeds in the dietary management of hyperlipidaemia. *Am. J. Clin. Nutr.* **38**, 567–573.

Judd, P. A., Kay, R. M., Truswell, A. S., (1976): Cholesterol-lowering effect of lignin in rats. *Proc. Nutr. Soc.* **35**, 73A.

Judd, P. A., Truswell, A. S. (1981): The effect of rolled oats on blood lipids and faecal steroid excretion in man. *Am. J. Clin. Nutr.* **34**, 2061–2067.

Judd, P. A., Truswell, A. S. (1982): Comparison of the effects of high- and low-methoxyl pectins on blood and faecal lipids in man. *Br. J. Nutr.* **48**, 451–458.

Judd, P. A. (1982): The effects of high intakes of barley on gastrointestinal function and apparent digestibility of dry matter, nitrogen and fat in human volunteers. *J. Plant Foods* **4**, 79–88.

Judd, P. A., Leeds, A. R., Ellis, P. R., Apling, C., Jepson, E. (1983): A new guar bread: an effective hypocholesterolaemic agent in subjects with hypercholesterolaemia. *Proc. Nutr. Soc. Engl.* **42**, 120A.

Judd, P. A., Truswell, A. S. (1985): The hypocholesterolaemic effects of pectins in rats. *Br. J. Nutr.*, **53**, 409–425.

Kaur, A. P., Bhat, C. M., Godara, R. B. (1981): Effect of cellulose on serum lipids in adolescent girls. *J. Hum. Nutr.* **35**, 456–460.

Kay, R. M. (1976): Pectin and serum-cholesterol. *Lancet* **2**, 799.

Kay, R. M., Truswell, A. S. (1977a): Effect of wheat fibre on gastrointestinal function, plasma lipids and steroid excretion in man. *Br. J. Nutr.* **37**, 227–235.

Kay, R. M., Truswell, A. S. (1977b): Effect of citrus pectin on blood lipids and faecal steroid excretion in man. *Am. J. Clin. Nutr.* **30**, 171–175.

Kay, R. M., Strasberg, S. M., Petruka, C. N., Wayman, M. (1979): Differential absorption of bile acids by lignins. In *Dietary fibres, chemistry and nutrition* ed G. E. Inglett, S. I. Falkehag, pp. 57–66. New York: Academic Press.

Kay, R. M., Truswell, A. S. (1980): Dietary fiber: effects on plasma and biliary lipids in man. In *Medical aspects of dietary fiber* ed G. A. Spiller, R. M. Kay, pp. 153–173. Plenum: New York and London.

Kay, R. M., Sabry, Z., Czisma, A. (1980): Multivariate analysis of diet and serum lipids in normal men. *Am. J. Clin. Nutr* **33**, 2566–2572.

Kelsay, J. L., Clark, W. M., Herbst, B. J., Prather, E. S. (1981): Nutrient utilisation by human subjects consuming fruits and vegetables as sources of fibre. *J. Agric. Fd. Chem.* **29**, 461–465.

Keys, A., Fidanza, F., Keys, M. H. (1955): Further studies on serum cholesterol of clinically healthy men in Italy. *Voeding* **16**, 492–497.

Keys, A., Anderson, J. T., Grande, F. (1960): Diet-type (fats constant) and blood lipids in man. *J. Nutr.* **70**, 257–266.

Keys, A., Grande, F., Anderson, J. T. (1961): Fiber and pectin in the diet and serum cholesterol concentration in man. *Proc. Soc. Exp. Biol. Med.* **106**, 555–558.

Keys, A., Anderson, J., Grande, F. (1965): Serum cholesterol response to changes in the diet. IV. Particular saturated fatty acids in the diet. *Metabolism* **14**, 776–787.

Kies, C., Fox, H. M. (1977): Dietary hemicellulose interactions influencing serum lipid patterns and protein nutritional status of adult men. *J. Fd Sci.* **42**, 440–443.

Kirby, R. W., Anderson, J. W., Sieling, B., Rees, E. D., Chen, W. J. L., Miller, R. E., Kay, R. M. (1981): Oat bran selectivity lowers serum low-density lipoprotein concentration: studies of hypercholesterolemic men. *Am. J. Clin. Nutr.* **34**, 824–929.

Kretsch, M. J., Crawford, L. K., Calloway, D. A. (1979): Some aspects of bile acid and urobilinogen excretion and faecal elimination in men given a rural Guatemalan diet and egg formulas with and without added oat bran. *Am. J. Clin. Nutr.* **32**, 1492–1496.

Langley, N. J., Thye, F. W. (1977): The effect of wheat bran and/or citrus pectin on serum cholesterol and triglycerides in middle aged men. *Fed. Proc.* **36**, 1118, Abstract.

Letchford, P., Zabroja, R., Arthur, J., Farrell, D. J. (1978): Manipulation of plasma cholesterol in man and its suppression. *Proc. Nutr. Soc. Australia* **3**, 97.

Leveille, G. A., Sauberlich, H. E. (1966): Mechanism of the cholesterol-depressing effect of pectin in the cholesterol-fed rat. *J. Nutr.* **88**, 209–214.

Levine, A. S., Silvis, S. E. (1980): Absorption of whole peanuts, peanut oil and peanut butter. *New Engl. J. Med.* **303**, 1729–1733.

Lewis, B., Chait, A., Oakley, C. M., Wooten, D. P., Krikler, D. M., Onitiri, A., Sigurdsson, S., February, A. (1974): Serum lipoprotein abnormalities in patients with coronary heart disease. *Br. Med. J.* **3**, 489–493.

Lewis, B., Hammett, F., Katan, M., Kay, R. M., Merkx, I., Nobels, A., Miller, N. E., Swan, A. V. (1981): Towards an improved lipid-lowering diet: additive effects of changes in nutrient intake. *Lancet* **2**, 1310–1313.

Liebman, M., Smith, M. C., Iverson, J., Thye, F. W., Hinkle, D. E., Herbert, W. G., Ritchey, S. J., Driscoll, J. A. (1983): Effects of coarse wheat bran fiber and exercise on plasma lipids and lipoproteins in moderately overweight men. *Am. J. Clin. Nutr.* **37**, 71–81.

Lindegärde, F., Larsson, L. (1984): Effects of a concentrated bran fibre preparation on HDL-cholesterol in hypocholesterolaemic men. *Hum. Nutr. Clin. Nutr.* **38C**, 39–46.

Lopez, A., Hopson, J., Krehl, W. A. (1968): Effect of dietary pectin on plasma and fecal lipids. *Fed. Proc.* **27**, 495, Abstract.

Luyken, R., Pikaar, N. A., Polman, H., Schippers, F. (1962): The influence of legumes on the serum cholesterol level. *Voeding* **23**, 447–453.

Luyken, R., de Wijn, J. F., Pikaar, N. A., Van der Meer, R. (1965): De invloed van havermont op het serum-cholesterolgehalte van het bloed. *Voeding* **26**, 229–244.

McDougall, R. M., Yakymyshyn, L., Walker, K., Thurston, O. G. (1978): Effects of wheat bran on serum lipoproteins and biliary lipids. *Can. J. Surg.* **21**, 433–438.

Malholtra, S. L. (1967): Serum lipids, dietary factors and ischemic heart disease. *Am. J. Clin. Nutr.* **20**, 462–474.

Marks, V., Turner, D. S. (1977): The gastrointestinal hormones with particular reference to their role in the regulation of insulin secretion. *Essays Biochem.* **3**, 109–152.

Mathur, K. S., Khan, M. A., Sharma, R. D. (1968): Hypocholesterolaemic effect of Bengal gram: a long-term study in man. *Br. Med. J.* **1**, 30–31.

Mathur, M. S., Singh, F., Chadda, V. S. (1977): Effect of bran on blood lipids. *J. Assn. Physns India* **25**, 275–278.

Miettinen, R. A., Tarpila, S. (1977): Effect of pectin on serum cholesterol, fecal bile acids and biliary lipids in normolipidemic and hyperlipidemic individuals. *Clin. Chim. Acta* **79**, 471–477.

Miettinen, T. A. (1980): Effects of dietary fiber on serum lipids and cholesterol metabolism in man. In *Atherosclerosis, V (Proc.)*, ed A. M. Gotto, L. C. Smith, B. Allen, pp. 311–315. New York: Springer-Verlag.

Miettinen, T. A. (1983): Effects of dietary fiber on cholesterol metabolism in man. In *Fibre in human and animal nutrition*, ed G. Wallace, L. Bell, *Roy. Soc. N.Z. Bull.* **20**, 173–177.

Miranda, P. M., Horwitz, D. L. (1978): High fiber diets in the treatment of diabetes mellitus. *Ann. Int. Med.* **88**, 482–486.

Mokady, S. (1974): Effect of dietary pectin and algin on the biosynthesis of hepatic lipids in growing rats. *Nutr. Metab.* **16**, 203–207.

Morgan, L. M., Goulder, I. J., Tsiolakis, D., Marks, V., Alberti, K. G. M. M. (1979): The effect of unabsorbable carbohydrates on gut hormones. *Diabetologia* **17**, 85–89.

Morrison, W. R., Mann, D. L., Soon, W., Coventry, A. M. (1975): Selective extraction and quantitative analysis of non-starch and starch lipids from wheat flour. *J. Sci. Fd Agric.* **26**, 507–521.

Munoz, J. M., Sanstead, H. H., Jacob, R. A., Logan, G. M., Reck, S. J., Klevay, L. M., Dinitzis, F. R., Inglett, G. F., Shuey, W. C. (1979*a*): Effects of some cereal brans and TVP on plasma lipids. *Am. J. Clin. Nutr.* **32**, 580–592.

Munoz, J. M., Sandstead, H. H., Jacob, R. A. (1979*b*): Effects of dietary fibre on glucose tolerance of normal men. *Diabetes* **28**, 496–502.

Oliver, M. F. (1984): Hypercholesterolaemia and coronary heart disease: an answer. *Br. Med. J.* **1**, 423–424.

Palmer, G. H., Dixon, D. G. (1968): Effect of pectin dose on serum cholesterol levels. *Am. J. Clin. Nutr.* **18**, 437–442.

Persson, I., Raby, K. N., Fønns-Bech, P., Jensen, E. (1975): Bran and blood lipids. *Lancet* **2**, 1308.

Pfeffer, P. E., Doner, L. W., Hoagland, P. D., McDonald, C. G. (1981): Molecular interactions with dietary fibre components. Investigation of the possible association of pectin and bile acids. *J. Agric. Fd. Chem.* **29**, 455–461.

Phillips, R. L., Lemon, F. R., Beeson, W. L., Kuzma, J. W. (1978): Coronary heart disease mortality among Seventh-Day Adventists with differing dietary habits: a preliminary report. *Am. J. Clin. Nutr.* **31**, Suppl. S191–198.

Prather, E. S. (1964): Effect of cellulose on serum lipids in young women. *J. Am. Diet. Ass.* **45**, 230.

Preece, I. A., Hobkirk, R. (1953): Non starch polysaccharides of cereal grains III Higher molecular gums of common cereals. *J. Inst. Brew.* **59**, 385–392.

van Raaij, J. M. A., Katan, M. B., Hautvast, J. G. A. J., Hermus, R. J. J. (1981): Effects of casein versus soy protein diets on serum cholesterol and lipoproteins in young healthy volunteers. *Am. J. Clin. Nutr.* **34**, 1261–1271.

van Raaij, J. M. A., Katan, M. B., West, C. E., Hautvast, J. G. A. J. (1982): Influence of diets containing casein, soy isolate and soy concentrate on serum cholesterol and lipoproteins in middle-aged volunteers. *Am. J. Clin. Nutr.* **35**, 925–934.

Raymond, T. L., Connor, W. E., Liu, D. S., Warner, S., Fry, M. M., Connor, S. L. (1977): The interaction of dietary fibres and cholesterol upon the plasma lipids and lipoproteins, sterol balance, and bowel function in human subjects. *J. Clin. Invest.* **60**, 1429–1437.

Rivellese, A., Riccardi, G., Giaco, A., Pacioni, D., Gebivesem, S., Mattioli, P. L., Mancini, M. (1980): Effect of dietary fibre on glucose control and serum lipoproteins in diabetic patients. *Lancet* **2**, 447–450.

Robertson, J., Brydon, W. G., Tadesse, K., Wenham, P., Walls, A., Eastwood, M. A. (1979): The effect of raw carrot on serum lipids and colon function. *Am. J. Clin. Nutr.* **32**, 1889–1892.

Rosenberg, S., Andersen, J. O. (1982): The effect of antibiotics on some lipid metabolism parameters in rats receiving cornstarch, potato flour or pectin in the diet. *Acta Agric. Scand.* **32**, 321–340.

Royal College of Physicians of London and the British Cardiac Society (1976): *Prevention of coronary heart disease. J. Roy. Coll. Physns.* **10**, 9.

Sacks, F. M., Castelli, W. P., Donner, A., Kass, E. M. (1975): Plasma lipids and lipoproteins in vegetarians and controls. *New Engl. J. Med.* **292**, 1148–1151.

Salvioli, G. R., Salati, R., Lugli, R. (1980): Effect of bran on serum lipoprotein and on fecel bile acids and neutral sterols. In *Diet and drugs in atherosclerosis* ed E. Noseda, B. Lewis, R. Paoletti, pp. 29–33. New York: Raven Press.

Sandberg, A. T. S., Ahderinne, R., Anderson, H., Hallgren, B., Hutten, L. (1983): The effect of citrus pectin on the absorption of nutrients in the small-intestine. *Hum. Nutr. Clin. Nutr.* **37C**, 171–184.

Schnell, M., Pacy, J., Judd, P. A. (1985): The effect of guar gum on chylomicron size and composition in rats. *Proc. Nutr. Soc.* **44**, 17A.

Schwandt, P., Richter, W. O., Weisweiler, P. (1981): Soybean protein and plasma cholesterol. *Atherosclerosis* **40**, 371–372.

Schwandt, P., Richter, W. O., Weisweiler, P., Neureuther, G. (1982): Cholestyramine plus pectin in treatment of patients with familial hyper-cholesterolemia. *Atherosclerosis* **39**, 379–383.

Schweizer, T. F., Bekhechi, A. R., Koellreutter, B., Reimann, S., Pometta, D., Bron, B. A. (1983): Metabolic effects of dietary fiber from dehulled soybeans in humans. *Am. J. Clin. Nutr.* **38**, 1–11.

Shurpalekar, K. S., Doraiswamy, T. R., Sunderavalli, O. E., Rao, M. N. (1971): Effect of inclusion of cellulose in an 'atherogenic' diet on the blood lipids of children. *Nature* **232**, 554–555.

Sirtori, C. R., Gatti, E., Mantero, O., Conti, F., Agradi, E., Tremoli, E., Sirtori, M., Fraterrigo, L., Tavazzi, L., Kritchevsky, D. (1979): Clinical experience with the soybean protein diet in the treatment of hypocholesterolemia. *Am. J. Clin. Nutr.* **32**, 1645–1658.

Sirtori, C. R., Descovich, G., Noseda, G. (1980): Textured soy protein and serum cholesterol. *Lancet* **1**, 149.

Southgate, D. A. T., Durnin, J. V. G. A. (1970): Calorie conversion factors. An experimental reassessment of the factors used in calculating the energy value of human diets. *Br. J. Nutr.* **24**, 517–535.

Stanley, M. M., Paul, D., Gacke, D., Murphy, J. (1972): Effect of cholestyramine, metamucil and cellulose on fecal bile acid excretion in man. *Gastroneterology* **65**, 889–894.

Stasse-Wolthuis, M., Katan, M. B., Hermus, R. J. J., Hautvast, J. G. A. J. (1979): Increase of serum cholesterol in man fed a bran diet. *Atherosclerosis* **34**, 87–91.

Stasse-Wolthuis, M., Albers, H. F. F., van Jeveren, J. G. C. Wil de Jong, J., Hautvast, J. G. A. J., Hermus, R. J. J., Katan, M. B., Brydon, W. C., Eastwood, M. A. (1980): Influence of dietary fiber from vegetables and fruits, bran or citrus pectin on serum lipids, fecal lipids and colonic function. *Am. J. Clin. Nutr.* **33**, 1745–1756.

Story, J. A., Kelley, M. J. (1982): Dietary fibre and lipoproteins. In *Dietary fibre in health and disease*, ed G. V. Vahouney, D. Kritchevsky, pp. 229–236. New York and London: Plenum Press.

Story, J. A., Thomas, J. N. (1982): Modification of bile acid spectrum by dietary fiber. In *Dietary fiber in health and disease*, ed G. V. Vahouney, D. Kritchevsky, pp. 193–202. New York and London: Plenum Press.

Tarpila, S., Miettinen, T. A. (1977): Effects of plantaco fibre on serum lipids and fecal composition in hypercholesterolaemic patients. *Scand. J. Gastroenterol.* **12**, (S.45) 105.

Tarpila, S., Miettinen, T. A., Metsaranto, L. (1978): Effects of bran on serum cholesterol, faecal mass, fat, bile acids and neutral steroids and biliary lipids in patients with diverticular disease of the colon. *Gut* **19**, 137–145.

Tarpila, S., Miettinen, T. A. (1980): Effects of guar gum and high fibre diet on serum lipoproteins, cholesterol absorption and fecal steroids. *Scand. J. Gastroenterol.* **15**, Abst. 14.

Thiffault, C., Belanger, M., Pauliot, M. (1970): Traitment de l'hyperlipoprotinémie essentielle de type II par un nouvel agent therapeutique, la Celluline. *Can Med Ass Jl.* **103**, 165–166.

Trowell, H. C. (1972): Ischaemic heart disease and dietary fibre. *Am. J. Clin. Nutr.* **25**, 926–932.

Trowell, H. C., Painter, N., Burkitt, D. P. (1974): Aspects of the epidemiology of diverticular disease and ischaemic heart disease. *Am. J. Dig. Disease* **19**, 864–873.

Truswell, A. S., Kay, R. M. (1975): Absence of effect of wheat bran on blood lipids. *Lancet* **1**, 922.

Tsai, A. C., Mott, E. L., McOwen, G. M., Benninck, M., Lo, G. S., Steinke, F. (1983): Effects of soy polysaccharide on gastrointestinal functions, nutrient balance, steroid excretions, glucose tolerance, serum lipids and other parameters in humans. *Am. J. Clin. Nutr.* **38**, 504–511.

Tuomilehto, J., Karrttunen, P., Vinni, S., Kostianinen, E., Uusitupa, M., (1983): A double-blind evaluation of guar gum in patients with dyslipidaemia. *Hum. Nutr.: Clin. Nutr.* **37C**, 109–116.

Vahouney, G. V. (1982): Dietary fibers and intestinal absorption of lipids. In *Dietary fiber in health and disease*, ed G. V. Vahouney, D. Kritchevsky, pp. 203–227. New York and London: Plenum Press.

Walker, A. R. P., Arvidsson, U. B. (1954): Fat intake, serum cholesterol concentration and atherosclerosis in the South African Bantu. *J. Clin. Invest.* **33**, 1358–1365.

Walters, R. L., McLean Baird, I., Davies, P. S., Hill, M. J., Drasar, B. S., Southgate, D. A. T., Green, J., Morgan, B. (1975): Effects of two types of dietary fibre on faecal steroid and lipid excretion. *Br. Med. J.* **2**, 536–538

Wells, A. F., Ershoff, B. H. (1961): Beneficial effects of pectin in prevention of hypercholesterolaemia and increase in liver cholesterol in cholesterol-fed rats. *J. Nutr.* **74**, 87–92.

Wirth, A., Middelhoff, G., Bracuning, C. L., Schlierf, G. (1982): Treatment of familial hypercholesterolaemia with a combination of Bezafibrate and guar. *Atherosclerosis* **45**, 291–297.

World Health Organisation (1982): *Prevention of coronary heart disease.* Report of a WHO Expert Committee. Tech. Rep. Ser. No. 678. Geneva: WHO.

Wu, A. L., Bennet-Clark, S., Holt, P. R. (1980): Composition of lymph chylomicrons from proximal and distal rat small intestine. *Am. J. Clin. Nutr.* **33**, 582–589.

Zavoral, J. H., Hannan, P., Fields, D. J., Hanson, M. N., Frantz, I. D., Kuba, K., Elmer, P., Jacobs, D. R. (1983): The hypolipidaemic effect of locust bean food products in familial hypercholesterolaemic adults and children. *Am. J. Clin. Nutr.* **38**, 285–294.

3
Dietary fibre and gallstones

Patricia A. Judd

Introduction

Epidemiological and experimental evidence is consistent with the hypothesis proposed by Heaton (1973) that consumption of fibre-depleted carbohydrate favours the formation of cholesterol-rich gallstones. A decade later it is still not clear, however, whether overnutrition consequent on consumption of a fibre-depleted diet (Heaton, 1973*a*) is the major cause or whether dietary fibre *per se* has a particular protective effect.

Development of the cholesterol gallstones commonly found in Western populations occurs when cholesterol precipitates from super-saturated (lithogenic) gall-bladder bile. Patients with gallstones also have a reduced bile-acid pool of around 1.5–2.0 g compared to the normal population level of 3–5 g (Sherlock, 1981; Vlahcevic *et al.*, 1976). This in itself may be a factor contributing to the formation of supersaturated bile.

Cholesterol secretion into bile is excessive in many patients with gallstones, possibly due to an increase in cholesterol synthesis (Nestel *et al.*, 1973; Grundy *et al.*, 1984). 3-Hydroxy-3-methylglutaryl coenzyme A (HMGCoA) reductase is the rate-limiting enzyme in hepatic cholesterol synthesis and overactivity of this enzyme has been suggested as a causal factor (Coyne *et al.*, 1976). The enzyme is stimulated by insulin and its activity is increased in obesity. Chenodeoxycholic acid, a primary bile acid, has been shown to reduce the activity of HMGCoA reductase (Coyne *et al.*, 1976) and has been used as a treatment for gallstones.

The cause of the reduced bile acid pool in patients with gallstones is not clear but it is thought to be due to reduced bile acid synthesis in the liver. Cholesterol 7-α-hydroxylase, the main rate-limiting enzyme in bile acid synthesis, is less active in patients with gallstones than control patients. Diet, and dietary fibre in particular, could therefore be involved in the aetiology of gallstones, both via effects on energy intake and obesity and by its ability to modify bile acid metabolism.

Refined carbohydrate, fibre and obesity

Cholesterol-rich gallstones are commonly associated with hyperglycaemia (and diabetes mellitus) and hypertriglyceridaemia as well as obesity (Heaton, 1973, 1979; Bennion & Grundy, 1975; Angelin, 1977; Ponz de Leon *et al.*, 1978) and consumption of refined carbohydrates has been suggested as a causative factor — both because this leads to high energy intake and because of the low levels of dietary fibre (Heaton, 1972; 1973*a*).

French workers have consistently implied that excessive energy intake is an important factor in the aetiology of gallstones (Sarles *et al.*, 1970; 1971; 1978*a*;

1978*b*), but three other studies have contradicted this (Wheeler *et al.*, 1970; Burnett, 1971; Costé *et al.*, 1979). A fourth contradictory study suggested that although female patients with gallstones were heavier than controls, their energy intake was lower (Smith & Gee, 1979). The authors linked this with the idea that fasting causes the production of a more lithogenic bile which is relieved by eating (Northfield & Hofmann, 1975; Larusso *et al.*, 1974).

Many of these studies have been criticised in a recent paper from Australia (Scragg *et al.*, 1984*a*). This describes a case-control study where 297 patients who had only recently developed gallstones (and theoretically, therefore, not changed their diets due to the disease) were compared with both hospital and community controls. Obesity was found to be associated with development of the disease only in young women (<50) but high intakes of energy and fat were a risk factor for young people of both sexes. Heaton (1984), reviewing the paper, suggested that the lack of association with obesity in men, despite the evidence that obese men have supersaturated bile (Bennion & Grundy, 1975; Mabee *et al.*, 1976) may be explained by the use of Quetelet's Index (weight/height^2) — which does not measure 'fatness' as such — as the measure of obesity.

Dietary fibre intake in the Australian study (Scragg *et al.*, 1984*a*) was negatively associated with gallstones, ie there was a suggestion that it had a protective effect. This supported an earlier report from Thornton *et al.* (1983) where patients with probable gallstones ate alternatively refined and unrefined carbohydrate diets (randomly assigned, with 6 weeks on each diet). On the refined diet, energy and sugar intakes were higher and dietary fibre intakes lower, and resulted in higher bile cholesterol saturation. In order to distinguish between the effects of refined sugar and fibre a second study (Werner *et al.*, 1984) was carried out.

In this case, patients with supersaturated bile took either a high (112 g/day) or low (14 g/day) sucrose diet for 6-week periods. Dietary fibre intake was 18.7 ± 1.3 g on the low sugar diet and 15.5 ± 0.7 g/day on the high sugar diet ($P < 0.01$). The results showed no difference in the lipid composition of bile, suggesting that dietary fibre and not the lower sucrose intake was the protective factor in the previous experiment.

The Adelaide study (Scragg *et al.*, 1984*a*), however, did produce evidence for the hypothesis that refined sugar is implicated in the development of gallstones — independently of obesity. Heaton (1984) suggested — commenting on Scragg *et al.*, 1984*a* — that sucrose may therefore act by stimulating insulin secretion, as insulin stimulates cholesterol synthesis *in vitro* (Bhathena, Avignon & Schreiner, 1974), and people with high sugar intakes sometimes have raised plasma insulin levels. A subsequent report from the Adelaide group (Scragg *et al.*, 1984*b*) has confirmed that higher plasma insulin levels were associated with increased risk of gallstones. In this study, although patients had higher sucrose intakes than controls, the effect of insulin appeared to be independent of all dietary variables.

Together with these observations, it is worth noting that some foods containing dietary fibre and some water-soluble components of the dietary fibre complex have been shown to reduce post-prandial insulin responses in man (Allbrink *et al.*, 1979; Jenkins *et al.*, 1977). This may therefore be one route by which high fibre intakes protect against gallstones.

Wheat bran

The cholesterol-saturation (or lithogenic) index of bile is a measure based on the molar ratios of bile acids, cholesterol and phospholipids — an index of greater than 1 indicating that formation of gallstones is likely (Thomas & Hofman, 1973). Several studies have demonstrated that addition of relatively large amounts of wheat bran to the diet of patients with gallstones reduces the cholesterol-saturation index of bile if this is initially raised. If it is normal, however, no such effect is shown.

Thus, an average of 33 g (range 20–100 g) of wheat bran eaten for 6–10 weeks significantly improved cholesterol saturation in patients with gallstones and an initial index of 1.5 (Pomare *et al.*, 1976). A similar quantity of bran consumed for 2 months reduced the saturation index in patients with an initial level >1, but those patients with a normal cholesterol saturation index demonstrated no change (Watts *et al.*, 1978). This lack of effect in normal subjects was also demonstrated by Wicks and co-workers (1978). Larger doses of bran had similar effects, eg McDougall and co-workers (1978) feeding an average of 50 g wheat bran per day demonstrated a reduction in the lithogenic index from 1.35 to 0.71 in patients, but no effect in control subjects. One other study has failed to show any effect of high doses of wheat bran, even when initial cholesterol-saturation index was high (Tarpila *et al.*, 1978).

In those experiments where the lithogenic index has fallen during consumption of wheat bran, this has usually been accompanied by changes in the biliary bile-acid spectrum. The changes have been described in detail by Story & Thomas (1982), but can be summarized as an increase in the proportion of chenodeoxycholic acid and a decrease in deoxycholate content of the bile.

As chenodeoxycholate inhibits cholesterol synthesis by altering the activity of HMGCoA reductase — the rate-limiting enzyme in cholesterol synthesis (Coyne *et al.*, 1976; Cooper, 1976) — and has also been shown to inhibit cholesterol absorption in man (Ponz de Leon, 1979) and animals (Wilson, 1972), these changes could be significant in the aetiology of gallstones. Chenodeoxycholic acid is currently used as a drug for the treatment of gallstones (Hofman, 1980).

It has been speculated that the changes in bile acid composition when wheat bran is fed might be due to reduced production of deoxycholate in the colon (Pomare *et al.*, 1973). This might be due to alterations in colonic flora with fewer bacteria able to dehydroxylate bile salts or to changes in the colonic environment which inhibit the enzyme 7-α-dehydroxylase. Changes in transit time and bulkier, more dilute colonic contents might also result in reduced contact between bile salts and bacteria — a mechanism which has also been suggested to be protective against large bowel cancer (Hill *et al.*, 1971).

A further suggestion is that reduced absorption of the dihydroxy bile acids (deoxycholic and lithocholic) produced in the colon may be part of the mechanism. Certain types of dietary fibre or fibre components have been shown to increase faecal bile acid excretion and reduce plasma cholesterol levels, but wheat fibre has repeatedly been shown to be ineffective in this respect (see Chapter 2).

Effect of components of dietary fibre

Pectin, a non-cellulosic polysaccharide which does increase faecal bile acid excretion, does not appear to have significant effects on biliary bile acid composition. Twelve grams of pectin daily for four weeks (Hillman *et al.*, 1983) had no significant effects and doses of up to 50 g per day for two weeks appeared to increase biliary deoxycholate rather than chenodeoxycholate (Miettinen & Tarpila, 1977). Results in the latter experiment were inconsistent and not statistically significant, however, and as with bran, the supersaturated bile in one subject returned to within normal limits after treatment with pectin.

Hillman and co-workers (1983) also studied another dietary fibre component, cellulose, at a dose of 15 g per day for four weeks and showed no significant changes in biliary composition.

Mixed high fibre diets

Increasing dietary fibre intakes from mixed food sources has also shown varying effects. Thornton *et al.* (1983) demonstrated a reduction in lithocholic index from 1.5 ± 0.10 on a 'refined' diet to 1.2 ± 0.12 on an 'unrefined' diet containing fibre from various food sources. This is a less pronounced change than that produced by feeding wheat bran and Heaton (1984) has suggested that there may be a threshold intake of fibre which must be attained before pronounced changes in biliary composition are seen.

Tarpila & Miettinen (1983) studied 34 middle-aged men on their normal diets and subsequently on high or low fibre diets for two months. Cholesterol-saturation index was unchanged on the high fibre diet, but biliary chenodeoxycholate levels fell as deoxycholate increased. The authors state that measurement of faecal β-sitosterol products indicated reduced bacterial activity during consumption of this particular high fibre diet. However, this study, together with observations of populations in the South Pacific and New Zealand (NZ) may suggest explanations for some of the different results.

Pomare (1983) describes a study comparing 25 healthy Tongan women living on an island in the South Pacific with 24 Tongans who had lived in New Zealand for an average of 5 years, 25 New Zealand Europeans and 19 New Zealand Maoris. Dietary fibre intakes and sources are shown in the Table. The Tongan islanders had extremely high intakes of dietary fibre — largely from roots and tubers and with relatively little supplied by cereals compared to the New Zealand groups. Their diet therefore contained large quantities of fermentable non-cellulosic polysaccharides in the form of pectins and hemicellulose. Biliary bile acid studies showed results opposite to those produced by bran-feeding — but similar to the study of Miettinen & Tarpila (1977) using pectin — ie significantly higher levels of deoxycholate and lower levels of chenodeoxycholate.

Pomare suggested that changes in the environment in the large intestine caused by different rates of fermentation of dietary fibre may be responsible for the differing effects of fibre components and foods containing fibre. Breakdown of bile acids in the colon is closely related to the activity of 7-α-dehydroxylase and the bacteria producing it. This enzyme is inhibited by pH less than 6.5 and Pomare suggested that the presence of slowly degraded fibres such as bran (or cellulose)

Table. *Dietary fibre intakes and sources in Tongan islanders, NZ Tongans, NZ Europeans and NZ Maoris* (From Pomare, 1983)

| | Tongan islanders (n = 25) | | New Zealand populations | | |
			Tongan (n = 25)	European (n = 25)	Maori (n = 25)
Dietary fibre intake (g)	71			18	
Sources	% of total	g	% of total	g	
Root veg	65*	45	?	?	
Fruit	31	22	20	4	
Cereals	2	2	32	6	
Leafy greens	2	2	34	6	

*Largely taro, cassava, yam and breadfruit.

may result in sustained reductions of colonic pH and inhibit the production of deoxycholic acid. High intakes of rapidly fermentable polysaccharides such as those eaten by the Tongan islanders may result in excessive degradation of bile acids and an increase in biliary deoxycholate.

Pomare's hypothesis may be borne out by the observations in Finland (Miettinen, 1983) where the high fibre diet (27 g per day) was said to be relatively high in soluble non-cellulosic polysaccharides from oat products, although the fact that Miettinen reported reduced bacterial activity in the colon appears to contradict the idea.

It may also appear that, as viscous polysaccharides such as pectins and hemicellulose appear to bind bile acids and cause increased faecal excretion of metabolites, the increase in biliary deoxycholate may be partly due to the presence of increased substrate for bacterial action.

Conclusions

The original essentially simple hypothesis of a link between dietary fibre and gallstones, ie that a low level of the former leads to the latter, is still not matched by a simple understanding of what causes this effect. It may result from some direct action of dietary fibre or its components or may be due to the interaction of these with other dietary components. Or it may be that dietary fibre has no direct role and it is overnutrition associated with low fibre intake which is the aetiological factor.

Many factors, including the type of fibre, the level at which it is fed, and the period of time required for changes in biliary composition to occur, may result in problems in interpreting results. However, an additional line of enquiry, both promising and inconvenient as far as an understanding of the link between dietary fibre and gallstones is concerned, is the possible role of fermentation of fibre in the colon of the individual.

References

Allbrink, M. J., Neuman, T., Davidson, P. C. (1979): Effect of high and low-fiber diets on plasma lipids and insulin. *Am. J. Clin. Nutr.* **32**, 1486–1491.

Angelin, B. (1977): Cholesterol and bile acid metabolism in normo- and hyperlipoproteinaemia. *Acta Med. Scand.* **610** (Suppl.), 1–40.

Bennion, L. J., Grundy, S. M. (1975): Effects of obesity and caloric intake on biliary lipid metabolism in man. *J. Clin. Invest.* **56**, 996–1011.

Bhathena, S. J., Avignan, J., Shreiner, M. E. (1974): Effect of insulin on sterol and fatty acid synthesis and hydroxymethylglutaryl CoA reductase activity in mammalian cells grown in culture. *Proc. Natl. Acad. Sci. USA* **71**, 2174–2178.

Burnett, W. (1971): The epidemiology of gallstones. *Tijdschr, Gastroenterol.* **14**, 79–89.

Cooper, A. D. (1976): The regulation of 3-hydroxy-3-methyl-glutaryl coenzyme A reductase in the isolated perfused rat liver. *J. Clin. Invest.* **57**, 1461–1470.

Coste, T., Karsenti, P., Berta, J-L., Cubeau, J., Guilloud-Bataille, M. (1979): Facteurs diététiques de la lithaise bilaire: comparaison de l'alimentation d'un groupe de lithiasiques à l'alimentation d'un group temoin. *Gastroenterologie Clin. Biol.* **3**, 655–658.

Coyne, M. J., Benorris, G. G., Goldstein, L. I., Schoenfield, L. J. (1976): Effect of chenodeoxycholic acid and phenobarbital on the rate-limiting enzymes of hepatic cholesterol and bile acid synthesis in patients with gallstones. *J. Lab. Clin. Med.* **87**, 281–291.

Grundy, S. M., Duane, W. C., Adler, R. D., Aron, J. M., Metzger, A. L. (1974): Biliary lipid outputs in young women with cholesterol gallstones. *Metabolism* **23**, 67–73.

Heaton, K. W. (1972): Cholelithiasis and cholecystitis. In *Bile salts in health and disease*, pp. 151–163. Edinburgh and London: Churchill Livingstone.

Heaton, K. W. (1973*a*): The epidemiology of gallstones and suggested aetiology. *Clin. Gastroenterol.* **2**, 67–83.

Heaton, K. W. (1973*b*): Food fibre as an obstacle to energy intake. *Lancet* **2**, 1418–1421.

Heaton, K. W. (1979): Diet and gallstones, pp. 371–389. In *Gallstones. Hepatology — research and clinical issues*, 4, ed M. M. Fisher, C. A. Goresky, E. A. Shaffer, S. M. Strasburg. New York: Plenum Press.

Heaton, K. W. (1984): The sweet road to gallstones. *Br. Med. J.* **288(1)**, 1103–1104.

Hill, M. J., Crowther, J. S., Drasar, B. S., Hawkesworth, G., Aries, V., Williams, R. E. O. (1971): Bacteria and aetiology of cancer of large bowel. *Lancet* **1**, 95–100.

Hillman, L. C., Peters, S. G., Pomare, E. W. (1983): Effects of pectin and cellulose on biliary composition and bile salt metabolism. In *Fibre in human and animal nutrition*, ed G. Wallace, L. Bell. *Royal Soc. NZ. Bull.* **20**, 205.

Hofman, A. F. (1980): The medical treatment of gallstones: a clinical application of the new biology of bile acids. In *The Harvey Lectures, Vol. 74*, pp. 23–48. New York: Academic Press.

Jenkins, D. J. A., Leeds, A. R., Gassull, M. A., Cochet, B., Alberti, K. G. M. M. (1977): Decrease in post-prandial insulin concentrations by guar and pectin. *Ann. Intern. Med.* **86**, 20–23.

Larusso, N. F., Korman, M. E., Hofmann, N. E., Hofmann, A. F. (1974): Dynamics of the enterohepatic circulation of bile acids — post-prandial serum concentrations of conjugates of cholic acids in healthy chole-cystectomised patients and patients with bile acid malabsorption. *New Engl. J. Med.* **291**, 689–692.

McDougall, R. M., Yaymyshyn, L., Walker, K., Thurston, O. G. (1978): Effect of wheat bran on serum lipoproteins and biliary lipids. *Can. J. Surg.* **21**, 433–435.

Miettinen, T. A. (1983): Effects of dietary fibre on cholesterol metabolism in man. In *Fibre in human and animal nutrition*, ed G. Wallace, L. Bell. *Roy. Soc. NZ Bull.* **20**, 173–177.

Miettinen, T. A., Tarpila, S. (1977): Effect of pectin on serum cholesterol, fecal bile acids and biliary lipids in normolipidaemic and hyperlipidaemic individuals. *Clin. Chim. Acta.* **79**, 471–477.

Nestel, P. J., Schriebman, P. H., Ahrens, E. H. (1973): Cholesterol metabolism in human obesity. *J. Clin. Invest.* **52**, 2389–2397.

Northfield, T. C., Hofmann, A. F. (1975): Biliary lipid output during three meals and an overnight fast. I. Relationship to bile salt pool size and cholesterol saturation of bile in gallstone and control subjects. *Gut* **16**, 1–11.

Pomare, E. W. (1983): Fibre and bile acid metabolism. In *Fibre in human and animal nutrition*, ed G. Wallace, L. Bell. *Roy. Soc. NZ Bull.* **20**, 177–182.

Pomare, E. W., Heaton, K. W., Low-Beer, T. S., Espiner, H. J. (1976): The effect of wheat bran upon bile salt metabolism and upon the lipid composition of bile in gallstone patients. *Am. J. Dig. Dis.* **21**, 521–526.

Ponz de Leon, M., Ferenderes, R., Carulli, N. (1978): Bile lipid composition and bile acid pool size in diabetics. *Am. J. Dig. Dis.* **23**, 710–716.

Ponz de Leon, M., Carulli, N., Loria, P., Iori, R., Zironi, F. (1979): The effect of chenodeoxycholic acid on cholesterol absorption. *Gastroenterology* **77**, 223–230.

Sarles, H., Hauton, J., Planche, N. E., Lafont, H., Gérolami, A. (1970): Diet, cholesterol gallstones and composition of bile. *Am. J. Dig. Dis.* **15**, 251–260.

Sarles, H., Crotte, C., Gérolami, A., Mulé, A., Domingo, N., Hauton, J. (1971): The influence of calorie intake and of dietary protein on the bile lipids. *Scand. J. Gastroenterol.* **6**, 189–191.

Sarles, H., Gérolami, H., Bord, A. (1978a): Diet and cholesterol gallstones. *Digestion* **17**, 128–134.

Sarles, H., Gérolami, A., Cros, R. C. (1978b): Diet and cholesterol gallstones. A multicenter study. *Digestion* **17**, 121–127.

Scragg, R. K. R., McMichael, A. J., Baghurst, P. A. (1984a): Diet, alcohol and relative weight in gallstone disease: a case-control study. *Br. Med. J.* **1**, 1113–1119.

Scragg, R. K. R., Calvert, G. D., Oliver, J. R. (1984b). Plasma lipids and insulin in gallstone disease: a case control study. *Br. Med. J.* **2**, 521–525.

Sherlock, S. (1981): Gallstones and inflammatory gall bladder diseases. In *Diseases of the liver and biliary system*, pp. 476–498. Oxford: Blackwell Scientific.

Smith, D. A., Gee, M. I. (1979): A dietary survey to determine the relationship between diet and cholelithiasis. *Am. J. Clin. Nutr.* **32**, 1519–1526.

Story, J. A., Thomas, J. N. (1982): Modification of bile acid spectrum by dietary fiber. In *Dietary fiber in health and disease*, ed G. V. Vahouney, D. Kritchevsky, pp. 193–201. New York: Plenum Press.

Tarpila, S., Miettinen, T. A. (1983): Effects of dietary fibre on serum, biliary and faecal lipids in middle-aged men. In *Fibre in human and animal nutrition* ed G Wallace, L. Bell. *Roy. Soc. NZ Bull* **20**, 207.

Tarpila, S., Miettinen, T. A., Metsäranta, L. (1978): Effects of bran on serum cholesterol, faecal mass, fat, bile acids and neutral sterols and biliary lipids in patients with diverticular disease of the colon. *Gut* **19**, 137–145.

Thomas, P. J., Hofmann, A. F. (1973): A simple calculation of the lithogenic index of bile: expressing biliary lipid composition on rectangular co-ordinates. *Gastroenterology* **65**, 698–700.

Thornton, J. R., Emmet, P. M., Heaton, K. W. (1983): Diet and gallstones: effects of refined and unrefined carbohydrate diets on bile cholesterol saturation and bile acid metabolism. *Gut* **24**, 2–6.

Vlahcevic, Z. R., Bell, C. C. Jr, Buhac, I. (1970): Diminished bile acid pool size in patients with gallstones. *Gastroenterology* **59**, 165–173.

Watts, J. McK., Jablonski, P., Toouli, J. (1978): The effect of added bran to the diet on the saturation of bile in people without gallstones. *Am. J. Surg.* **135**, 321–324.

Werner, D., Emmet, P. M., Heaton, K. W. (1984): Effects of dietary sucrose on factors influencing cholesterol gallstone formation. *Gut* **25**, 269–274.

Wheeler, M., Hills, L. L., Laby, B. (1970): Cholelithiasis: a clinical and dietary survey. *Gut* **11**, 430–437.

Wicks, A. C. B., Yeates, J., Heaton, K. W. (1978): Bran and bile: a time course of changes in normal young men given a standard dose. *Scand. J. Gastroenterol.* **13**, 289–292.

Wilson, J. D. (1972): The role of bile acids in the overall regulation of steroid metabolism. *Archs Intern. Med.* **130**, 493–505.

4
Fibre and diabetes — new perspectives

David B. Peterson

Introduction

The high prevalence of diabetes and certain other diseases in Western society has been attributed in part to a low intake of dietary fibre. The epidemiological evidence for this as a causative factor in diabetes has been reviewed by Mann (1983). Total energy intake may turn out to be more important. The corollary of the dietary fibre hypothesis, that a higher national intake of fibre will reduce the incidence and ultimately the prevalence of diabetes, remains untested. It may well remain so, as recent research suggests that the former straightforward distinction made between dietary fibre and digestible carbohydrate is no longer valid, and they cannot be considered as separate components of the diet. The very diversity of what we understand by dietary fibre makes it difficult to say what sort of foods are lacking in our diets that could account for the development of diabetes in susceptible individuals. As will be seen, however, the clinical use of high fibre/high carbohydrate diets in the treatment of diabetes is now well-established. The construction of such diets is by no means simple, and is a prime issue in current research.

It is widely believed that tighter control of blood glucose fluctuations and a lowering of lipid levels will lessen the risk of developing the late complications of diabetes. There has always been a search for foods that have least impact on blood glucose levels. The historical use of low carbohydrate content diets in diabetes was based on empirical observations, when no other treatment was available. West (1973) pointed out the contradictions in using a low carbohydrate diet some years ago, but only recently has there been a change towards recommending a diet high in unrefined carbohydrate and low in fat.

The selection of appropriate carbohydrate foods has become a key issue. It was assumed previously that foods high in fibre as determined by chemical analyses would be the most effective in controlling blood glucose levels. It is now recognised that the fibre and carbohydrate components in a food have separate influences on metabolism. The paradox is that they cannot be considered separately within natural foods; the very physical form of a food influences its metabolic effects. Individual foods have been intensively studied, and although no hard and fast guidelines are available, we are nearer now to defining foods according to their clinical effects rather than making predictions from food analysis tables.

The role of fibre supplements has also been under scrutiny recently. Attention has again focussed on the viscous gums, particularly guar, now that commercial preparations are available. The poor palatability of guar has not yet been overcome completely, but there are exciting developments and its future in the diabetic diet seems assured in one form or another.

Clinical trials with high fibre diets

It is just a few years since the first clinical trials of high fibre diets in diabetes, earlier work having focussed on changes in the carbohydrate content of the diet. The studies of Anderson and colleagues with a variety of high fibre diets seemed encouraging (Kiehm *et al.*, 1976, Anderson & Ward, 1978, Anderson & Chen, 1979). They suffered the drawbacks of being metabolic ward studies and having test diets of extremely high carbohydrate and fibre content. Some investigators have used formula diets (Brunzell *et al.*, 1974) to look at the effect of digestible carbohydrate, and although hardly physiological they emphasised the problem of the separate influences of fibre and carbohydrate, which is examined in the next section.

Following this groundwork there were attempts to use high fibre diets containing real foods to answer criticisms about their practical relevance (Simpson *et al.*, 1979*a,b*; Monnier *et al.*, 1981). Though more realistic in terms of foods and carbohydrate content (usually 55–60 per cent energy), there was criticism and doubt expressed about the application of such diets to all diabetics (Reaven, 1980). In particular, the reductions in blood glucose achieved were very modest and there was a suggestion of adverse effects on blood lipids. At that time most high fibre/high carbohydrate diets relied on cereal fibre almost exclusively. Simpson and colleagues (1979*a*) used wholemeal bread to provide over 40 per cent of daily energy, and one can indeed question the practicality of changing large numbers of diabetics to such a diet, in spite of early enthusiasm (Mann, 1980).

The solution to this problem lay in earlier work by Jenkins and colleagues who had shown the potent hypoglycaemic and hypolipidaemic effects of guar and other viscous gums (Jenkins *et al.*, 1976; 1978*b*). These gums had been investigated as discrete 'fibre supplements' and it took a while to realise the potential of gel-forming fibres in natural foods, particularly pulses or legumes, for the diabetic diet. It was only by increasing both leguminous and cereal sources of fibre in the high carbohydrate diet that dramatic benefits were found. With such a diet, Simpson and colleagues (1981) found reductions in both basal and postprandial blood glucose levels for the first time.

The growing body of evidence in favour of high fibre/high carbohydrate diets in diabetes led to organisations in many Western countries publishing similar specific recommendations on the ideal diabetic diet (Nuttall, 1980; Special Report Committee, 1981; British Diabetic Association, 1982). These essentially included an increased intake of unrefined carbohydrate foods of legume and cereal origin, rich in all types of fibres, to provide 50–55 per cent of daily energy intake, with a concomitant reduction in total fat to about 30–35 per cent of daily energy intake. Restriction of total energy intake for the obese and general avoidance of simple sugars remained as ground-rules.

That such a diet was practicable and palatable was by no means universally accepted (Anon, 1983), despite various practical strategies offered (Geekie *et al.*, 1981). It is only a recent succession of trials that seems to have convinced

48

physicians and dietitians. High fibre/high carbohydrate diets have now been tested in most diabetic patient groups. Both Type 1 (insulin-dependent) and Type 2 (non-insulin-dependent) patients seem to benefit (Simpson *et al.*, 1981; 1982*b*). Simpson's trials in Oxford were on well controlled patients, but Lousley and colleagues (1984) subsequently showed that poorly controlled diabetics can also respond to such diet measures. It is still unsettled whether or not obese diabetics will benefit. Compliance is always a problem with this group, and assessment of any satiating effect of fibre is difficult. Certainly glycaemic control can be improved in the short term, even in the severely obese (Hoffmann *et al.*, 1984) and without weight loss. Even difficult to follow-up rural outpatients in South Africa have been shown to benefit from a high fibre/high carbohydrate diet (Rosman *et al.*, 1983). Another group in Oxford have found quite acceptable wholefood diets for children (Kinmonth *et al.*, 1982), endorsed in the paediatric world (Rayner, 1982). High fibre diets and fibre supplements have been applied successfully in pregnancy, when glycaemic control is so important (Ney *et al.*, 1982; Fraser *et al.*, 1983).

There is no reason to doubt the efficacy and practicality of high fibre diets using available foods, although long-term compliance still requires further testing. The metabolic benefits extend beyond glycaemic and lipid improvements to effects on haemostasis (Simpson *et al.*, 1982*a*), suggesting a lower risk of developing thrombotic vascular complications.

Studies with soluble fibre supplements

Soluble fibres in the form of viscous gums require special mention as they have been extensively investigated, can be extremely effective, and numerous commercial preparations are now available recommended for use in diabetes. Most are granulated preparations of guar gum, a galactomannan, although konjac (glucomannan) is also available. Jenkins and colleagues were the first to demonstrate the ability of guar to attenuate the rise in blood glucose after glucose and carbohydrates (Jenkins *et al.*, 1976). Subsequent work showed that insulin levels also rose less after guar in both healthy and non-insulin-dependent diabetic subjects. All the early studies were of acute meal tests and no conclusions about long-term effects could be made.

Most clinical studies have used granulated guar preparations, but some have tested guar food products. To be active clinically, guar preparations need to be of high viscosity and preferably mixed with food (see next section, on Mechanisms). To solve the mixing problem Jenkins produced a guar crispbread (Jenkins *et al.*, 1978*b*), but this early attempt was highly unpalatable. Other work suggested that supplements in general were unlikely to encourage patient compliance (Cohen & Martin, 1979). Recent efforts to produce acceptable guar food products have been more successful (Ellis *et al.*, 1981, and see Chapter 8 this volume). Guar-containing wheat bread has been shown to be active in non-insulin-dependent diabetics (Peterson *et al.*, 1984) and, perhaps equally important, to be palatable. Other studies with guar biscuits (Smith *et al.*, 1982) and bread (Vaaler *et al.*, 1983) have been metabolically successful though it is not clear whether the foods were acceptable. No guar foods are commercially available and their role has yet to be fully defined.

Few long-term studies have adequately characterised the physical qualities of the guar gum used, making it difficult to generalise about the applications of guar in diabetes. Nevertheless, two interesting recent studies showed improvements in overall glycaemic control as well as more striking changes in blood cholesterol, representing a double benefit for diabetics (Aro *et al.*, 1981; Smith & Holm, 1982). Of particular note is the fact that most of the glycaemic improvement was due to reductions in the basal blood glucose levels. When allowance is made for the difference in basal glucoses after guar and placebo, no change is seen in the post-prandial increments. At present there is no explanation for this, but 'suitable' guar preparations can undoubtedly improve diabetic control in selected patients. No studies to date have allowed us to define which groups of diabetics will benefit most from guar, nor what are the qualities of the most effective gum, as there is such variation between preparations.

Mechanisms of action of dietary fibre in diabetes

The separate effects of fibre and carbohydrate on glycaemic control
Any explanation of the beneficial effects of a high fibre diet must address the part played by digestible carbohydrate, which is also increased on such a diet. Changes in the proportions of other nutrients may also contribute; such as the lower fat content or the presence of 'anti-nutrients' such as lectins and saponins in the fibre itself. In fact, fat ingestion with carbohydrate can reduce the glycaemic response to a meal (Collier *et al.*, 1984), although the long-term relevance of this is uncertain.

Early work with high carbohydrate formula diets showed improvements in blood glucose levels in the virtual absence of fat and fibre when compared to a low carbohydrate/high fat diet (Brunzell *et al.*, 1974; Anderson & Chen, 1979). The importance of digestible carbohydrate had been mooted by Himsworth in the 1930s, but adequate documentation had to wait 50 years. Metabolic ward studies by Rivellese and her colleagues apparently showed that dietary fibre is responsible for improved glycaemia independent of carbohydrate content (Rivellese *et al.*, 1980, Riccardi *et al.*, 1984). Three diets were given for 10-day periods: high carbohydrate with high or low fibre and low carbohydrate/low fibre. The effect of fibre was exclusively on post-prandial not fasting blood glucose levels. In addition, increasing the carbohydrate had very little effect on glucose levels at any time. Another metabolic ward study (Karlstrom *et al.*, 1984) using two low carbohydrate diets, one with added cereal fibre (wheat and rye), showed reductions in post-prandial glycaemia, with only a small effect on fasting levels. An earlier acute meal study, however, showed no change in blood glucose response after removing fibre from various cereal foods (Jenkins *et al.*, 1981), the suggestion being that fibre contributes little to the benefits of long-term high carbohydrate diets.

Regardless of this evidence from short-term studies, there is no substitute for long-term diet studies which have all shown separate effects from increasing both carbohydrate and fibre. The early studies in Oxford (Simpson *et al.*, 1979*a,b*) showed overall reductions in daily blood glucose levels, comparing a high carbohydrate/high fibre to a low carbohydrate/low fibre diet, each taken for six weeks. This was due almost entirely to an improvement in fasting levels, and post-prandial increments were little affected. These studies used cereal fibre (mainly wholemeal bread) as the source of fibre. It was only when leguminous foods were used to provide soluble fibre as well that improvements were found in

50

both fasting and post-prandial blood glucose levels (Simpson *et al.*, 1981). Further review (Simpson *et al.*, 1982*b*) showed that an increase in carbohydrate led to lower fasting glucose levels even when fibre intake remained the same. It may be that fibre has to be part of a high carbohydrate diet to be effective, as evidence from a somewhat flawed acute study suggests that fibre has little effect when added to a low carbohydrate diet (Jenkins *et al.*, 1980*a*).

Looking critically at evidence from long-term diet studies we can conclude that the increase in digestible carbohydrate accounts for most of the reduction found in fasting blood glucose levels, and that fibre is mainly responsible for reductions in post-prandial rises in glucose (Monnier *et al.*, 1981; Kinmonth *et al.*, 1982). In addition, cereal fibre is much less potent than soluble fibre of leguminous origin in lowering post-prandial levels. For maximum improvement both fibre and carbohydrate need to be increased (Manhire *et al.*, 1981; Simpson *et al.*, 1981). However, their relative contributions to this improvement are by no means clear, nor are the mechanisms involved.

High fibre diets
The data available on the metabolic effects of high fibre diets are purely descriptive. All explanations of mechanisms remain incomplete and circumstantial. Acute meal tests confirmed that fibre delays the absorption of carbohydrates without causing actual malabsorption, detected by breath hydrogen measurements (Jenkins *et al.*, 1976; 1978*a*). It is likely that this effect continues in the long term, given the persistent reductions found in post-prandial glucose levels. This is due to decreased absorption from the gut rather than increases in peripheral glucose utilisation or uptake by the liver (Wahren *et al.*, 1982).

The physical nature of the fibre in a food also seems to affect the rate of digestion and absorption. With soluble fibre supplements intimate mixing with carbohydrate is vital for effectiveness (Jenkins *et al.*, 1979*a*). Conversely, removal of fibre can lead to an increased rate of carbohydrate absorption. In two classic studies (Haber *et al.*, 1977; Bolton *et al.*, 1981) apples were given either whole, puréed or as juice. Increasing disruption or removal of the fibre resulted in higher blood glucose levels. Presumably fibre can obstruct the access of carbohydrate to the digestive processes in the gut. Soluble fibre seems the most effective in this respect (Jenkins *et al.*, 1976; Simpson *et al.*, 1981).

The physical form of the carbohydrate in a food seems to be equally important. The rate of digestion and subsequent rise in blood glucose is affected by the chemical chain length (Wahlqvist *et al.*, 1978) and even by the degree of branching (Goddard *et al.*, 1984) of the starch molecules. Indeed, it has been suggested that in leguminous foods the physical structure may be more important than the viscosity of the fibre in determining the rate of digestion of the carbohydrate (Wong and O'Dea, 1983). The overall importance of the physical structure of a food in determining the glycaemic response is confirmed by studies on the influence of various food preparation (grinding, blending, etc.) and cooking methods (O'Dea *et al.*, 1980; Bolton *et al.*, 1981; Jenkins *et al.*, 1982*b*).

The conclusion from studies of food form is that the digestibility of starch is possibly the main determinant of the final glycaemic response. Individual foods differ widely, but some with a particular combination of starch and fibre, such as legumes, can produce favourable acute responses implying poor digestibility. This concept may not fully explain the benefits of high carbohydrate/high fibre diets, but it serves as a way of selecting appropriate foods for such diets (Jenkins *et al.*, 1980*b*; 1982*b,c,d*; Thorne *et al.*, 1983; and see section on 'Food selection' below).

A variety of metabolic changes have been described in association with a high fibre diet. In addition to lower blood glucose levels, lower insulin levels are found in normal subjects and in non-insulin-dependent diabetics (Jenkins *et al.*, 1976; Kay *et al.*, 1981; and many others). Urinary C-peptide levels are also reduced on a high fibre diet (Burke *et al.*, 1982). This represents enhanced sensitivity to insulin and there is a number of possible explanations. In acute tests, reductions have been found in the insulinogenic hormones GIP and glucagon (Miranda & Horwitz, 1978; Morgan *et al.*, 1979; Kay *et al.*, 1981). Intermediary metabolites (ketone bodies) are also reduced (Jenkins *et al.*, 1979*b*). Increased insulin receptor binding has been reported in adipocytes and monocytes (Ward *et al.*, 1982; Hjollund *et al.*, 1982; Pedersen *et al.*, 1983), which could explain the reduced insulin resistance.

A number of workers have attempted dynamic studies of glucose kinetics to try and pinpoint the mechanisms responsible for increased insulin sensitivity, but the results have been conflicting and inconclusive (Hall *et al.*, 1980; Nestel *et al.*, 1984). Suggestions that other gut-related hormones, such as somatostatin, may be involved in modulating insulin production still await a definitive long-term study. The hormonal side is certainly worth pursuing further, unlike acute clamp studies which merely record other measures of insulin resistance. Investigating this aspect of metabolism is difficult and even more speculative in insulin-dependent diabetics. The conclusion must be that the mechanisms of action of high fibre diets remain unclear. Insulin sensitivity and glucose turnover are both improved by unknown factors.

Soluble fibre supplements
Results from long-term studies with guar have been somewhat conflicting, perhaps because of marked differences in the physical characteristics of the preparations used (O'Connor *et al.*, 1981). Aro and colleagues showed primarily a reduction in basal glycaemia on long-term guar, with little effect on post-prandial increments (Aro *et al.*, 1981). In acute studies the reductions in post-prandial blood glucose and insulin levels are well-documented, and guar has also been shown to reduce stimulatory gut hormones such as GIP and glucagon (Morgan *et al.*, 1979). However, no causal link between these changes and lower insulin levels has yet been described. It does appear that intact neuroendocrine connections are necessary for soluble fibre at least to be effective. In diabetics with autonomic neuropathy affecting the gut guar (admittedly in a low dose) fails to improve glucose tolerance, in a comparison with normal subjects and diabetics without this complication (Levitt *et al.*, 1980).

Delayed absorption of carbohydrates, inferred from the results of acute studies, cannot be the only mechanism operating during chronic administration and the full explanation must be more complex. Guar probably acts at several stages in the process of carbohydrate digestion and absorption. It was suggested originally that guar delays gastric emptying (Holt *et al.*, 1979). There was some controversy about this study (Taylor, 1979; Leeds 1979) and other studies either contradicted this (Wilmhurst & Crawley, 1980; Leatherdale *et al.*, 1982; Rainbird *et al.*, 1982) or produced conflicting results within one group (Blackburn *et al.*, 1984). Rainbird's study using the pig as a human model (Leeds *et al.*, 1980) was the first invasive study and suggested acceleration of gastric emptying.

On balance, it seems that guar causes some delay in gastric emptying, but that this does not correlate with any effects on the blood glucose response to a liquid test meal (Ray *et al.*, 1983; Blackburn *et al.*, 1984). As the liquid and solid phases of a meal leave the stomach at different rates, it may not be appropriate to extrapolate from such experiments to the *in vivo* situation. The action of guar may be greatly influenced by whether it is given as a liquid or solid supplement to a meal.

The effectiveness of guar preparations seems to depend largely on their highly viscous nature when hydrated (Jenkins *et al.*, 1978*a*; O'Connor *et al.*, 1981). Although the importance of viscosity is not in doubt, the precise reasons remain unconfirmed. Blackburn and colleagues (1984) have suggested that the convective mixing currents set up by intestinal contractions are reduced by guar, thus limiting access of oligosaccharides and carbohydrates to digestive enzymes and absorption sites. Their study used healthy volunteers in whom isolated segments of intestine were perfused with liquid test meals; though the conditions were as near *in vivo* as possible, they must be interpreted with caution. No changes could be measured in the unstirred layer when guar was infused, suggesting that an effect of guar on this layer is less relevant than was previously thought (Johnson & Gee, 1981). It seems to be the effect on the viscosity of the gut contents as a whole that is really important.

Regardless of viscosity, the effect of guar is greatly reduced if it is taken separately from food. This becomes more marked the greater the interval between the two (Jenkins *et al.*, 1979*a*). As the timing of the dose is so critical, guar should ideally be intimately mixed with carbohydrate (Jenkins *et al.*, 1979*a*; Wolever *et al.*, 1979). Nevertheless, it has been shown that guar with a test meal can also improve glucose tolerance four hours later (Jenkins *et al.*, 1980*b*). This is analogous to the basal changes found on a high fibre diet, and may account for the long-term adaptation found in Aro's study (Aro *et al.*, 1981), where basal rather than incremental blood glucose values are reduced.

Although guar and carbohydrate are fully mixed only in a food, the absorption of other carbohydrates taken in a mixed meal may not be equally delayed. However, it seems worthwhile incorporating guar in foods, as a recent study suggests that lower doses of guar are then required than with a granulate (Peterson *et al.*, 1984). It is uncertain just how low a dose of guar can be effective. A study in healthy volunteers showed that a very low dose of guar (2.5 g) could be metabolically active, and also found an apparent threshold effect beyond which increased amounts of guar had no extra effect (Smith *et al.*, 1983). The mechanism for this was not suggested and it may not apply to diabetics with elevated basal glucose levels.

A final possibility is that soluble fibre may have a useful role in obese diabetics, by increasing feelings of satiety when incorporated into meals (Van Itallie, 1978). It probably has more effect than cereal fibre. There is a complex interaction of fibre with hunger and satiety and as yet there have not been any well-designed long-term studies to investigate this.

It is of great importance to know the most appropriate foods and the correct amount of carbohydrate to choose for maximum benefit in the diabetic diet. A classification of foods according to glycaemic response is required, to allow us to safely encourage a high intake of carbohydrate and fibre. The choice would ideally be based on a sound knowledge of the mechanisms of action of fibre. Unfortunately this remains incomplete and reliance has had to be placed on methods of testing individual foods. Conventional food tables do not help, as it has been shown that fibre content does not necessarily reflect the influence a particular food has on post-prandial glycaemia (Jenkins *et al.*, 1981*a,b*; Ionescu-Tirgoviste *et al.*, 1983).

Jenkins' group has paid a great deal of attention to this problem and developed the concept of the 'glycaemic index', where a food is graded by expressing the area under the blood glucose curve after a 50 g carbohydrate portion as a percentage of the response to the equivalent amount of a reference carbohydrate, either glucose or white bread (Jenkins *et al.*, 1981*a* and 1983*b*). In this way a league table can be created, ranking foods according to their clinical effects. This followed earlier pioneering work, looking at clinical responses rather than figures from food analysis tables (Schauberger *et al.*, 1977; Crapo *et al.*, 1980, 1981). Pulses and legumes have the lowest glycaemic indices, only 20–40 per cent that of bread (Jenkins *et al.*, 1981*a* and 1983*b*), which supports the results of diet studies using beans (Rivellese *et al.*, 1980; Simpson *et al.*, 1981).

This approach is certainly useful in confirming foods that are particularly effective, such as pulses or beans, but care is needed not to extrapolate too far as the evidence is contradictory. High fibre foods such as wholemeal bread that have been successfully used in diet studies (Simpson *et al.*, 1979*a* and 1979*b*) turn out to have unacceptably high glycaemic indices, similar to simple sugars (Jenkins *et al.*, 1981*a* and 1983*b*). White and wholemeal breads have the same glycaemic index and yet small amounts of added wheat bran can have metabolic benefits after a short period (Miranda & Horwitz, 1978). White spaghetti has a lower glycaemic index than white or wholemeal breads which are identical (Jenkins *et al.*, 1983*a*). Jenkins interprets this as a lack of effect of the fibre in wholemeal bread, in contrast to the potent influence of the physical form of pasta.

There are many limitations of acute tests of single foods and the situation can be quite different within a mixed meal (Bantle *et al.*, 1983) and with long-term use. Bantle *et al.* showed that, in a high fibre meal, added simple sugars (sucrose and fructose) and starches (potato and wheat) produce similar glycaemic responses. Other nutrients can obviously delay the absorption of a range of carbohydrates and reduce the glycaemic responses to a similar extent.

It has been postulated that the key factor determining the glycaemic response is the digestibility of a carbohydrate. Foods such as bread and potato are rapidly digested causing higher blood glucose and insulin levels than less digestible foods like lentils (Jenkins *et al.*, 1982*c,d*). This would account for the influence of physical form, when grinding and blending can render a food more digestible (Haber *et al.*, 1977; O'Dea *et al.*, 1980; Jenkins *et al.*, 1982*b*). Searching for a laboratory model to predict the glycaemic index and digestibility of foods, Jenkins developed an *in vitro* system, where foods are incubated in digestive juices under standard conditions inside a dialysis bag. The rate of glucose production is reflected by the glucose collected in the medium surrounding the bag (Jenkins *et al.*, 1980*b* and 1982*c*). There was a strong correlation with the *in vivo* blood glucose changes.

Legumes appear to be the best sources of high fibre foods for diabetics. Their digestibility and fibre content are such as to make their benefits the greatest and also the most prolonged, even affecting second meal tolerance 4 hours later (Jenkins *et al.*, 1982*a*). The appropriate choice of foods has been well reviewed recently (Mann, 1984). It is quite clear that there are discrepancies between acute and chronic diet study results, and Mann rightly urges caution in relying solely on acute tests. There is no substitute for long-term feeding studies, but it is difficult to assess a large number of individual foods in such a manner. The digestibility approach will probably remain useful and should be further improved, perhaps by incorporation of mixed meal studies. Even so, the implications of Bantle's study of simple sugars in a high fibre meal (Bantle *et al.*, 1983) cannot be accepted until diabetics have been assessed on a long-term high fibre diet containing sugar. Tests of the practicality of the published current diet recommendations (eg Nuttall *et al.*, 1983) certainly support the results of the experimental studies on which they are based and diabetics can feel quite clear about the best diet to try and follow.

Summary

Recent work using dietary fibre in natural foods has led to dramatic changes in the advice given to diabetic patients on the best diet to follow. Fibre is no longer seen as a distinct entity from the digestible carbohydrate in a food. The physical form of a carbohydrate food and the intimacy with which it is mixed with fibre, as well as the method of cooking, can all affect the glycaemic response. Various techniques are being developed to try and predict which foods are most useful for diabetic patients; further food testing is still required, however, before we can understand fully the principles that govern the responses to fibre and carbohydrate. We still remain some way from a clear picture of the mechanisms of action of fibre in diabetes. Delayed absorption of carbohydrate and increased insulin sensitivity are only part of a complex story. The concept of overall digestibility as a practical guide to choosing foods seems worth pursuing.

The actions of fibre supplements of viscous gums such as guar are better understood, although we are still some way from a full explanation. Their effects on gut motility and access of carbohydrates to digestive processes can all be measured. It is likely that parallels will soon be found in the actions of the other types of food fibres. There is no agreement yet on the precise place of gums in diabetes therapy. This is partly a reflection of the variety of preparations available, all of which face the problems of poor palatability, and uncertainties about the correct timing and mode of administration. Palatability may be conquered by the development of various foods containing guar, but the problems of availability and cost are still some way from being solved.

By following the current recommendations for a high fibre intake from cereal and leguminous sources diabetics can achieve an improvement in metabolic control. The ideal amount and type of fibre and carbohydrate content in the diet is still unsettled. Undoubtedly, there is now a need for an agreed methodology for assessing foods, and the further development of 'league tables' according to clinical responses. Finally, there can be no substitute for practical feeding studies, which are far more informative than acute tests, even though the latter point us in the right direction. Further information on the effects of fibre on satiety and limiting energy intake is particularly needed. It is justifiable to hope that the present heightened awareness of the importance of nutritional aspects of diabetes therapy will help to reduce the occurrence of long-term complications.

Acknowledgement — The support of a Medical Research Council Training Fellowship is gratefully acknowledged.

References

Anderson, J. W., Ward, K. (1978): Long-term effects of high carbohydrate, high fiber diets on glucose and lipid metabolism. A preliminary report on patients with diabetes. *Diabetes Care* **1**, 77–82.

Anderson, J. W., Chen, W. L. (1979): Plant fiber: carbohydrate and lipid metabolism. *Am. J. Clin. Nutr.* **32**, 346–363.

Anon. (1983): High-carbohydrate, high-fibre diets for diabetes mellitus (Editorial). *Lancet* **1**, 741–742.

Aro, A., Uusitupa, M., Voutilanien, E., Hersio, K., Korhonen, T., Siitonen, O. (1981): Improved diabetic control and hypocholesterolaemic effect induced by long-term dietary supplementation with guar gum in type 2 (insulin-independent) diabetes. *Diabetologia* **21**, 29-33.

Bantle J. P, Laine, J. C., Castle, G. W., Thomas, J. W., Hoogwerf, B. J., Goetz, F. C. (1983): Post-prandial glucose and insulin responses to meals containing different carbohydrates in normal and diabetic subjects. *New Engl. J. Med.* **309**, 7–12.

Blackburn, N. A., Redfern, J. S., Jarjis, H., Holgate, A. M., Hanning, I., Scarpello, J. H. B., Johnson, I. T., Read, N. W. (1984): The mechanism of action of guar gum in improving glucose tolerance in man. *Clin. Sci.* **66**, 329–336.

Bolton, R. P., Heaton, K. W., Burroughs, L. F. (1981): The role of dietary fiber in satiety, glucose and insulin: studies with fruits and fruit juices. *Am. J. Clin. Nutr.* **34**, 211–217.

British Diabetic Association (1982): Dietary recommendations for the 1980s. *Hum. Nutr: Appl. Nutr.* **36**, 378–386.

Brunzell, J. D., Lerner, R. L., Porte, D., Bierman, E. L. (1974): Effect of a fat free high carbohydrate diet on diabetic subjects with fasting hyperglycaemia. *Diabetes* **23**, 138–142.

Burke, B. J., Hartog, M., Heaton, K. W., Hooper, S. (1982): Assessment of the metabolic effects of dietary carbohydrate and fibre by measuring urinary excretion of C-peptide. *Hum. Nutr.: Clin. Nutr.* **36C**, 373–380.

Cohen, M., Martin, F. I. R. (1979): Guar crispbread in the diabetic diet. *Br. Med. J.* **2**, 616–617.

Collier, G., O'Dea, K. (1982): Effect of physical form of carbohydrate on the post-prandial glucose, insulin, and gastric inhibitory polypeptide responses in type 2 diabetes. *Am. J. Clin. Nutr.* **36**, 10–14.

Collier, G., McLean, A., O'Dea, K. (1984): Effect of co-ingestion of fat on the metabolic responses to slowly and rapidly absorbed carbohydrates. *Diabetologia* **26**, 50–54.

Crapo, P. A., Kolterman, O. G., Waldeck, N., Reaven, G. M., Olefsky, J. M. (1980): Postprandial hormonal responses to different types of complex carbohydrate in individuals with impaired glucose tolerance. *Am. J. Clin. Nutr.* **33**, 1723–1728.

Crapo, P. A., Insel, J., Sperling, M., Kolterman, O. G. (1981): Comparison of serum glucose, insulin, and glucagon responses to different types of complex carbohydrates in noninsulin-dependent diabetic patients. *Am. J. Clin. Nutr.* **34**, 184–190.

Ellis, P. R., Apling, E. C., Leeds, A. R., Bolster, N. R. (1981): Guar bread: acceptability and efficacy combined. Studies on blood glucose, serum insulin and satiety in normal subjects. *Br. J. Nutr.* **46**, 267–276.

Fraser, R. B., Ford, F. A., Milner, R. D. G. (1983): A controlled trial of high dietary fibre intake in pregnancy — effects on plasma glucose and insulin levels. *Diabetologia* **25**, 238–241.

Greekie, M., Eaton, J., Simpson, H., Mann, J. I. (1981): Will diabetes accept an increase in dietary carbohydrate? *Diabetologia* **21**, 507.

Goddard, M. S., Young, G., Marcus, R. (1984): The effect of amylose content on insulin and glucose responses to ingested rice. *Am. J. Clin. Nutr.* **39**, 388–392.

Haber, G. B., Heaton, K. W., Murphy, D., Burroughs, L. F. (1977): Depletion and disruption of dietary fibre; effects on satiety, plasma glucose and serum insulin. *Lancet* **2**, 679–682.

Hall, S. E. H., Bolton, T. M., Hetenyi, G. (1980): The effects of bran on glucose kinetics and plasma insulin in non-insulin-dependent diabetes mellitus. *Diabetes Care* **3**, 520–525.

Hjollund, E., Pedersen, O., Richelsen, B., Beck-Nielsen, H., Schwartz-Sorensen, N. (1983): Increased insulin binding to adipocytes and monocytes and increased insulin sensitivity of glucose transport and metabolism in adipocytes from non-insulin-dependent diabetics after a low-fat/high-starch/high-fiber diet. *Metabolism* **32**, 1067–1075.

Hoffman, C. R., Fineberg, S. E., Howey, D. C., Clark, M. C., Pronsky, Z. (1984): Short-term effects of a high-fiber, high-carbohydrate diet in very obese diabetic individuals. *Diabetes Care* **5**, 605–611.

Holt, S., Heading, R. C., Carter, D. C., Prescott, L. F., Tothill, P. (1979): Effect of gel fibre on gastric emptying and absorption of glucose and paracetamol. *Lancet* **1**, 636–639.

Ionescu-Tirgoviste, C., Popa, E., Sintu, E., Mihalache, N., Cheta, D., Mincu, I. (1983): Blood glucose and plasma insulin responses to various carbohydrates in type 2 (non-insulin dependent) diabetes. *Diabetologia* **24**, 80–84.

Jenkins, D. J. A., Goff, D. V., Leeds, A. R., Alberti, K. G. M. M., Wolever, T. M. S., Gassull, M. A., Hockaday, T. D. R. (1976): Unabsorbable carbohydrates and diabetes: decreased post-prandial hyperglycaemia. *Lancet* **2**, 172–174.

Jenkins, D. J. A., Wolever, T. M. S., Leeds, A. R., Gassull, M. A., Haisman, P., Dilawari, J., Goff, D. V., Metz, G. L., Alberti, K. G. M. M. (1978a): Dietary fibres, fibre analogues, and glucose tolerance: importance of viscosity. *Br. Med. J.* **1**, 1392–1394.

Jenkins, D. J. A., Wolever, T. M. S., Nineham, R., Taylor, R., Metz, G. L., Bacon, S., Hockaday, T. D. R. (1978b): Guar crispbread in the diabetic diet. *Br. Med. J.* **2**, 1744–1746.

Jenkins, D. J. A., Nineham, R., Craddock, C., Craig-McFeely, P., Donaldson, K., Leigh, T., Snook, J. (1979a): Fibre and diabetes. *Lancet* **1**, 434–435.

Jenkins, D. J. A., Hockaday, T. D. R., Wolever, T. M. S., Nineham, R., Goff, D. V., Haisman, P., Charnock, R., Taylor, R. H., Bacon, S. (1979b): Dietary fibre and ketone bodies: reduced urinary 3-hydroxybutyrate excretion in diabetics on guar. *Br. Med. J.* **2**, 1555.

Jenkins, D. J. A., Wolever, T. M. S., Bacon, S., Nineham, R., Lees, R., Rowden, R., Love, M., Hockaday, T. D. R. (1980a): Diabetic diets: high carbohydrate combined with high fiber. *Am. J. Clin. Nutr.* **33**, 1729–1733.

Jenkins, D. J. A., Wolever, T. M. S., Taylor, R. H., Ghafari, H., Jenkins, A. L., Barker, H., Jenkins, M. J. A. (1980b): Rate of digestion of foods and post-prandial glycaemia in normal and diabetic subjects. *Br. Med. J.* **2**, 14–17.

Jenkins, D. J. A., Wolever, T. M. S., Nineham, R., Sarson, D. L., Bloom, S. R., Ahern, J., Alberti, K. G. M. M., Hockaday, T. D. R. (1980c): Improved glucose tolerance four hours after taking guar with glucose. *Diabetologia* **19**, 21–24.

Jenkins, D. J. A., Wolever, T. M. S., Taylor, R. H., Barker, H., Fielden, H., Baldwin, J. M., Bowling, A. C., Newman, H. C., Jenkins, A. L. Goff, D. V. (1981a): Glycaemic index of foods: a physiological basis for carbohydrate exchange. *Am. J. Clin. Nutr.* **34**, 362–366.

Jenkins, D. J. A., Wolever, T. M. S., Taylor, R. H., Barker, H. M., Fielden, H., Gassull, M. A. (1981b): Lack of effect of refining on the glycaemic response to cereals. *Diabetes Care* **4**, 509–513.

Jenkins, D. J. A., Wolever, T. M. S., Taylor, R. H., Griffiths, C., Krzeminska, K., Lowrie, J. A., Bennett, C. M., Goff, D. V., Sarson, D. L., Bloom, S. R. (1982a): Slow release dietary carbohydrate improves second meal tolerance. *Am. J. Clin. Nutr.* **35**, 1339–1346.

Jenkins, D. J. A., Thorne, M. J., Camelon, K., Jenkins, A., Rao, A. V., Taylor, R. H., Thompson, L., Kalmusky, J., Reichert, R., Francis, T. (1982b): Effects of processing on digestibility and the blood glucose response: a study of lentils. *Am. J. Clin. Nutr.* **36**, 1093–1101.

Jenkins, D. J. A., Ghafari, H., Wolever, T. M. S., Taylor, R. H., Jenkins, A. L., Barker, H. M., Fielden, H., Bowling, A. C. (1982c): Relationship between rate of digestion of foods and post-prandial glycaemia. *Diabetologia* **22**, 450–455.

Jenkins, D. J. A., Taylor, R. H., Wolever, T. M. S. (1982d): The diabetic diet, dietary carbohydrate and differences in digestibility. *Diabetologia* **23**, 477–484.

Jenkins, D. J. A., Wolever, T. M. S., Jenkins, A. L., Lee, R., Wong, G. S., Josse, R. (1983*a*): Glycemic response to wheat products: reduced response to pasta but no effect of fiber. *Diabetes Care* **6**, 155–159.

Jenkins, D. J. A., Wolever, T. M. S., Jenkins, A. L., Thorne, M. J., Lee, R., Kalmusky, J., Reichert, R., Wong, G. S. (1983*b*): The glycaemic index of foods tested in diabetic patients: a new basis for carbohydrate exchange favouring the use of legumes. *Diabetologia* **24**, 257–264.

Johnson, I. T., Gee, J. M. (1981): Effect of gel-forming gums on the intestinal unstirred layer and sugar transport in vitro. *Gut* **22**, 398–403.

Karlstrom, B., Vessby, B., Asp, N-G., Boberg, M., Gustafsson, I-B., Lithell, H., Werner, I. (1984): Effects of an increased content of cereal fibre in the diet of type 2 (non-insulin-dependent) diabetic patients. *Diabetologia* **26**, 272–277.

Kay, R. M., Grobin, W., Track, N. S. (1981): Diets rich in natural fibre improve carbohydrate tolerance in maturity-onset, non-insulin dependent diabetics. *Diabetologia* **20**, 18–21.

Kiehm, T. G., Anderson, J. W., Ward, K. (1976): Beneficial effects of a high carbohydrate, high fiber diet on hyperglycemic diabetic men. *Am. J. Clin. Nutr.* **29**, 895–899.

Kinmonth, A-L., Angus, R. M., Jenkins, P. A., Smith, M. A., Baum, J. D. (1982): Wholefoods and increased dietary fibre improve blood glucose control in diabetic children. *Archs Dis. Child.* **57**, 187–194.

Leatherdale, B. A., Green, D. J., Harding, L. K., Griffin, D., Bailey, C. J. (1982): Guar and gastric emptying in non-insulin dependent diabetes. *Acta Diabetol. Lat.* **19**, 339–343.

Leeds, A. R. (1979): Gastric emptying, fibre and absorption. *Lancet* **1**, 872–873.

Leeds, A. R., Kang, S. S., Low, A. G., Sambrook, I. E. (1980): The pig as a model for studies on the mode of action of guar gum in normal and diabetic men. *Proc. Nutr. Soc.* **39**, 44A.

Levitt, N. S., Vinik, A. I., Sive, A. A., Child, P. T., Jackson, W. P. U. (1980): The effect of dietary fiber on glucose and hormone responses to a mixed meal in normal subjects and in diabetic subjects with and without autonomic neuropathy. *Diabetes Care* **3**, 515–519.

Lousley, S. E., Jones, D. B., Slaughter, P., Carter, R. D., Jelfs, R., Mann, J. I. (1984): High carbohydrate-high fibre diets in poorly controlled diabetes. *Diabetic Medicine* **1**, 21–25.

Manhire, A., Henry, C. L., Hartog, M., Heaton, K. W. (1981): Unrefined carbohydrate and dietary fibre in treatment of diabetes mellitus. *J. Hum. Nutr.* **35**, 99–101.

Mann, J. I. (1980): Diet and diabetes. *Diabetologia* **18**, 89–95.

Mann, J. I. (1983): In *Diabetes in epidemiological perspective*, ed J. I. Mann, K. Pyorala, A. Teuscher, pp. 122–139. London: Churchill Livingstone.

Mann, J. I. (editorial) (1984): What carbohydrate foods should diabetics eat? *Br. Med. J.* **288**, 1025–1026.

Miranda, P. M., Horwitz, D. L. (1978): High fiber diets in the treatment of diabetes mellitus. *Ann. Int. Med.* **88**, 482–486.

Monnier, L. H., Blotman, M. J., Colette, C., Monnier, M. P., Mirouze, J. (1981): Effects of dietary fibre supplementation in stable and labile insulin-dependent diabetics. *Diabetologia* **20**, 12–17.

Morgan, L. M., Goulder, T. J., Tsiolakis, D., Marks, V., Alberti, K. G. M. M. (1979): The effect of unabsorbable carbohydrate on gut hormones: modification of postprandial GIP secretion by guar. *Diabetologia* **17**, 85–89.

Nestel, P. J., Nolan, C., Bazelmans, J., Cook, R. (1984): Effects of a high-starch diet with low or high fibre content on postabsorptive glucose utilization and glucose production in normal subjects. *Diabetes Care* **7**, 207–210.

Ney, D., Hollingsworth, D. R., Cousins, L. (1982): Decreased insulin requirement and improved control of diabetes in pregnant women given a high-carbohydrate, high-fiber, low-fat diet. *Diabetes Care* **5**, 529–533.

Nuttall, F. Q. (1980): Dietary recommendations for individuals with diabetes mellitus 1979: summary of report from the Food and Nutrition committee of the American Diabetic Association. *Am. J. Clin. Nutr.* **33**, 1311–1312.

Nuttall, F. Q. (1983): Diet and the diabetic patient. *Diabetes Care* **6**, 197–207.

Nuttall, F. Q., Mooradian, A. D., DeMarais, R., Parker, S. (1983): The glycemic effect of different meals approximately isocaloric and similar in protein, carbohydrate, and fat content as calculated using the ADA exchange lists. *Diabetes Care* **6**, 432–435.

O'Connor, N., Tredger, J., Morgan, L. (1981): Viscosity difference between various guar gums. *Diabetologia* **20**, 612–615.

O'Dea, K., Nestel, P. J., Antonoff, L. (1980): Physical factors influencing post-prandial glucose and insulin responses to starch. *Am. J. Clin. Nutr.* **33**, 760–765.

Pedersen, O., Hjollund, E., Lindskov, H. O., Helms, P., Sorensen, N. S., Ditzel, J. (1982): Increased insulin receptor binding to monocytes from insulin-dependent diabetic patients after a low-fat, high-starch, high-fiber diet. *Diabetes Care* **5**, 284–291.

Peterson, D. B., Ellis, P. R., Baylis, J. M., Frost, P. G., Leeds, A. R., Jepson, E. M. (1984): Effects of guar on diabetes and lipids — food and pharmacology compared. *Diabetologia* **27**, 319A.

Rainbird, A. L., Low, A. G., Sambrook, I. E. (1982): Lack of effect of guar gum on gastric emptying in pigs. *Procs. Nutr. Soc.* **42**, 24A.

Ray, T. K., Mansell, K. M., Knight, L. C., Malmud, L. S., Owen, O. E., Boden, G. (1983): Long-term effects of dietary fiber on glucose tolerance and gastric emptying in non-insulin dependent patients. *Am. J. Clin. Nutr.* **37**, 376–381.

Rayner, P. H. (editorial). (1982): Diet for diabetic children: a change in emphasis. *Archs Dis. Child.* **57**, 487–489.

Reaven, G. M. (1980): How high the carbohydrate? *Diabetologia* **19**, 409–413.

Riccardi, G., Rivellese, A., Pacioni, D., Genovese, S., Mastranzo, P., Mancini, M. (1984): Separate influence of dietary carbohydrate and fibre on the metabolic control in diabetes. *Diabetologia* **26**, 116–121.

Rivellese, A., Riccardi, G., Giacco, A., Pacioni, D., Genovese, S., Mattioli, P. L., Mancini, M. (1980): Effect of dietary fibre on glucose control and serum lipoproteins in diabetic patients. *Lancet* **2**, 447–450.

Rosman, M. S., Smith, C. J., Jackson, W. P. U. (1983): The effect of long-term high-fibre diets in diabetic outpatients. *S. Afr. Med. J.* **63**, 310–313.

Schauberger, G., Brinck, U. C., Guldner, G., Spaethe, R., Niklas, L., Otto, H. (1977): Exchange of carbohydrates according to their effects on blood glucose. *Diabetes* **26**, 415.

Simpson, H. C. R., Simpson, R. W., Lousley, S., Carter, R. D., Geekie, M., Hockaday, T. D. R., Mann, J. I. (1981): A high carbohydrate leguminous fibre diet improves all aspects of diabetic control. *Lancet* **1**, 1–5.

Simpson, H. C. R., Mann, J. I., Chakrabarti, R., Imeson, J. D., Stirling, Y., Tozer, M., Woolf, L., Meade, T. W. (1982a): Effect of high-fibre diet on haemostatic variables in diabetes. *Br. Med. J.* **284**, 1608.

Simpson, H. C. R., Carter, R. D., Lousley, S., Mann, J. I. (1982b): Digestible carbohydrate — an independent effect on diabetic control in type 2 (non-insulin dependent) diabetes. *Diabetologia* **23**, 235–239.

Simpson, R. W., Mann, J. I., Eaton, J., Moore, R. A., Carter, R., Hockaday, T. D. R. (1979a): Improved glucose control in maturity-onset diabetes treated with high-carbohydrate-modified fat diet. *Br. Med. J.* **1**, 1753–1756.

Simpson, R. W., Mann, J. I., Eaton, J., Carter, R. D., Hockaday, T. D. R. (1979b): High carbohydrate diets and insulin-depeendent diabetics. *Br. Med. J.* **2**, 523–525.

Smith, C. J., Rosman, M. S., Levitt, N. S., Jackson, W. P. (1982): Guar biscuits in the diabetic diet. *S. Afr, Med. J.* **61**, 196–198.

Smith, C., Rosman, M. S., Levitt, N. S., Jackson, W. P. U. (1985): The use of guar gum in the diabetic diet. In *Diabetes and nutrition* International Proceedings of 1st Intl Conference on Diet and Nutrition, Tel Aviv 1983, ed C. Horwitz. London: John Libbey.

Smith, U., Holm, G. (1982): Effect of a modified guar gum preparation on glucose and lipid levels in diabetics and healthy volunteers. *Atherosclerosis* **45**, 1–10.

Special Report Committee of the Canadian Diabetes Association. (1981): 1980 guidelines for the nutritional management of diabetes mellitus. *J. Can. Diab. Ass.* **42**, 110–118.

Taylor, R. H. (1979): Gastric emptying, fibre and absorption. *Lancet* **1**, 872.

Thorne, M. J., Thompson, L. U., Jenkins, D. J. A. (1983): Factors affecting starch digestibility and the glycemic response with special reference to legumes. *Am. J. Clin. Nutr.* **38**, 481–488.

Vaaler, S., Hanssen, K. F., Dahl-Jorgensen, K., Frolich, W., Aaseth J., Odegaard, B., Aagenaes, O. (1983): Improvement in long-term diabetic control after high fibre (bran and guar) diets. *Diabetologia* **25**, 200.

Van Itallie, T. B. (1978): Dietary fiber and obesity. *Am. J. Clin. Nutr.* **31**: Suppl 10; 43–52.

Wahlqvist, M. L., Wilmshurst, E. G., Murton, C. R., Richardson, E. N. (1978): The effect of chain length on glucose absorption and the related metabolic response. *Am. J. Clin. Nutr.* **31**, 1998–2001.

Wahren, J., Juhlin-Dannfelt, A., Bjorkman, O., DeFronzo, R., Felig, P. (1982): Influence of fiber ingestion on carbohydrate utilization and absorption. *Clin. Physiol.* **2**, 315–321.

Ward, G. M., Simpson, R. W., Simpson, H. C., Naylor, B. A., Mann, J. I., Turner, R. C. (1982): Insulin receptor binding increased by high carbohydrate low fat diet in non-insulin-dependent diabetics. *Eur. J. Clin. Invest.* **12**, 93–96.

West, K. M. (1973): Diet therapy: an analysis of failure. *Ann. Intern. Med.* **79**, 425–434.

Wilmhurst, P., Crawley, J. C. W. (1980): The measurement of gastric transit time in obese subjects using 24Na, and the effects of energy content and guar gum on gastric emptying and satiety. *Br. J. Nutr.* **44**, 1–6.

Wolever, T. M. S., Taylor, R., Goff, D. V., Ahern, J. (1979): Fibre and diabetes. *Lancet* **1**, 435.

Wong, S., O'Dea, K. (1983): Importance of physical form rather than viscosity in determining the rate of starch hydrolysis in legumes. *Am. J. Clin. Nutr.* **37**, 66–70.

5
Dietary fibre in obesity

Marcin Krotkiewski and Ulf Smith

Introduction

Fibre was long considered uninteresting from a nutritional point of view. In the beginning of the 1970s interest was rekindled by the observations of Burkitt and Trowell, discussed elsewhere in this book, that certain disorders typical of the affluent countries, like diabetes and coronary heart disease, were considerably less common in the rural areas of Africa. It was suggested that the different dietary habits in the industrial countries played an important role, and the well-known 'fibre hypothesis' about the relationship between the dietary fibre intake and the incidence of these disorders was then formulated.

Dietary fibre, defined on physiological grounds according to Trowell, is made up of the polysaccharides and lignin from plant material which are resistant to hydrolysis by the digestive enzymes. However, the colonic bacterial flora is capable of fermenting some complex fibres and their derivatives and of producing short-chain fatty acids and intestinal gas. The degree of fermentation varies between different subjects, probably due to differences in the colonic flora. Taken together, however, the digestion of fibre is normally limited and fibres are generally recognised as poor sources of dietary energy (Ali *et al.*, 1981). Food rich in dietary fibre is generally calorically less dense than food with a low fibre content. This aspect, as well as some other properties to be discussed, makes dietary fibre interesting and potentially important with regard to the development and treatment of obesity.

The potential importance of dietary fibre in relation to obesity has recently been discussed by several investigators (Cleave, 1977; Heaton, 1973, 1978; Southgate, 1973; van Itallie, 1978). Possible mechanisms through which fibre can influence or, possibly, prevent the development of obesity and/or facilitate weight reduction are summarized in the Table. In general, dietary fibre may influence the physical properties of food in such way that satiety is favoured and caloric intake reduced. The gastrointestinal effects are also important, not least in preventing the constipation commonly seen during caloric restriction. In addition, the effects of certain fibres on metabolism appear extremely useful since they may reduce the risk of some of the medical problems of obesity, such as lipid abnormalities and propensity to diabetes.

Dietary fibre, food intake and satiety

One of the most obvious and potentially important effects of dietary fibre in relation to obesity is its ability to reduce the caloric density of food. Thus, if the total amount of food ingested remains the same, fibre-rich food should lead to a predictable

Table. Potential importance of dietary fibre in relation to obesity

1. Fibre, with its low caloric availability and capacity to bind water, offers considerable opportunity for caloric dilution of foods.
2. Fibre-rich diets stimulate chewing and increase the time required for the consumption of the meal. It remains in the mouth longer, allowing more time for the development of a feeling of satisfaction. Food intake may, therefore, be interrupted earlier.
3. The gut-filling properties and the chewing required during ingestion of fibre may trigger afferent signals inducing satiety.
4. The effect of fibre in slowing the rate of gastric emptying may reduce hunger and prolong the feeling of satiety.
5. Fibre causes a slight malabsorption of, above all, fatty acids and bile acids.
6. Fibre can influence the release of certain gastrointestinal hormones which may lead to lower insulin levels and attenuated hunger.
7. Fibre can improve both glucose tolerance and insulin sensitivity which may influence hypothalamic centres involved in hunger regulation.
8. Fibre increases the passage rate and peristalsis in the terminal part of the large intestine and markedly increases the faecal volume, thereby preventing constipation. The laxative properties of fibre are particularly important during weight reduction with a low caloric diet, which by itself reduces the faecal volume.

weight loss. If the most important effect of fibre is to reduce the caloric density of the food, all dietary fibres should have the same efficacy. However, recent studies strongly suggest that the gel-forming fibres, such as guar gum and pectin, are more potent in promoting a weight reduction than the non-gel-forming fibres like bran. This difference is probably due to some specific properties of the gel-forming fibres such as their ability to reduce the rate of gastric emptying, lower the insulin levels etc.

The potential effectiveness in obesity of a modest caloric dilution of food *per se* is probably limited. Animal experiments have shown that the food ingestion frequently becomes increased so that the body weight is unchanged or only slightly decreased. Similar findings have also been reported in man (Campbell *et al.*, 1971; Spiegel, 1973). However, a marked caloric dilution is able to reduce the total intake and lead to a clear weight reduction in experimental animals (Peterson & Baumgardt, 1971; Adolph, 1974; O'Hea, 1974). One example of this is the finding that rats fed a 'snack' diet of calorically dense, low fibre food such as nuts, chips, chocolate biscuits, become obese. However, the rats rapidly reduce weight again when they are fed their ordinary laboratory chow which is considerably less calorically dense and more fibre-rich than the 'snack' food.

There is also clear evidence in man that appropriate food dilution can be an important factor for weight reduction. Haber *et al.* (1977) reported that satiety was more pronounced when the same meal was ingested as an apple rather than as apple puree or apple juice. Covert replacement of sucrose by an artificial low-calorie sweetner like aspartame leads to a reduced caloric intake which is maintained throughout the observation period (Porikos *et al.*, 1977). Methyl cellulose and guar gum (10 g) reduced the food intake in healthy volunteers by around 10 per cent (Shearer, 1976). A clear weight reduction has also been reported in a long-term study of females supplementing their diet with 15 g guar gum (Tuomilehto *et al.*, 1980).

Mickelsen *et al.* (1979) found a high-fibre bread aided weight loss during an energy-restricted diet. The subjects eating the high-fibre bread also reduced their caloric intake to a slightly greater extent than those eating the regular white bread.

Mickelsen (1980) also recently reported that the high-fibre bread when included in the food ration to experimental animals supported a much lower weight gain than a food ration containing regular white bread.

Krotkiewski (unpubl. observations) found in a 2 months' cross-over study that supplementing a normal diet with fibre biscuits containing 40 per cent oat bran led to a weight reduction in obese patients. In a longitudinal study, 54 obese patients were given an energy-reduced diet of 1000 kcal/day supplemented with 24 g NDF fibre in the form of oat bran biscuits. A control group of 42 obese patients were given the same diet, but without the fibre supplementation. The weight reduction was significantly greater in the fibre group (5.1 ± 1.7 kg per week) than in the group without the fibre supplementation (3.8 ± 1.8 kg per week). The withdrawal rate was also significantly lower in the fibre group than in the control group (24 *vs* 36 per cent after 20 weeks).

Similar results have also been reported in a group of overweight patients treated with 10 g guar gum twice daily before the two main meals (Krotkiewski, 1984). The patients given guar gum showed a significantly greater weight reduction than during the period when they were given regular commercially available wheat bran taken in the same way.

However, it should be pointed out that, in general, the studies in man have not been strictly controlled. It is, thus, not possible to decide whether, or to what extent, the total food intake was reduced and, if so, whether the fibre intake caused nausea or other side-effects which could be of importance for the weight reduction. Such carefully controlled studies are required to clearly delineate the importance and role of dietary fibre in obesity. It is also not clear whether 'pure' fibre supplements to the diet are more or less effective than a more complete change in the diet towards an increased consumption of fibre-rich foods. It is our impression from treating several hundred obsese patients that the compliance with the treatment is superior for fibre supplements than for a regimen where a more profound change in the dietary composition is instituted, even though the latter may be more appealing. Over a long-term range, however, the fibre supplements may help to motivate patients to increase their fibre intake and permit a gradual change in their dietary habits.

High-fibre foods have in general a substantially greater satiety effect in human subjects than low-fibre foods (Haber *et al.*, 1977; Grimes & Gordon, 1978; Kay, 1978; Bolton *et al.*, 1981; Wilmhurst & Crawley, 1980). In the bread studies of Mickelsen *et al.* (1979) practically all subjects felt hungry at the beginning of the study. A reduction of the hunger sensation toward the end of the study was generally reported, but those on the high-fibre bread were the least hungry at any point in time. Grimes & Gordon (1978) also reported that in ten of 12 subjects, white bread was less effective in reaching a point of comfortable fullness than a wholemeal bread.

Krotkiewski (1984) reported a significant reduction of hunger when the diet was supplemented with 10 g guar gum as compared to obese women taking 10 g wheat bran in the same way. The reduction in hunger was also seen when the subjects were maintained on a long-term weight reducing diet of 1000 kcal (unpubl. observations).

In conclusion, most studies, albeit mostly over short-term periods, support the importance of fibre-rich foods or fibre supplementation in obesity. It is unlikely that the effect of fibre is only due to a dilution of the caloric content. Fibre, and particularly the gel-forming fibres, appear to induce an increased satiety which may be due to an effect on gastric emptying. In support of this, it was recently demonstrated that a

fibre has a unique profile and should be widely advocated in the treatment of obesity. Such an effect may indeed prevent or delay the development of manifest diabetes.

An additional property of gel-forming fibres which is beneficial to obese individuals is their lipid-lowering effect. Several studies have shown that gel-forming fibres reduce the LDL-cholesterol while the HDL-cholesterol remains essentially unchanged (Jenkins *et al.*, 1979; Smith & Holm, 1982). Similar findings have also recently been reported in obese subjects (Krotkiewski, 1984). This effect may be largely due to an increased faecal elimination of fat and bile salts. Most studies indicate that the VLDL-triglycerides remain unchanged. Taken together, an increased intake of dietary fibre, particularly gel-forming fibre, offers an interesting and promising therapeutic approach to obesity. Their effects include a way to achieve weight reduction *per se* and also to alleviate some important deleterious effects of obesity on metabolism.

Conclusion

The importance of dietary fibre with respect to obesity is still unclear as only a few studies have addressed this issue. However, the results obtained in studies of non-obese individuals are promising and interesting. An increased intake of dietary fibre, particularly of a gel-forming fibre like guar gum, appears capable of facilitating weight reduction and may in future be demonstrated to prevent weight gain. Concomitantly, an increased intake of gel-forming fibre leads to lower lipid levels and an improved glucose tolerance. An increased intake of a gel-forming fibre like guar gum seems to be one of the most interesting therapeutic approaches to obesity today. This possibility should be further evaluated in carefully controlled clinical trials.

References

Adolph, E. F. (1974): Urges to eat and drink in rats. *Am. J. Physiol.* **151**, 110.

Ali, R., Staub, H., Coccodrilli, G. Jr., Schaubacher, L. (1981): Nutritional significance of dietary fiber. Effect on nutrient biovailability and selected gastrointestinal functions. *J. Agric. Fd Chem.* **29**, 465.

Bolton, R. P., Heaton, K. W., Buroughs, L. F. (1981): The role of dietary fiber in satiety, glucose and insulin: Studies with fruit and fruit juices. *Am. J. Clin. Nutr.* **34**, 211.

Campbell, R. G., Haskin, S. A., Van Itallie, T. B. (1971): Studies of food intake regulation in man. Responses to variation in nutritive density in lean and obese subjects. *New Engl. J. Med.* **285**, 1402.

Cleave, T. L. (1977): Over-consumption, now the most dangerous cause of disease in Westernized countries. *Publ. Hlth* **91**, 127.

Evans, E., Miller, D. S. (1975): Bulking agents in the treatment of obesity. *Nutr. Metab.* **18**, 199.

Garrison, M. V., Reel, R. L., Fawley, P., Breidenstem, C. P. (1978): Comparative digestibility of acid detergent fiber by laboratory albino and wild polynesian rats. *J. Nutr.* **108**, 191.

Grimes, D. S., Gordon, C. (1978): Satiety value of wholemeal and white bread. *Lancet* **2**, 106.

Haber, G. R., Heaton, K. W., Murphy, D., Burroughs, L. F. (1977): Depletion and disruption of dietary fiber effects on satiety, plasma-glucose and serum insulin. *Lancet* **2**, 679.

Heaton, K. W. (1973): Food fiber as an obstacle to energy intake. *Lancet* **2**, 1418.

Heaton, K. W. (1978): Fibre, satiety and insulin — a new approach to over-nutrition and obesity. In *Dietary fibre: Current developments of importance of health*, ed K. W. Heaton, pp. 141–150. London: John Libbey.

Holt, S., Heading, R. C., Carter, D. C., Prescott, L. F., Tothill, P. (1979): Effect of gel fibre on gastric emptying and absorption of glucose and paracetamol. *Lancet* **2**, 636.

Jenkins, D. J. A., Wolever, T. M. S., Leeds, A. R., Gassull, M. A., Haisman, P., Dilawari, J., Goff, D., Metz, G. L., Alberti, K. G. M. M. (1978): Dietary fibres, fibre analogues, and glucose tolerance: importance of viscosity. *Br. Med. J.* **1**, 1392.

Jenkins, D. J. A., Leeds, A. R., Slavin, B., Mann, J., Jepson, E. M. (1979): Dietary fiber and blood lipids — Reduction of serum cholesterol in type II hyperlipidemia by guar gum. *Am. J. Clin. Nutr.* **32**, 16.

Jenkins, D., Wolever, T., Taylor, R., Barker, H., Fielden, H. (1980): Exceptionally low blood glucose response to dried beans: comparison with other carbohydrate foods. *Br. Med. J.* **281**, 578.

Johnson, I., Gee, J. M. (1981): Effect of gel-forming gums on the intestinal unstirred layer and sugar transport *in vitro*. *Gut 22*, 398.

Kay, R. M. (1978): Food form, postprandial glycemia and satiety. *Am. J. Clin. Nutr.* **31**, 738.

Keim, K., Kies, C. (1979): Effects of dietary fiber on nutritional status of weanling mice. *Cereal Chem.* **56**, 73.

Krotkiewski, M., Björntorp, P., Sjöström, L., Smith, U. (1983): Impact of obesity on metabolism in men and women. Importance of regional adipose tissue distribution. *J. Clin. Invest.* **72**, 1150.

Krotkiewski, M. (1984): Effect of guar on body weight, hunger ratings and metabolism in obese subjects. *Br. J. Nutr.* **52**, 97.

Mickelsen, O., Makdani, D. P., Cotton, R. H., Titcomb, S. T., Colmey, J. C., Gatty, R. (1979): Effects of a high fiber bread on weight loss in college-age males. *Am. J. Clin. Nutr.* **32**, 1703.

Mickelsen, O. (1980): Prevention and treatment of obesity. In *Nutrition, physiology and obesity*, ed R. Schemmel, pp. 167–184. Boca Raton, Florida: CRC Press.

Morgan, L. M., Goulder, T. J., Triolakis, D., Marks, V., Alberti, K. G. M. M. (1979): The effect of unabsorbable carbohydrate on gut hormones. *Diabetologia* **17**, 85.

O'Hea, K. E., Aldis, A. E., Skidmore, G. B., Smith, B. H. *et al.* (1974): Effect of dietary dilution on food intake, weight gain, plasma glucose and insulin and adipose tissue insulin sensitivity in rats. *Comp. Biochem. Physiol.* **48A**, 21.

Peterson, A. D., Baumgardt, B. R. (1971*a*): Food and energy intake of rats fed with diets varying in energy concentration and density. *J. Nutr.* **101**, 1057.

Peterson, A. D., Baumgardt, B. R. (1971*b*): Influence of level of energy demand on the ability of rats to compensate for diet dilution. *J. Nutr.* **101**, 1069.

Porikos, K. P., Booth, B., Van Itallie, T. B. (1977): Effect of covert nutritive dilution on the spontaneous food intake of obese individuals: A pilot study. *Am. J. Clin. Nutr.* **30**, 1638.

Rao, A. U., Bright-See, E. (1979): Effect of graded amounts of dietary pectin on growth parameters of rats. *Nutr. Rep. Intern.* **19**, 411.

Sandberg, A., Ahderinne, R., Andersson, H., Hallgren, B., Hultén, L. (1983): The effect of citrus pectin on the absorption of nutrients in the small intestine. *Hum. Nutr.: Clin. Nutr.* **37C**, 171.

Shearer, R. S. (1976): Effects of bulk producing tablets on hunger intensity and dieting patients. *Curr. Ther. Res.* **19**, 431.

Smith, U., Holm, G. (1982): Effect of a modified guar gum preparation on glucose and lipid levels in diabetics and healthy volunteers. *Atherosclerosis* **45**, 1.

Southgate, D. A. T., Durnin, J. V. G. A. (1970): Caloric conversion factors. An experimental reassessment of the factors used in the calculation of the energy values of human diets. *Br. J. Nutr.* **24**, 517.

Southgate, D. A. T. (1973): Fiber and other unavailable carbohydrates and their effects on the energy value of the diet. *Proc. Nutr. Soc.* **32**, 131.

Southgate, D. A. T. (1978): Dietary fiber analyses and food sources. *Am. J. Clin. Nutr.* **31**, 107.

Spiegel, T. S. (1973): Caloric regulation of food intake in man. *J. Comp. Physiol. Psychol.* **84**, 24.

Sullivan, A. C., Triscari, J., Comai, K. (1978): Caloric compensatory responses to diets containing either nonabsorbable carbohydrate or lipid by obese and lean Zucker rats. *Am. J. Clin. Nutr.* **31**, 261.

Tuomiletho, J., Voutilainen, E., Huttunen, J., Vinni, S., Homan, K. (1980): Effect of guar gum on body weight and serum lipids in hypercholesterolemic females. *Acta Med. Scand.* **208**, 45.

Van Itallie, T. B. (1978): Dietary fibre and obesity. *Am. J. Clin. Nutr.* **31**, 43.

Vohra, P., Shariff, G., Fratzer, F. H. (1979): Growth inhibitory effect of some gums and pectin for Tribolium Castaneum larvae, chickens and Japanese quail. *Nutr. Rep. Intern.* **19**, 463.

Wilmshurst, P., Crawley, J. C. W. (1980): The measurement of gastric transit time in obese subjects using ^{24}Na and the effects of energy content and guar gum on gastric emptying and satiety. *Br. J. Nutr.* **44**, 1.

6
Dietary fibre supplements and weight reduction

Kjeld R. Ryttig

Introduction

Overweight is a commonly occurring disorder in the industrialised countries (van Itallie, 1978). The frequency of overweight is growing rapidly and is probably caused by changes in eating habits, decreased physical activity and by economic and social factors. The possibility that dietary fibre could influence body weight was proposed by Cleave in 1957.

In recent years there has been a considerable reduction in consumption of fibre (Trygg, 1976) together with a changed pattern in fibre intake: a slight increase in fibre originating from fruits and vegetables, but a bigger decrease in fibre originating from cereals.

An enhancement of dietary fibre intake may prevent development of overweight or be of value as part of a diet during weight reduction. This enhancement can be accomplished in two distinctly different ways: by changing eating pattern towards food rich in dietary fibre or by making use of commercially available fibre preparations.

As the beneficial effects of fibre-rich food have already been dealt with (Chapter 5), fibre supplements only will be considered below.

Mild overweight

Unfortunately only a few well-controlled investigations with placebo have been carried out under double-blind conditions.

One controlled investigation was performed in a slimming club in Norway (Solum, 1983). Fifty-three slightly overweight participants were enrolled in a weight-reducing programme consisting of a daily energy intake of approx 1100 kcal per day. In addition to the restricted diet 30 participants received 16 fibre tablets consisting of fibre from grain (80 per cent) and citrus (20 per cent)*. Twenty-three participants received identical-looking placebo tablets. Allocation to treatments was made on a random basis. The participants were weighed every week for an **8-week** period. Some of them had their blood pressure measured at the same time.

The two groups were initially comparable, median weight 72.8 kg (fibre group) versus 70.5 kg (placebo group) ($P = 0.47$). After 8 weeks the corresponding figures were 69.8 kg (fibre group) versus 69 kg (placebo group). The median weight

---

*The fibre tablets are produced by Farma Food A/S Copenhagen. Each tablet contains 44 per cent dietary fibre (AOAC 84).

reduction in the fibre group was 2.8 kg *vs* 1.5 kg in the placebo group. The difference was statistically significant ($P = 0.04$).

There was a tendency towards a lower blood pressure in the fibre-treated group.

This investigation was followed up by another well-controlled investigation in a slimming club regimen (Ryttig, Larsen & Hægh, 1984). A total of 90 slightly overweight (>115 per cent of ideal body weight) participants were included. The trial was performed as a randomised, double-blind investigation with parallel groups. The subjects were given a diet with an energy content of about 1200 kcal per day. In addition to the diet the participants were on a random basis, given seven fibre tablets or identical-looking placebo tablets approx 30 min before each of four daily meals. The tablets were taken with at least 300 ml of water. The participants were weighed weekly for 12 weeks.

The two groups were initially comparable. Both groups lost weight during treatment ($P < 0.01$). At the end of 11 weeks of treatment the average weight loss in the placebo group was 4.2 kg *vs* 6.3 kg in the fibre group. The difference of 2.1 kg was statistically significant ($P = 0.01$). This investigation revealed another piece of important information: the probability of adherence to a diet was significantly ($P = 0.05$) higher in the fibre-treated group compared with placebo. This was evident after 4 weeks of treatment.

The possible effect of the fibre tablets in lowering blood pressure led us to investigate this effect more closely (Solum *et al.*, 1985). Seventy-one slightly overweight (>115 per cent of ideal body weight) women were included in a double-blind, placebo-controlled study for 12 weeks. They were all treated with a weight-reducing diet with an energy content of about 1200 kcal/day. Additionally 37 received 20 fibre tablets and the remaining 34 identical-looking placebo tablets.

Nearly all patients were considered normotensive (<160/95 mmHg) at the beginning of the trial.

Mean systolic and diastolic blood pressure were initially significantly lower ($P < 0.02$) in the fibre group (123/84 mmHg) compared to the placebo group (142/95 mmHg). Despite that fact, the blood pressure was significantly reduced ($P < 0.01$) in the fibre-treated group (114/75 mmHg) compared to the placebo group where the blood pressure remained nearly unchanged (142/91 mmHg). In this study a statistically significant ($P < 0.01$) weight reduction in both groups was found. The mean reduction after 12 weeks of treatment was 7.6 kg in the fibre group versus 6.1 kg in the placebo group. The difference between the groups was found to be significant ($P = 0.03$).

Blood lipids (serum total triglyceride and serum total cholesterol) were checked in some of the participants. There was a significant ($P < 0.02$) reduction of triglyceride and cholesterol in both groups. No significant differences between the groups were detected at any time. The reduction in serum triglyceride and cholesterol could be due to either the weight reduction or the fibre supplement as such.

The beneficial effect of a dietary fibre supplement of 4.3 g and 7.6 g to slightly overweight persons has thus been confirmed in the above mentioned studies.

Moderate and severe overweight
Where there is a beneficial effect from using a fibre supplement to moderate and

severe overweight people has not yet been fully elucidated. The following study looked at weight loss and blood pressure.

Sixty patients, more than 20 per cent above ideal weight, in an obesity unit of a hospital were included in a double-blind, randomized trial (Rössner *et al.*, 1985). Before entering the study each patient had his diet checked by a nutritionist. Four 24-hour recalls were performed during the treatment period.

All patients were placed on a diet of approx. 1400 kcal per day. In addition the patients received either 18 fibre tablets or identical-looking placebo tablets, on a random basis. Patients were seen regularly at 2-week intervals for 2 months. The two groups were initially comparable with regard to weight, 94.5 kg in the fibre group *vs* 93.9 in the placebo group. Both groups lost weight during treatment ($P <$ 0.01). Median weight loss in the fibre group was slightly, but insignificantly higher, 7 kg *vs* 6 kg. The fibre group showed a significant reduction in blood pressure ($P <$ 0.05), from 131/83 to 121/78 mmHg.

In a subsequent study in the same clinic on the same patient material, but with an energy intake of approx. 1800 kcal per day, the amount of fibre was enhanced from approx. 5 to 6.5* g per day. This supplement produced a statistically significant ($P = 0.04$) weight reduction of 6.2 kg in the fibre-treated group compared to 4.1 kg in the placebo group, during a treatment period of 3 months. In the fibre-treated group a statistically significant reduction ($P < 0.05$) in diastolic blood pressure from 86 to 81 mmHg was also noted.

Discussion and conclusion

The evidence suggests that a dietary fibre supplement can facilitate weight reduction in grade I obesity (BMI 25 to 30). The additional weight loss is probably achieved by a reduction in hunger feelings and a better adherance to the prescribed diet. The question of energy utilisation has not been highlighted in these studies, but trials aiming at an investigation of energy balance with and without a fibre supplement are in progress. A reduced energy utilisation could be a reason for a greater weight reduction.

As regards the reducing effect on blood pressure of the fibre supplement the mode of action is not established. A part of the effect could be due to the weight reduction. This is probably the case with regard to changes in systolic blood pressure (SBP), as the fall in SBP is correlated very well with changes in weight.

The fall in diastolic blood pressure (DBP) takes place within the first 2 weeks of treatment and then DBP remains nearly unchanged during the rest of the treatment period.

According to Fagerberg (1984) restricted energy intake alone did not reduce blood pressure; simultaneous restriction of sodium was required. The reduction in blood pressure reported elsewhere in this chapter could have been linked to spontaneous sodium restriction, but unfortunately a sodium balance study was not performed in the above mentioned weight reduction investigations.

The beneficial effects of a fibre supplement on grade II obesity (BMI 30 to 40) is not as marked as in grade I, although a high intake of a fibre supplement has been

---

*Another not yet marketed fibre tablet formulation produced by Farma Food A/S Copenhagen. Each tablet contains 60 per cent dietrary fibre (AOAC. 84).

70

shown to facilitate a weight reduction in this type of obesity. Further research is needed to clarify the role of fibre supplements in this area.

References
Cleave, T. L. (1957): *Fat consumption and coronary disease*. Bristol: John Wright.
Fagerberg, B. (1984): On the hypotensive response to weight reduction. Göteborg: Thesis.
Rössner, S., von Zweigbergk, D., Öhlin, A., Ryttig, K. R. : Weight loss with dietary fibre supplementation: result of two double-blind randomized long-term studies. To be published.
Ryttig, K. R., Larsen, S., Hægh, L. (1984): Treatment of slightly to moderate overweight persons: a double-blind, placebo-controlled investigation with diet and fibre tablets (Dumovital). *Tidsskr. Nor. Laegeforen* **104**, 989–91.
Solum, T. T. (1983): Fibre tablets, Dumovital, as a means to achieve weight reduction. *Tidsskr. Nor. Laegeforen* **103**, 1707–8.
Solum, T. T., Ryttig, K., Solum, E., Larsen, S. (1985): The influence of a low fat, high fibre diet on blood pressure, serum lipids and body weight in slightly to moderately overweight persons: A randomized double-blind placebo-controlled investigation with diet and fibre tablets (Dumovital). Submitted to Tidsskr Nor Laegeforen.
Trygg, K. (1976): Plantefiber i norsk kosthold. *Tidskr Nor. Laegeforen* **103**, 1707–08.
van Itallie, T. B. (1978): Dietary fibre and obesity. *Am. J. Clin. Nutr.* **31**, s 43.

7
Fibre and mineral absorption

Barbara F. Harland and Eugene R. Morris

It is now recognised that inclusion of dietary fibre in the diet is essential for optimum nutritional health. Continued research will provide the answers: 'how much?' and 'what kinds?' A complication to the resolution of these two questions is that foods or diets high in dietary fibre may alter mineral metabolism. A further complication is the natural presence of phytate in most high fibre fruits, vegetables and whole grains. Phytate, too, binds minerals making them unavailable to the body. Present information is insufficient to indicate how serious the problem may be except in instances of high intakes of whole grain cereals, legumes, or wheat bran. This brief summary of some recently published human studies pertinent to the question, 'Does dietary fibre affect the absorbability of minerals?', provides the answer, 'yes' — and points to phytate as the primary cause of alteration of mineral metabolism on high fibre diets, rather than fibre itself.

Introduction

Over the past several decades, information has proliferated on the physiological functions of minerals in living organisms. The effects in humans of frank deficiencies of some minerals, iron and zinc for example, are known and readily recognised. The effects of marginal deficiencies are less well understood and possibly not even recognised at the present time. Thus, the ability of the diet to provide an adequate input of the inorganic nutrients is of concern to nutritionists. The minerals in diets and foods that are high in dietary fibre are suspected to be of marginal bioavailability in comparison with diets low in dietary fibre. This is true of foods high in phytate as well. Because of the complexities of dietary fibre analyses and because of the various physical and chemical conditions which may alter fibre/phytate/mineral interactions, the picture is not totally clear. Studies have been selected for presentation in this paper which contribute to our understanding of this very intricate problem. Some reviews on the topic include Cummings (1978), Kelsay (1981, 1982), Hallberg (1981) and Forbes & Erdman (1983).

Metabolic balance studies

I. Van Dokkum *et al.* (1982) provided 12 young adult men with a basal omnivore diet that supplied 7 g daily of neutral detergent fibre (NDF), exclusive of NDF from bread. Bread prepared from white flour was consumed for 20 days, followed by bread containing coarse wheat bran for the same length of time, giving total intakes of 9 and 22 g of NDF, respectively. Approximately 25 and 69 per cent, respectively, of the total NDF intakes were derived from the white and coarse bran breads. The white flour bread was not fortified. Mean mineral intakes, faecal excretion and balances are summarized in Table 1. Although intakes of each of the five elements measured were significantly greater when coarse bran bread was consumed, balance values for Mg, Fe, Zn and Cu did not differ by type of bread. The mean Ca

Table 1. *Intake, faecal excretion and balance of human subjects consuming white or coarse bran bread. Values are means (mg/d). Adapted from Van Dokkum et al. (1982).*

	White flour bread	Coarse bran bread
NDF intake (g/d)	9	22
Calcium		
Intake	956	1003*
Faecal excretion†	717 (0.75)	836* (0.83)
Balance	14	−42
Magnesium		
Intake	213	373*
Faecal excretion†	105 (0.49)	240* (0.64)
Balance	−8	−3
Iron		
Intake	8.3	12.2*
Faecal excretion†	7.4 (0.89)	11.4* (0.93)
Balance	0.8	0.7
Zinc		
Intake	9.0	11.3*
Faecal excretion†	8.9 (0.99)	11.1* (0.98)
Balance	−0.6	−0.4
Copper		
Intake	1.24	1.48*
Faecal excretion†	0.97 (0.78)	1.18* (0.80)
Balance	0.22	0.25

* Means significantly different, ($P < 0.01$).
† Fractional faecal excretion, ie faecal excretion/intake, is given in parentheses

balance was negative when the coarse bran bread was consumed, but not significantly less than when white bread was consumed. Faecal excretion of each of the elements, however, was significantly greater when consuming the coarse bran bread. Also, the calculated fractional faecal excretion of Ca, Mg and Fe was greater when the coarse bran bread was consumed.

II. Sandberg *et al.* (1982) compared the apparent absorption of Ca, Mg, Zn and Fe in ileostomy patients given either a low fibre or a wheat bran supplemented diet. Undigested bran components were found to be excreted by these patients on the day of consumption, avoiding problems in demarcating faeces corresponding to period of intake (Sandberg *et al.*, 1981). A constant low fibre diet was given to 11 patients for 5 days followed by 2 days free choice, then 5 days supplemented with 16 g wheat bran daily. Ileostomy fluid and excreta were collected during the last 3 days of each test period. Mean intakes, mg/d, on the low fibre diet were: Ca 1270, Mg 219, Zn 12.9 and Fe 10.6, and increased by 24, 73. 0.3 and 2.2 mg, respectively, when supplemented with the wheat bran. During bran supplementation, the relative apparent absorption of Zn decreased by approximately 50 per cent, of Mg by 15 per cent, both significantly different ($P < 0.01$), while Ca decreased only slightly, and Fe increased. The amount of each element recovered from the ileostomy fluid was significantly greater ($P < 0.02$) when the wheat bran was consumed. Apparent balances were positive for the four elements during each test period.

III. Andersson *et al.* (1983) studied the effect on mineral balance of three levels of non-starch polysaccharides from wheat bran while maintaining constant mineral and phytate intakes. Inorganic salts of Ca, Fe and Zn and Na phytate were added to white and brown bread to provide the amounts of these elements and of phytic acid present in wholemeal bread. Six volunteers consumed a 3-day rotating menu for 72 days, each type of bread being consumed for 24 consecutive days, assigned in random order. The bread, 200 g daily, was consumed at breakfast. The amounts (g/d) of non-starch polysaccharide provided by 200 g of bread were: white 3.3, brown 10.9, and wholemeal 18.7. The calculated total dietary fibre intakes were: white 16.1, brown 23.7 and wholemeal 31.5. Metabolic balance data were presented for the last 12 days of each 24-day diet treatment. Total intakes of Ca, Zn and Fe were the same for each diet, 1400, 11 and 15 mg/d. Faecal excretion and balance of Ca, Zn and Fe were not changed by the type of bread consumed. The fractional faecal excretion of Mg increased from 68 per cent when white bread was consumed to 74 and 76 per cent when brown or wholemeal bread was consumed. Although the total faecal excretion of Mg was greater than intake, and increased when brown or wholemeal bread was eaten, balance was not affected by the type of bread. Overall mean balance values were: Ca 140, Zn 0.5, Fe 1.4 and Mg −20 mg/d.

IV. In another study, despite a substantially increased Ca intake, four young men were in negative Ca balance — 77 mg/d — when their high protein diet included wholemeal crispbread, compared with a mean balance of 32 mg/d without the crispbread (Cummings *et al.*, 1979*a*). There was no change in urinary Ca excretion, the negative balance resulting from increased faecal Ca excretion. Calculated dietary fibre intake was 53.2 g/d when the crispbread was consumed, more than twice the amount without the bread. Phytate intake was not determined. However, when the addition of dietary pectin was tested (36 g/d for 6 wk), pectin was found to be completely metabolized in the human gut and Ca balance remained unchanged (Cummings *et al.*, 1979*b*).

V. The effect of whole or dephytinized bran on mineral balance of adult men was examined (Morris *et al.*, 1980; Morris & Ellis, 1982, 1983, 1985). Wheat bran was incubated in a water suspension to allow the endogenous phytase to hydrolyze the phytate. The entire incubation mixture was then freeze-dried and the product was baked into muffins at the same level as in untreated wheat bran muffins. Mineral intakes were thus the same for each type of muffin (as in Table 2, above). For both muffin diets, analysed NDF was approximately 16 g/d. (NDF was the same for each type of muffin as well). Phytic acid intake differed 10-fold (2 g/d for whole wheat bran, 0.2 g/d for the dephytinized bran muffins). Muffins were consumed for two, 15-day periods, consisting of three consecutive repeats of a 5-day menu cycle; five volunteers in the sequence, whole to dephytinized muffins, and five volunteers in the opposite sequence. All stools were collected and composites were made of days 1 through 5, and 6 through 15 for each dietary treatment. Urine was collected for

74

Table 2. Type of bran muffin and apparent absorption of minerals (mg/d). Mean intakes (mg/day) Zn 17.0, Fe 21.7, Mn 10.6, Cu 1.91, Ca 1100, Mg 553; (g/day) NDF 16, phytic acid: 2.0, (whole bran), 0.2 (dephytinized bran). Adapted from Morris *et al* (1980): Morris & Ellis (1982, 1983, 1984).

	Chronological days of study			
	1–5	6–15	16–20	21–30
		Group A (N = 5)		
	Whole bran muffins		*Dephytinized bran muffins*	
Zn	−1.4	3.2	1.8	2.4
Fe	−3.0[a]	2.2	1.3[a]	2.8
Mn	−2.0[a]	1.3	1.1[a]	1.2
Cu	0.53	0.66	0.59	0.69
Ca	148[a]	399	382[a]	416
Mg	140[a]	137[b]	250[a]	191[b]
		Group B (n = 5)		
	Dephytinized bran muffins		*Whole bran muffins*	
Zn	1.2	2.4	0.9	3.0
Fe	0.0	1.1	−0.3	3.5
Mn	0.0	0.4	−0.5	1.5
Cu	0.56	0.43	0.40	0.51
Ca	196	321	174	343
Mg	199	205[b]	195	152[b]

[a,b] Means significantly different by paired t-test ($P < 0.05$).

days 6 through 15, only. For the total 15 days of each dietary treatment, the mean apparent absorption of Zn, Fe, Mn and Cu was the same, regardless of the type of muffin consumed. Apparent absorption of Ca and Mg was greater when the dephytinized muffins were consumed (40 and 70 mg, respectively). However, when the apparent absorption values were examined chronologically (Table 2) a different pattern emerged. During the first 5 days, when the whole bran muffins were consumed, apparent mean daily absorption of Zn, Fe and Mn was much less than for the subsequent 10 days (more of these elements was excreted in faeces). Except that the values were positive, the same pattern appeared for Ca, and to a lesser degree, for Cu and Mg. When dephytinized bran muffins were consumed, apparent absorption values also tended to be lower the first 5 days than for the subsequent 10 days. However, the amplitude of difference was less and the overall values were positive for the trace elements Zn, Fe and Mn. Some individuals in Group B (the sequence of consumption, dephytinized to whole bran muffins) secreted more in the faeces than was consumed during days 1 through 5.

Apparent balances over the last 10 days of each dietary treatment were not significantly affected by the type of muffin, tended to be positive overall, and for Zn, Fe, Mn, Cu and Ca, were greatest when the whole bran muffins were consumed. Although phosphorus values are not presented in Table 2, a significantly greater percentage of total P consumed during the whole bran muffin periods was excreted in the stools. Urinary P during the dephytinized bran muffin periods was sufficiently great that P balance between dietary regimens did not differ. The mean recovery of phytate in the stool was 80 per cent while consuming the whole wheat bran muffins.

VI. Fruits and vegetables are excellent sources of dietary fibre. Kelsay *et al.*, (1979*a,b*) compared the effect of daily intakes of 4.6 or 23.8 g of NDF. The high fibre diet contained fruits and vegetables, the low fibre diet, the fruit and vegetable juices. Each diet was consumed for 26 days by 12 adult men in a crossover experimental design. During the final week of each dietary regimen, samples of diet, stools and urine were collected for analysis. The low fibre diet was supplemented with inorganic compounds of Mg, Fe and Cu to provide intakes equivalent to the high fibre diet. Fractional faecal excretion of Ca, Mg, Fe, Cu and Zn was significantly increased and balance of these elements was negative when the high fibre diet was consumed. Apparent absorption values for Fe and P did not differ between diets. The high fibre diet included spinach, and the possible role of oxalate in spinach was implicated as a contributor to the negative mineral balances. In a subsequent experiment (Kelsay & Prather, 1983) the presence of spinach in the diet was shown to contribute to negative balances for Mg and Zn.

VII. After 5 weeks in a group of 62 young, healthy volunteers, neither the addition of pectin (28 g/d) nor wheat bran (36 g/d) to a high fibre diet, rich in vegetables and fruits, had any negative effect on apparent balances of Ca or Mg (Stasse-Wolthuis *et al.*, 1980).

VIII. Morris *et al.* (1984, 1985) conducted an experiment to determine the effect on apparent mineral balance of feeding three levels of phytate supplied by a basal diet and two levels of sodium phytate incorporated into muffins — see Table 3. Twelve adult men in a randomized crossover design consumed controlled diets repeated in 5-day menu cycles for 45 days. There was no overall effect of increasing levels of phytate on Fe, Mn and Cu. However, there was a tendency for decreased apparent absorption of Zn, and Mg and Ca apparent absorption were decreased by one-half and one-sixth, respectively, as dietary phytate was increased to the highest level.

Isotope studies

I. In the studies reported above, subjects consumed whole foods in settings as nearly 'life-like' as could be arranged without compromising a controlled experiment. In the following study (Turnlund *et al.*, 1984), young men were confined to a metabolic ward, and fed a liquid formula diet containing alpha-cellulose as the fibre source and sodium phytate. Zn-67, a stable isotope, was added to the formulae and zinc absorption was measured by faecal monitoring of Zn-67. The study was conducted to determine whether the high fibre, or the phytate, or both, would result in inhibition of zinc absorption. Average zinc absorption decreased from 34.0 per cent (basal diet) to 33.8 per cent with 0.5 g/kg body weight of alpha-cellulose. When 2.34 g of sodium phytate were added to the basal formula, absorption decreased to 17.5 per cent.

II. In another isotope study conducted by Sandstrom *et al.* (1980), Zn-65 and whole

Table 3. *Overall daily apparent mineral balance (apparent min. bal.) in adult men consuming three levels of phytate.* Adapted from Morris *et al.* (1984, 1985).

Element	Intake (mg/d)	Mean daily apparent min. bal. (3 phytate levels, g)		
		(0.5)	(1.7)	(2.9)
Fe	12.9	−0.8	−1.3	−0.7
Zn	10.6	0.7	0.3	0.2
Mn	4.0	−0.7	−0.3	−0.5
Cu	1.4	0.02	0.02	−0.02
Mg	254	4	6	−2
Ca	728	−23	−34	−82

body counting were employed to monitor zinc absorption in 35 women and 31 men, aged 19–61. Wheat flour of 100 per cent extraction as whole wheat bread, and of 72 per cent extraction as white bread, were incorporated into composite meals. In contrast to what might be expected, a lower absolute quantity of zinc was absorbed from the white bread meal than from the wholewheat bread meal. However, when both breads were enriched with zinc chloride, absorption was greater from the white bread meal. The addition of calcium in the form of milk products (milk and cheese) to the meal containing wholewheat bread improved the absorption of zinc. Other foods high in protein such as beef and egg were also found to enhance zinc absorption. It was theorized that an ample supply of proteins and/or peptides may facilitate zinc complexation and thus override the zinc-binding characteristics of fibre and/or phytate.

III. Cook *et al.* (1983) studied the absorption of radio-iron in normal males and females after adding bran, pectin or cellulose to muffins baked with wheat flour. Fifty mg of ascorbic acid was added to the meal to enhance iron absorption. Values were 2.26, 1.07, 1.89 and 2.26 per cent iron absorption from the plain muffins, bran muffins, pectin muffins and cellulose muffins, respectively. The significant differences were between the low absorption of iron from the bran muffins compared with the greater absorption from the plain and cellulose muffins. In another experiment when meals comprising a mixture of fruits, vegetables and grains were composited to contain 'low' or 'high' fibre, iron absorption from the low fibre diet was more than two-fold greater than from the high fibre diet (6.07 and 2.96 per cent, respectively). The authors concluded however, that fibre did not appear to be the major determinant of food iron availability in humans.

Mineral status in diabetics consuming high fibre diets

Beneficial effects of increased dietary fibre by way of a greater intake of complex carbohydrates have been reported for diabetics, but until the study of Vaaler *et al.* (1984), the effect of such a regimen on mineral status in diabetics had not been studied in depth. In three, 3-month periods (cross-over design) 28 diabetics receiving insulin twice a day consumed: (1) a low fibre diet, (2) a low fibre diet plus wheat bran bread, and (3) a low fibre diet plus guar gum bread. The following serum and urinary minerals were monitored: Ca, P as phosphate, Mg, Fe, Zn, Cu and Se. There were no changes in body weight or insulin dosages during the study.

Moreover, there were no changes in serum or urinary concentrations of any of the minerals.

A review of mineral binding by dietary fibre

The most comprehensive review of mineral binding by dietary fibre in humans has recently been published (Frolich, 1984). In Table 2 of her publication Frolich presents a summary of normal human studies of mineral bioavailability from cereals, encompassing the years 1942 to 1984. The following minerals were examined: Ca, Cl, Cu, Fe, K, Mg, Na, P and Zn. Of 55 human studies reported, metabolic balance as a result of ingesting fibre from cereals and grains became negative in 35, positive in two or remained unaltered in 18 studies. Table 4 of Frolich's publication lists human studies in which mineral bioavailability from unrefined cereal products was enhanced by the addition of certain foods other than those containing high fibre or phytate. Of 16 studies (in addition to those discussed above) absorption of Fe and/or Zn was increased by the addition of meat, fish, milk, fruit, fruit juice, orange juice, papaya, and ascorbic acid.

Beltsville year-long balance studies

At long last, self-selected dietary fibre intakes are presented in a normal American population who were studied for a year (Kelsay & Clark, 1984), Table 4. A group of 29 men and women collected duplicate portion dietary intakes for one week during each of the four seasons and contributed blood, urine and faecal samples during these same weeks. NDF intakes averaged 7.7 g/d for females and 9.5 g/d for males. These are reasonable fibre intakes, and yet, during the reporting periods, Ca, P and Mg balances were negative (Lakshmanan *et al.*, 1984*a,b*); iron balances were negative for the women (Miles *et al.*, 1984) and Zn, Cu and Mn balances were negative for both men and women (Patterson *et al.*, 1984). Mean phytic acid intake was 0.63 g/day. Only two men consumed more than 1 g/day (Ellis *et al.*, 1984). Although a close examination of the data revealed that, compared with the year's intakes, dietary intakes were under-consumed for the four reporting periods, one has reservations about recommending large increases in dietary fibre (and thus phytate) with the potential for mineral binding as demonstrated in some of the previous studies.

In vitro and animal studies

Invaluable contributions to our understanding of fibre/phytate/mineral interrelationships have been made by *in vitro* and animal studies. Reinhold *et al.* (1981) looked at iron binding in the presence of acid detergent and neutral detergent fibres with changes in iron concentration, pH, and the presence or absence of various quantities of inhibitors of iron binding. Fibre binding of iron was strongly inhibited by ascorbic, citric and phytic acids and by EDTA in low concentrations. Of several amino acids, cysteine inhibited iron binding most strongly; of minerals, calcium and phosphate were strong inhibitors. The authors theorised that most of the ingested non-haem iron combines with fibre unless it can be released by 'surges' of gastric acid, or inhibitors of binding. The inhibitors may release iron for absorption which may have been 'trapped' by dietary fibre.

Plants low in phytate bind calcium according to their uronic acid content (James *et al.*, 1978). Thus if small intestinal absorption of calcium has been reduced because of

Table 4. *Fibre intakes (mean values ± s.e.m) of 29 subjects for 1 wk during the four different seasons.* (Adapted from Kelsay & Clark, 1984).

	Spring	Summer	Autumn	Winter
CF(g/day)	3.74 ± 0.25	3.96 ± 0.28	3.89 ± 0.30	4.02 ± 0.31
NDF(g/day)	7.42 ± 0.75^a	$8.26 \pm 0.73^{a,b}$	$8.83 \pm 0.73^{b,c}$	9.52 ± 0.84^c
NDF/1000kcal	4.02 ± 0.39^a	$4.19 \pm 0.35^{a,b}$	$4.67 \pm 0.39^{b,c}$	5.10 ± 0.49^c
NDF/CF	1.95 ± 0.12^a	$2.10 \pm 0.10^{a,b}$	$2.30 \pm 0.09^{b,c}$	2.34 ± 0.08^c

[a–c] Row means followed by the same superscript are not significantly different at the 5% level according to Duncan's multiple range comparisons. CF = crude fibre.

complexation with the non-cellulosic fraction of fibre, all is not lost. There can be subsequent release of Ca for absorption by the lower bowel, a function of the colonic microbial population. Microbial fermentation affects primarily the non-cellulosic polysaccharides, resulting in the fermentation of over 80 per cent of the uronic acids, and the release of Ca for absorption.

Naturally present soluble ligands were shown to play a major role in the *in vitro* bioavailability indices of Ca, Mg, Cu and Zn by Lyon (1984).

Plant cell wall components possess different cation exchange capacities. Compared with the strong bonding capabilities of lignin and the Maillard products resulting from the browning process, cellulose has a relatively low binding capacity for minerals (McBurney *et al.*, 1984).

When phytate hydrolysis can be effected by fermentation (certain yeast phytases are more effective than the phytase from wheat), minerals, formerly bound by the phytate become available for absorption. Research is being conducted to discover the mineral binding properties of phytate hydrolysis products (Frolich & Asp, 1984).

An animal study (Ballam *et al.*, 1984) showed that when dietary calcium intakes of chickens were low, there was greater hydrolysis of the phytate molecule than when calcium intakes were high (except when the diet contained rice bran). In this experiment, phytate hydrolysis was affected more by the level of dietary calcium than by either the level of phytate or fibre fed in the diet.

Phytate: mineral molar ratio

It is believed by many that a tool for estimating the mineral binding effect of phytate which is naturally present in most high fibre foods is the phytate:mineral molar ratio. If the ratio is low (10 or less for zinc: Oberleas & Harland, 1981; Oberleas 1983*a,b*; Morris & Ellis, 1983); zinc status should not be compromised. However, the higher the phytate:zinc molar ratio, the greater the risk of zinc deficiency. Calcium level is known to influence the phytate:zinc molar ratio in *in vitro* and animal studies (Oberleas & Moody, 1981; Morris & Ellis, 1983 & Davies *et al.*, 1984). In order to overcome high phytate:zinc molar ratios, the phytate may be decreased (Harland & Harland, 1980*a*) or the amount of zinc may be increased by the consumption of foods high in zinc (Harland & Peterson, 1980*b*). For a discussion of the important considerations when contending with fibre/phytate interrelationships, see Harland & Prosky (1979). The phytate:mineral molar ratio has received research emphasis primarily with respect to zinc and iron. Further research will confirm its usefulness as an estimation of the bioavailability of other minerals.

Discussion

One must be cautious when extrapolating *in vitro* or animal data to humans. Fibre fractions behave differently when isolated from their food matrices or from the milieu of the gut, as does phytate, and as do minerals. The immediate effect of a high fibre and thus frequently a high phytate intake is to put the system into apparent negative balance until mineral reserves are mobilized, or the absorptive and excretory mechanisms may adapt, by absorbing more and/or excreting less. When an individual has been eating a nutritious diet and his mineral stores are optimal, and if he continues to consume a wide variety of foods to meet his nutritional needs, his health should not be jeopardized by a reasonable increase in dietary fibre intake. Nutrient interactions are vastly complex. It is not just the interactions between fibre or phytate and minerals, but the presence of other foods in various stages of digestion and absorption which eventually influence bioavailability of the nutrients. For example, five studies (49 subjects) were conducted by Hallberg & Rossander (1984) to improve the iron absorption from a 'simple Latin American meal' consisting of maize, rice and black beans. Various foods or compounds were added to the meals to enhance non-haem iron absorption: meat, soy protein, cauliflower as a source of ascorbic acid, citric acid and ferrous sulphate. By monitoring haemoglobin, haematocrit and whole body counting, it was found that all of the foods, with the exception of citric acid enhanced non-haem iron absorption.

Conclusion

A general recommendation for beneficial metabolic effects of increased dietary fibre could be approximately 2 tablespoons of wheat bran per day. The normal population with adequate nutrient status can likely accommodate this dietary fibre increase. Those at risk from increased fibre or phytate are individuals who do not, or cannot, select foods to meet their nutrient needs, or the special 'at-risk' groups such as children, pregnant or lactating women, and the elderly, who have additional nutrient demands of growth or altered metabolism.

References

Andersson, H., Navert, B., Bingham, S. A., Englyst, H. N., Cummings, J. H. (1983): The effects of breads containing similar amounts of phytate but different amounts of wheat bran on calcium, zinc, and iron balance in man. *Br. J. Nutr.* **50**, 503–510.

Ballam, G. C., Nelson, T. S., Kirby, L. K. (1984): Effect of fiber and phytate source and of calcium and phosphorus level on phytate hydrolysis in the chick. *Poult. Sci.* **63**, 333–338.

Cook, J. D., Noble, N. L., Morck, T. A., Lynch, S. R., Petersburg, S. J. (1983): Effect of fiber on nonheme iron absorption. *Gastroenterology* **85**, 1354–1358.

Cummings, J. H. (1978): Nutritional implications of dietary fiber. *Am. J. Clin. Nutr.* **31**, 521–529.

Cummings, J. H., Hill, M. J., Jivraj, T., Houston, H., Branch, W. J., Jenkins, D. J. A. (1979a): The effect of meat protein and dietary fiber on caloric function and metabolism. 1. Changes in bowel habit, bile acid excretion, and calcium absorption. *Am. J. Clin. Nutr.* **32**, 2086–2093.

Cummings, J. H., Southgate, D. A. T., Branch, W. J., Wiggins, H. S., Houston, H., Jenkins, D. J. A., Jivraj, T., Hill, M. J. (1979b): The digestion of pectin in the human gut and its effect on calcium absorption and large bowel function. *Br. J. Nutr.* **41**, 477–485.

Davies, N. T., Carswell, A. J. P., Mills, C. F. (1985): The effect of variation in dietary calcium intake on the phytate-zinc interaction in rats. In *Proceedings of trace element metabolism in man and animals* (TEMA-5). Aberdeen, Scotland. June 29–July 4, 1984. Edinburgh: Churchill Livingstone.

Ellis, R., Morris, E. R., Hill, A. D., Kelsay, J. L. (1984): Phytate, zinc, phytate:zinc molar ratio intakes and phytate balance of adult subjects consuming self-chosen diets. *Fed. Proc.* **43**, 851.

Forbes, R. M., Erdman, J. W., Jr. (1983): Bioavailability of trace mineral elements. *Ann Rev. Nutr.* **3**, 213–231.

Frolich, W. (1984): Bioavailability of minerals from unrefined cereal products: *in vitro* and *in vivo* studies. Department of Food Chem., Chem. Center, University of Lund, Lund, Sweden, S-220 07.

Frolich, W., Asp, N.-G. (1984): Minerals and phytate in the analysis of dietary fiber from cereals during the process of breadmaking. Part III. Ph.D. Thesis. Dept. of Food Chem., Chem. Center, U. of Lund, Lund, Sweden, S–220 07.

Hallberg, L. (1981): Bioavailability of dietary iron in man. *Ann. Rev. Nutr.* **1**, 123–147.

Hallberg, L., Rossander, L. (1984): Improvement of iron nutrition in developing countries: comparison of adding meat, soy protein, ascorbic acid, citric acid, and ferrous sulphate on iron absorption from a simple Latin American-type of meal. *Am. J. Clin. Nutr.* **39**, 577–583.

Harland, B. F., Harland, J. (1980): Fermentative reduction of phytate in rye, white and whole wheat breads. *Cereal Chem.* **57**, 226–229.

Harland, B. F., Peterson, M. (1980): Nutrient status of lacto-ovo vegetarian Trappist monks. *J. Am. Diet. Ass.* **72**, 259–264.

Harland, B. F., Prosky, L. (1979): Development of dietary fiber values for foods. *Cereal Foods World* **24**, 387–394.

James, W. P. T., Branch, W. J., Southgate, D. A. T. (1978): Calcium binding by dietary fibre. *Lancet* **1**, 638–639.

Kelsay, J. L. (1981): Effect of diet fiber level on bowel function and trace mineral balances of human subjects. *Cereal Chem.* **58**, 2–5.

Kelsay, J. L. (1982): Effects of fiber on mineral and vitamin bioavailability. In *Dietary fiber in health and disease*, ed G. V. Vahouny, D. Kritchevsky, pp. 91–103. New York: Plenum Press.

Kelsay, J. L., Behall, K. M., Prather, E. S. (1979a): Effect of fiber from fruits and vegetables on metabolic responses of human subjects. II Calcium, magnesium, iron, and silicon balances. *Am. J. Clin. Nutr.* **32**, 1876–1880.

Kelsay, J. L., Jacob, R. A., Prather, E. S. (1979b): Effect of fiber from fruits and vegetables on metabolic responses of human subjects. III. Zinc, copper, and phosphorus balances. *Am. J. Clin. Nutr.* **32**, 2307–2311.

Kelsay, J. L., Clark, W. M. (1984): Fiber intakes, stool frequency, and stool weights of subjects consuming self-selected diets. *Am. J. Clin. Nutr.* **40**, 1357–1360.

Kelsay, J. L., Prather, E. S. (1983): Mineral balances of human subjects consuming spinach in a low-fiber diet and in a diet containing fruits and vegetables. *Am. J. Clin. Nutr.* **38**, 12–19.

Lakshmanan, F. L., Rao, R. B., Church, J. P. (1984a): Calcium and phosphorus intakes, balances, and blood levels of adults consuming self-selected diets. *Am. J. Clin. Nutr.* **40**, 1368–1379.

Lakshmanan, F. L., Rao, R. B., Church, J. P. (1984b): Magnesium intakes, balances, and blood levels of adults consuming self-selected diets. *Am. J. Clin. Nutr.* **40**, 1380–1389.

Lyon, D. B. (1984): Studies on the solubility of Ca, Mg, Zn, and Cu in cereal products. *Am. J. Clin. Nutr.* **39**, 190–195.

McBurney, M. I., Van Soest, P. J., Chase, L. E. (1983): Cation exchange capacity and buffering capacity of neutral detergent fibres. *J. Sci. Fd Agric.* **34**, 910–916.

Miles, C. W., Collins, J. S., Holbrook, J. T., Patterson, K. Y., Bodwell, C. E. (1984): Iron intake and status of men and women consuming self-selected diets. *Am. J. Clin. Nutr.* **40**, 1393–1396.

Morris, E. R., Ellis, R. (1983): Dietary phytate/zinc molar ratio and zinc balance in humans. In *Nutritional bioavailability of zinc*, ed G. E. Inglett, pp. 159–172. ACS Symposium Series, No. 210. Washington, DC: American Chemical Society.

Morris, E. R., Ellis, R. (1985): Level of phytate intake and calcium nutriture of adult men consuming non-vegetarian diets. In *Nutritional bioavailability of calcium*, ed C. Kies. ACS Symposium Series, No. 275. Washington, DC: American Chemical Society.

Morris, E. R., Ellis, R. (1982): Phytate, wheat bran and bioavailability of dietary iron. In *Nutritional bioavailability of iron*, ed C. Kies, pp. 121–141. ACS Symposium Series, No. 203, Washington, DC: American Chemical Society.

Morris, E. R., Ellis, R., Hill, A. D., Cottrell, S., Steele, P., Moy, T., Moser, P. B. (1984): Trace element nutriture of adult men consuming three levels of phytate. *Fed. Proc.* **43**, 846.

Morris, E. R., Ellis, R., Hill, A. D., Steele, P., Cottrell, S. (1985): Magnesium and calcium nutriture of adult men consuming omnivore diets with three levels of phytate. *Fed. Proc.* **44**, In press.

Morris, E. R., Ellis, R., Steele, P., Moser, P. (1980): Trace element nutriture response of adult men consuming dephytinized or non-dephytinized wheat bran. In *Trace substances in environmental health XIV*, ed D. D. Hemphill, pp. 103–109. Columbia, Mo: University of Missouri.

Oberleas, D. (1983a): Phytate content in cereals and legumes and methods of determination. *Cereal Foods World*. **28**, 352–357.

Oberleas, D. (1983b): The role of phytate in zinc bioavailability and homeostasis. In. *Nutritional Bioavailability of Zinc*, ed G. E. Inglett, pp. 145–158. Washington, DC: American Chemical Society.

Oberleas, D., Harland, B. F. (1981): Phytate content on foods: effect of dietary zinc bioavailability. *J. Am. Diet. Ass.* **79**, 433–436.

Oberleas, D., Moody, N. (1981): *In vitro* interaction of phytate with trace elements. In *Trace element metabolism in man and animals (TEMA-4)*, ed J. McC. Howell, J. M. Gawthorne, C. L. White, pp. 129–132. Canberra, ACT 2601: Australian Academy of Science.

Patterson, K. Y., Holbrook, J. T., Bodner, J. E., Kelsay, J. L., Smith, J. C., Jr., Veillon, C. (1984): Zinc, copper and manganese intake and balance for adults consuming self-selected diets. *Am. J. Clin. Nutr.* **40**, 1397–1403.

Reinhold, J. G., Garcia, J. S., Garzon, P. (1981): Binding of iron by fiber of wheat and maize. *Am. J. Clin. Nutr.* **34**, 1384–1391.

Sandberg, A.-S., Andersson, H., Hallgren, B., Hasselblad, K., Isaksson, B. (1981): Experimental model for *in vivo* determination of dietary fibre and its effect on the absorption of nutrients in the small intestine. *Br. J. Nutr.* **45**, 283–294.

Sandberg, A.-S., Hasselblad, C., Hasselblad, K. (1982): The effect of wheat bran on the absorption of minerals in the small intestine. *Br. J. Nutr.* **48**, 185–191.

Sandstrom, B., Arvidsson, B., Cederblad, A., Bjorn-Rasmussen, E. (1980): Zinc absorption from composite meals. 1. The significance of wheat extraction rate, zinc, calcium, and protein content in meals based on bread. *Am. J. Clin. Nutr.* **33**, 739–745.

Stasse-Wolthuis, M., Albers, H. F. F., van Jeveren, J. G. C., WildeJong, J., Hautvast, J. G. A. J., Hermus, R. J. J., Katan, M. B., Brydon, W. G., Eastwood, M. A. (1980): Influence of dietary fiber from vegetables and fruits, bran or citrus pectin on serum lipids, fecal lipids and colonic function. *Am. J. Clin. Nutr.* **33**, 1745–1756.

Turnlund, J. R., King, J. C., Keyes, W. R., Bonnie Gong, M. A., Michel, M. C. (1984): A stable isotope study of zinc absorption in young men: effects of phytate and alpha-cellulose. *Am. J. Clin. Nutr.* **40**, 1071–1077.

Vaaler, S., Aaseth, J., Hanssen, K. F., Dahl-Jorgensen, K., Frolich, W., Odegaard, B., Agenaes, O. (1985): Trace elements in serum and urine of diabetes patients given bread enriched with wheat bran or guar gum. In *International symposium on trace element metabolism in man and animals*, TEMA-5, pp. 142–150. Edinburgh: Churchill Livingstone.

Van Dokkum, W., Wesstra, A., Schippers, F. A. (1982): Physiological effects of fibre-rich types of bread. 1. The effect of dietary fibre from bread on the mineral balance of young men. *Br. J. Nutr.* **47**, 451–460.

8
Fibre and food products

Peter R. Ellis

Introduction

It is generally well-accepted by nutritionists that dietary fibre has an important role to play in maintaining good health in the population as a whole. Concern about the lack of dietary fibre in the diet has prompted expert and official committees in Britain and other countries to recommend an increase in fibre consumption (Royal College of Physicians, 1981; NACNE, 1983; US Department of Agriculture, 1979). Fibre has the added status of being an effective form of therapy in a number of metabolic and gastrointestinal disorders (eg, diabetes and constipation).

The growing consumer awareness of the nutritional attributes of fibre has led to a greater demand for high-fibre commodities, and this is already having a profound effect on the food industry. However, the consumer can still be faced with the problem of identifying the major fibre-containing foods and knowing the types and levels of intake of fibre that are nutritionally beneficial. The difficulties experienced by nutritionists and food scientists in finding a suitable definition for dietary fibre and developing a reliable and accurate method for fibre analysis have probably contributed to this problem.

This chapter discusses the problems of defining dietary fibre and developing techniques for fibre analysis, lists the main sources of fibre in foodstuffs and reviews the current intake and recommended level of fibre in the UK. Much of the chapter is devoted to reviewing the types of high-fibre product that have been developed worldwide, but distinguishes between those products recommended for prophylactic use and those that can be used therapeutically in routine clinical practice.

Definition and analysis of dietary fibre

Definition

No precise and universally accepted definition of dietary fibre exists at the present time. The term dietary fibre, introduced 30 years ago by Hipsley (1953) and later resurrected by Trowell (1972), does not describe a single chemical component but represents a heterogeneous mixture of substances found mainly in the cell wall of plants (Royal College of Physicians, 1980; Heaton, 1983). The current and most popular definition is a physiological one, based on the way in which dietary fibre behaves in the human gastrointestinal tract. Trowell (1972) first defined dietary fibre as the skeletal remnants of the plant cells that are not hydrolysed by the alimentary enzymes of man. Trowell (1972, 1978) was referring here to the plant cell walls only, which structurally are made up of predominantly polysaccharide material and lignin (between 80–90 per cent in the mature cell wall; Southgate,

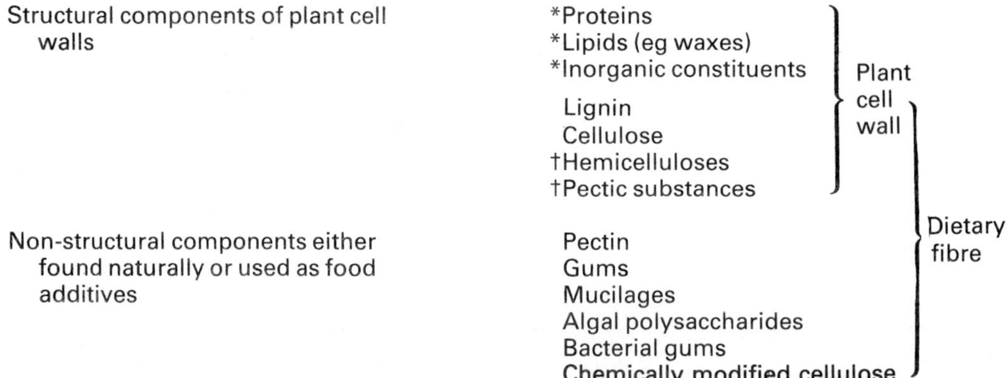

Table 1. *Components of dietary fibre*

Structural components of plant cell walls

*Proteins
*Lipids (eg waxes)
*Inorganic constituents
Lignin
Cellulose
†Hemicelluloses
†Pectic substances

Non-structural components either found naturally or used as food additives

Pectin
Gums
Mucilages
Algal polysaccharides
Bacterial gums
Chemically modified cellulose

Plant cell wall

Dietary fibre

*Fibre-associated substances.
†Hemicelluloses and pectic substances usually referred to as the non-cellulosic polysaccharides of the plant cell wall.

1982). Lignin is a name that describes a complex series of polymers of aromatic alcohols (phenylpropane units) in a three-dimensional structure (Southgate, 1976a). The original description of dietary fibre was, however, inadequate because it did not include indigestible components of the plant unassociated with the cell walls. These components are also polysaccharides which are structurally similar to many of the materials found in the plant cell wall and may be present naturally in plant foods or used as foods additives (Southgate, 1976a). Accordingly, Trowell *et al.* (1976) expanded the definition to include all plant polysacharides and lignin which are resistant to enzyme digestion. Table 1 contains a list of all the dietary fibre components and a number of indigestible non-carbohydrate substances (eg, protein) which may be an integral part of the plant cell wall structure or very closely associated with the structural elements of the wall (Southgate, 1976a). The chemical constituents present in the cell wall will vary depending on the type of plant tissue (Table 2). Thus, the overall composition of dietary fibre in the diet will vary according to the relative proportions of plant foods present. The detailed structure and composition of plant cell walls have been comprehensively reviewed by Selvendran (1983, 1984).

The present physiological definition of dietary fibre still has a number of deficiencies (Royal College of Physicians, 1980; Heaton, 1983). First, it focusses attention on the indigestibility of dietary fibre and ignores other physiological properties such as fibre's effect on the digestion and absorption of nutrients. Secondly, it implies that dietary fibre is unavailable for assimilation. There is evidence, however, that most forms of fibre are degraded by bacterial enzymes in the lower bowel, releasing short-chain fatty acids (eg acetic, propionic and butyric acids) which are absorbed and metabolized (Cummings, 1982). Thirdly, starch made resistant to α-amylase digestion by food processing (ie resistant starch) (Englyst, Wiggins & Cummings, 1982), and caramelization and Maillard polymers formed during the cooking of foods (Van Soest, 1978), may have similar

84

Table 2. *Components of dietary fibre of the major plant foods.* Information taken from Selvendran (1983, 1984).

Plant	Tissue types	Main constituent groups of dietary fibre polymers
Fruits and vegetables	Growing cells and parenchymatous tissues	Cellulose, hemicelluloses (eg, xyloglycans), pectic substances and some glycoproteins
	Lignified tissues	Cellulose, hemicellulose (eg, glucuronoxylans), lignin and some glycoproteins
	Cutinised tissues	Cutin and waxes
Cereals	Parenchymatous tissues	Arabinoxylans, β-D-glucans, cellulose, proteins and phenolic esters
	Lignified tissues	Glucuronoarabinoxylans, cellulose, lignin and phenolic esters and proteins
Seeds other than cereals (eg, leguminous seeds)	Parenchymatous tissues	Cellulose, hemicelluloses (eg, xyloglucans), pectic substances and glycoproteins
	Some cells with thickened walls (endosperm)	Hemicelluloses (mainly galactomannans) and some cellulose, pectic substances and glycoproteins

properties to dietary fibre. The limitations of Trowell's physiological definition are discussed in more detail elsewhere (Royal College of Physicians, 1980; Heaton, 1983).

A chemical and shortened definition, non-starch polysaccharides (NSP), has been suggested (Cummings, 1981) and is now frequently used for analytical purposes (Englyst *et al.*, 1982). NSP, the major fraction of dietary fibre, can be divided into cellulose and non-cellulosic polysaccharides (NCP), the latter containing the hemicelluloses, pectin, gums etc. (Southgate, Hudson & Englyst, 1978; Cummings, 1981).

Analysis
The quantitative analysis of such a complex mixture of NSP (and lignin if included) is fraught with problems and many of the technical difficulties are still unresolved (Southgate, 1976*b*; James & Theander, 1981). There are two approaches to dietary fibre analysis and the methods can be divided into two main groups: *gravimetric methods*—the dietary fibre is weighed after removing other components (eg protein and starch) in the food sample; *fractionation methods*—the components of dietary fibre are hydrolysed to their monomeric sugar residues, which are then assayed by colorimetry or gas-liquid chromatography (GLC). The fractionation methods give detailed information on all the components of dietary fibre.

Gravimetric methods. The detergent gravimetric methods (neutral and acid detergents) of Van Soest (1976) were developed, originally for animal feeds, to try and overcome the serious deficiencies of the crude fibre method, which markedly underestimates dietary fibre (Southgate, 1976*b*). The neutral detergent fibre (NDF) method was later modified to allow starch to be removed more easily from starchy foods (eg wheat flour), by including an α-amylase pre-incubation step

(Robertson & Van Soest, 1977; Schaller, 1977). However, one disadvantage of this procedure is that the water-soluble components of NSP are lost during detergent extraction (Southgate, 1976*b*). A number of enzymatic gravimetric methods have been used (Schweizer & Würsch, 1979; Asp & Johansson, 1981; Furda, 1981) and are based on the procedure used by Hellendoorn, Noordhoff & Slagman (1975) which involves the removal of protein and starch by enzyme hydrolysis. The Hellendoorn assay does not determine the water-soluble fraction of dietary fibre (Hellendoorn *et al.*, 1975), but the modified procedures include an alcohol precipitation stage to recover the soluble components (Schweizer & Würsch, 1979; Asp & Johansson, 1981; Furda, 1981). Schweizer & Würsch (1979) and Asp & Johansson (1981) utilized the physiological enzymes pancreatin and pepsin for their assays, whereas Furda (1981) employed the use of pure bacterial (*Bacillus subtilis*) protease and α-amylase. Recently, Asp *et al.* (1983) proposed a rapid enzyme assay (10–15 duplicate samples/day) for soluble and insoluble dietary fibre that overcomes the problems of long incubation times and laborious centrifugation procedures of previous enzyme methods.

Fractionation methods. For detailed information on the components of dietary fibre, fractionation methods have been employed (Southgate, 1976*b*; James and Theander, 1981). Southgate's procedure (Southgate, 1969, 1976*c*; Southgate *et al.*, 1976), a development of the unavailable carbohydrate method of McCance, Widdowson & Shackleton (1936), was the first real attempt to obtain information on the components of dietary fibre in food materials (Southgate *et al.*, 1976). Briefly, the method involves removing starch (by enzyme hydrolysis) from the food sample and separating the residue into cellulose, NCP and lignin. The polysaccharide fractions are then hydrolysed by acid into component sugars which are measured colorimetrically. This procedure has been criticized because of the incomplete removal of starch, the coprecipitation of a number of intracellular compounds with the cell wall material (Selvendran, Ring & DuPont, 1979*a*) and for the use of non-specific colorimetric methods for the measurement of individual sugars (Hudson & Bailey, 1980). In one collaborative study, a wide inter-laboratory variation in the values for total dietary fibre and fibre components was found (Southgate & White, 1981). It has also been reported that the original Southgate method markedly underestimated the pentose fraction of NCP in cereals (Wenlock, Buss & Agater, 1984; Wenlock, Sivell & Agater, 1985). This has been attributed, in part, to the presence of hemicellulases contaminating the takadiastase, the starch-digesting enzyme originally used in the Southgate procedure. Values for total dietary fibre using this method were incorporated into the UK food tables (Paul & Southgate, 1978), which are now under revision (see next section). Other fractionation methods employ the use of GLC for the separation and quantification of neutral sugars (alditol acetate derivatives) following starch removal (by enzyme hydrolysis) and hydrolysis of NSP (Selvendran, March & Ring, 1979*b*; Theander & Aman, 1979, 1982; Englyst *et al.*, 1982; Englyst *et al.*, 1983). The Englyst method includes a separate analysis for resistant starch as well as NSP (Englyst *et al.*, 1982; Englyst *et al.*, 1983). Lignin can be determined separately (Robertson & Van Soest, 1977), but many analysts choose not to determine it, mainly on the grounds that it is a minor component of the diet and it is difficult to analyse chemically.

86

To evaluate potential legislative methods for dietary fibre analysis, five methods including the Englyst fractionation procedure (Englyst *et al.*, 1982) and an Association of Official Analytical Chemists (AOAC) enzymatic technique (Prosky *et al.*, 1984) were tested in a collaborative trial in the UK organised by the Ministry of Agriculture, Fisheries and Food (MAFF) (Cummings, Englyst & Wood, in press). The Englyst method was found to be the most accurate and informative, but for statutory purposes none of the methods were considered to be satisfactory. The results of a second collaborative trial, using a simplified Englyst method (Englyst & Cummings, 1984) are awaited with interest. The results of the lignin analysis were highly variable; the Advisory Panel (organised by MAFF) recommended, therefore, that lignin should not be included in any method for dietary fibre determination. The AOAC enzymatic method (Prosky *et al.*, 1984) based on the work of Asp *et al.* (1983) and others (Schweizer & Würsch, 1979; Furda, 1981), and already undergoing collaborative trials in USA and Europe, was not a technique favoured by the Advisory Panel. The dietary fibre values obtained by this method were variable and significantly higher than those obtained by the Englyst procedure. The high values were probably due to the presence of enzyme-resistant substances other than NSP in the fibre residue (eg lignin, fibre-associated substances, Maillard products and resistant starch).

The choice of technique for dietary fibre analysis is dependent on what information is required. The Englyst procedure is useful for research workers who require detailed information on NSP in a food or mixed diet. For labelling and quality control purposes a food manufacturer requires a method giving total dietary fibre or, at the very most, values for the water soluble and insoluble fibre fractions. Such a method needs to be quick, simple, reliable and inexpensive. The rapid enzymatic assay proposed by Asp *et al.* (1983) may satisfy these criteria, but the technique would still need to be verified with a more detailed chemical method of analysis (Cummings *et al.*, in press).

Sources and intakes of dietary fibre

The major sources of dietary fibre are cereals and cereal products, nuts and certain vegetable and fruit commodities (eg beans, spinach and blackcurrants) (Table 3). Many of the vegetables, and most of the fruits (eg carrots, tomatoes and rhubarb) contain significant quantities of fibre on a dry weight basis, but also contain a high proportion of water which effectively dilutes the fibre content. Dried fruits (eg raisins and apricots) are a much more concentrated source of fibre. The fibre content of staple cereal foods, such as wheat bread and pasta, will vary depending on the extraction rate of flour used for making these products (ie wholemeal or 100 per cent extraction rate flour will provide the most dietary fibre). The dietary fibre values listed in Table 3 were taken from the British food composition tables (Paul & Southgate, 1978). Values for cellulose, NCP (hexoses, pentoses and uronic acids) and lignin in a wide range of commodities are listed elsewhere (Southgate *et al.*, 1976; Southgate, 1978). The MAFF are revising the food tables using an improved method based on the Southgate technique (Wenlock *et al.*, 1984; Wenlock *et al.*, 1985). The new values for total fibre and its components in 138 cereal products and cereal-containing meat products have just been published (Wenlock *et al.*, 1985). Some of these new values for total fibre are given in Table 3.

Table 3. *Typical dietary fibre and moisture contents of various food commodities (g/100 g food).*

Food	Food tables[a]		New values[b]	
	Water	Dietary fibre	Water	Dietary fibre
Breakfast cereals:				
All Bran	2.3	26.7	3.0	26.0
Weetabix	3.8	12.7	6.7	9.3
Cornflakes	3.0	11.0	3.6	8.4
Muesli	5.8	7.4	–	–
Rice Krispies	3.8	4.5	3.5	6.0
Bread:				
Wholemeal	40.0	8.5	39.6	8.2
Brown	39.0	5.1	37.6	6.8
White	39.0	2.7	40.2	4.1
Rye	–	–	37.4	6.4
Pasta (spaghetti):				
Wholemeal (raw)	–	–	9.8	5.6
White (raw)	–	–	10.5	12.7
Biscuits:				
Crispbread (rye)	6.4	11.7	5.6	12.8
Digestive (plain)	4.5	5.5	4.6	5.1
Chocolate	2.2	3.1	8.6	3.2
Cakes:				
Fruit types[c]	18–21	2–4	–	–
Plain (no fruit or filling)[c]	20.0	1–2	–	–
Vegetables:				
Haricot (boiled)	69.6	7.4	–	–
Peas (canned)	81.6	6.3	–	–
Spinach (boiled)	85.1	6.3	–	–
Tomatoes (raw)	93.4	2.3	–	–
Carrots (boiled)	91.5	3.1	–	–
Fruits:				
Blackcurrants (raw)	77.4	8.7	–	–
Rhubarb (raw)	94.2	2.6	–	–
Strawberries (raw)	88.9	2.2	–	–
Dried types[c]	15–18	7–24	–	–
Nuts:				
Peanuts (fresh)	4.5	8.1	–	–

[a]Paul & Southgate (1978); [b]Wenlock *et al.* (1985); [c]Range of values.

The high levels of fibre obtained for white bread compared to previous estimates were probably due to the presence of resistant starch (Wenlock *et al.*, 1985). Estimates of resistant starch have been reported by Englyst *et al.* (1982, 1983), who found significant amounts in processed foods such as cooked potatoes and cornflakes (Table 4). In the latter the level of resistant starch was higher than the total NSP. This may partly explain the very high levels of fibre determined in

Table 4. *Non-starch polysaccharides (NSP) of various food commodities (g/100 g dry matter).* RS = resistant starch. Data taken from Englyst *et al.* (1983) except the values for vegetables which are from Englyst *et al.* (1982).

Food	% Dry matter	Cellulose	Non-cellulosic polysaccharides		RS	Total NSP
			Sol.	Insol.		
Breakfast cereals:						
All bran	94.9	4.4	3.9	15.4	0.2	23.7
Weetabix	93.8	1.6	3.3	5.5	0.3	10.4
Cornflakes	94.9	0.3	0.2	0.2	3.1	0.7
Rice Krispies	95.2	0.4	0.2	0.3	0.2	0.9
Porridge oats	90.0	0.3	4.0	3.0	–	7.2
Bread:						
Wholemeal	60.4	1.5	2.6	5.5	0.8	9.6
Brown	58.7	1.1	2.3	3.9	0.9	7.3
White	60.7	0.1	1.9	0.6	1.2	2.6
Pasta (spaghetti):						
Wholemeal	90.1	1.8	2.4	5.8	0.2	10.0
White	90.1	0.2	1.9	1.0	0.2	3.0
Rice:						
Brown	86.0	0.7	0.1	1.2	–	2.0
White	87.4	0.2	0.1	0.2	–	0.6
Biscuits:						
Digestive	97.1	0.3	1.4	1.3	0.1	3.0
Flours and grain:						
Rye	86.6	1.4	4.6	7.7	0.2	13.7
Wholemeal wheat	88.0	1.6	2.6	6.0	0.1	10.2
Barley grain	87.1	1.4	3.9	6.5	–	11.8
Vegetables:						
Haricot beans (raw)	–	4.2	7.2	5.4	–	16.8
Cabbage (raw)	–	9.9	13.5	4.2	–	27.6
Raw potato	–	1.8	2.8	0.6	–	5.1
Cooked potato	–	1.6	2.6	0.6	2.1	4.8

cornflakes using the Southgate method (Table 3). Englyst *et al.* (1982, 1983) have also determined total soluble and insoluble fibre, as fractions of NCP. In some food commodities (eg, oats, barley, potatoes and cabbage) the soluble fraction can constitute more than 50 per cent of the total NSP (Table 4).

Estimates of the mean fibre intake in the British diet of about 20 g/person/day have been made based on National Food Survey records and using fibre values from the British food tables (Bingham, Cummings & McNeil, 1979; Bingham & Cummings, 1980). Recently, an *ad hoc* working party of the NACNE have recommended that the average fibre intake should be increased to 25 g/person/day during the 1980s and to 30 g/person/day by the mid–1990s and that this increase should come mainly from an increased consumption of wholegrain cereals (NACNE, 1983). It has been suggested, however, that a level of 30 g is not a realistic level for subgroups of the population with below average energy intake (Black, Ravenscroft & Sims, 1984).

Variations in total intake in Britain exist and can be attributed mainly to differences in energy intake (Bingham & Cummings, 1980). Perhaps it would be more appropriate for fibre intake to be calculated as a percentage of the energy intake. In a survey of the Cambridgeshire population, a variation of 8–32 g/day was reported (Bingham *et al.*, 1979). In vegetarians a range of 6–87 g/day was found (Gear *et al.*, 1979).

Cereals and vegetables contribute most of the total fibre in the diet, with vegetables being the major contributor (Bingham & Cummings, 1980). The contribution of fruit and cereal-containing meat products is relatively small (9 per cent). Bread still remains the most important staple food in Britain and contributes most of the cereal fibre in the diet, despite a 39 per cent reduction in total domestic* consumption (due to white bread alone) between 1956 and 1982 (MAFF, 1956–1982). Furthermore, since 1975 there has been a pronounced increase in the consumption of brown and wholemeal high-fibre breads. Recent figures indicate that the increase for the brown variety has levelled off and that wholemeal consumption has overtaken brown for the first time (MAFF, 1985). In total, brown and wholemeal breads now have a 21.5 per cent share of the domestic market compared to only 10 per cent in 1975 (MAFF, 1985).

There has also been a marked rise in the consumption of breakfast cereals since 1970, particularly the high-fibre varieties (Walker, 1984; Hilliam, 1984). Between 1981–1983 the volume sales of bran-enriched products and muesli have increased by 45 and 29 per cent respectively (Mintel, 1984). Another major area of change has been the increased sales of processed vegetables at the expense of fresh varieties (Walker, 1984). The consumption of baked beans (7.3 g fibre/100 g) has doubled since the 1950s. In 1981 the volume sales of baked beans, along with broad beans and butter beans, accounted for 44 per cent of all canned vegetable purchases (Economist Intelligence Unit, 1982).

High fibre foods for therapeutic use

Diabetes and hyperlipidaemia
The therapeutic benefits of dietary fibre in the treatment of diabetes and hyperlipidaemia are well known (Royal College of Physicians, 1980; Jenkins, Taylor & Wolever, 1982; Vahouny & Kritchevsky, 1982; Taylor, 1984). Evidence for the ameliorative effects of dietary fibre on carbohydrate and lipid metabolism and its mechanism of action are discussed in Chapters 2 & 4. In both these metabolic disorders the water-soluble types of fibre (eg, guar and pectin) have proved to be more clinically effective than the insoluble particulate fibres (eg, cellulose and wheat bran) (Lithell, Selinus & Vessby, 1984; Behall, Lee & Moser, 1984; Jenkins *et al.*, 1978*a*).

Clinicians have used two methods for the administration of fibre. The first method involves feeding patients fibre-rich foods, mainly from vegetable, cereal

---

*The fall in domestic consumption has been partly offset by an increase in bread eaten outside the home between 1965 and 1980 (from 10 to 20 per cent of total bread consumed) – N. Chamberlain, pers. commun.

90

listed
there
nutri
In
hydr
Visc
hype
was
here
been
Yagl
adhe
artifi
et al.
N
arou
infor
stud
with
brea
(Jen
pect
opti
to b
Spey
al.,
on i
form
I
chee
diab
(Tr
(197
gua
resp
dele
cou
Hov
a m
I
Col
use
Kh
whi
and
clin
dia

and fruit sources (Anderson, 1980; Mann, 1984; Kay & Truswell, 1980). Some clinicians have included substantial quantities of legumes in the experimental regimen and found significant improvements in their patients' carbohydrate and lipid metabolism (Mann, 1984; Rivellese *et al.*, 1980; Anderson & Chen, 1983). Oats (whole oats and oat bran), a particularly good source of water-soluble fibre (β-glucans), may also be beneficial to patients with carbohydrate and lipid disorders (Anderson, 1980; Chen, Anderson & Gould, 1981). In many of the diabetic studies high fibre was administered in conjunction with a high level of complex carbohydrate (starchy foods) which is now known to improve diabetic control (Mann, 1984; Anderson, 1980). This is probably achieved by certain types of carbohydrate being more slowly digested and absorbed ('lente' or slowly-absorbed carbohydrate), leading to a flattening of the postprandial glucose and insulin profiles (Jenkins *et al.*, 1982). This also explains the mechanism by which fibre exerts its beneficial effects on blood glucose homeostasis (Leeds, 1982). Bread, one of the major staple foods, is potentially a good source of dietary fibre for patients. However, evidence for the therapeutic effects of wholemeal wheat bread in diabetes is contradictory. In a study with healthy subjects, wholemeal wheat bread produced a lower glycaemic response than white bread (Thomas & Elchazly, 1976), but this effect was not confirmed in other studies either with healthy subjects (Jenkins *et al.*, 1981) or with diabetic patients (Jenkins *et al.*, 1983). Breads made with the high soluble fibre cereals, rye, barley and oats, may be more effective than wheat bread in lowering postprandial hyperglycaemia. Blood glucose concentrations and insulin requirements were reduced in insulin-dependent diabetics fed high rye bran crispbread (Nygren, Hallmans & Lithner, 1984). In a study with insulin and non-insulin-dependent diabetic patients, Finnish wholemeal rye bread induced a slower postprandial glycaemic response than a meal of white wheat bread (Heinonen, Korpela & Mantere, 1985). Part of this effect was probably due to the lower starch content of the rye bread. Many factors other than the quantity of soluble fibre in the wholegrain cereals (and other starchy foods) are thought to alter the rate of digestion and absorption of carbohydrate (starch). The type of starch (eg, ratio of amylose to amylopectin fractions), the particle size of cereal flour used in breadmaking, the baking/cooking conditions which may affect the degree of gelatinised starch (more susceptible to α-amylase attack), interactions of starch with proteins and lipids, and the formation of resistant starch could all affect the avaiiability of starch for digestion (Greenberg, 1976; Thorne, Thompson & Jenkins, 1983; Björck *et al.*, 1984*a*; Björck *et al.*, 1984*b*; Hagander *et al.*, 1985).

The alternative way to administer dietary fibre is to use a pharmacological method, an approach popularised by Jenkins and his co-workers in the UK. This method involves supplementing the patient's diet with concentrated forms of dietary fibre (Jenkins *et al.*, 1982; Peterson, 1984). The most potent therapeutic agents are the water-soluble gummy polysaccharides of which guar and pectin are the most widely used (Jenkins *et al.*, 1978*a*). In the case of guar it is administered in the raw form (usually as a granulated preparation; see Chapter 4) or as a guar-containing food product. Guar and many other types of gum are used worldwide as thickening and stabilising agents in a wide variety of food products (eg, mayonnaise and ice cream) (Glicksman, 1979), but the amounts used (<1 per cent of food weight) are probably insignificant from a physiological point of view.

Ispaghula). The therapeutic effectiveness of cereal fibre concentrates or foods is dependent on the quality of the fibre. The ability of wheat bran to increase faecal weight, reduce transit time and intraluminal pressure in the colon is diminished if the bran is milled to a fine particle size (Kirwan *et al.*, 1974; Smith, Drummond & Eastwood, 1981; Heller *et al.*, 1980). Also, raw bran is more effective in improving colonic function compared to an equivalent amount of cooked bran (All-Bran) (Wyman *et al.*, 1976). But reducing the particle size of wheat bran may improve the structural quality and palatability of certain high-fibre cereal products (eg, bread and cakes) (Pomeranz *et al.*, 1977; Rajchels, Zabik & Everson, 1975; Springsteen, Zabik & Shafer, 1977) and cooking would certainly improve bran's palatability. Patients are more likely, therefore, to adhere to a high-fibre regimen if the food is enjoyable to eat.

High-fibre foods for prophylactic use
The recent interest in the nutritional benefits of dietary fibre arose mainly from the epidemiological observations of workers like Burkitt and Trowell (Burkitt & Trowell, 1975). They claimed that a diet rich in dietary fibre is protective against a range of diseases prevalent in Western communities (eg diabetes, atherosclerosis, diverticular disease, large bowel cancer, etc.) and that in some instances a diet lacking in dietary fibre is a causative factor in the development of the disease (eg, diverticular disease) (Burkitt & Trowell, 1975; Southgate, 1982). Although the clinical role of dietary fibre in certain disorders is now well-established, the prophylactic benefits are not well-defined and there is a lack of experimental data to support the epidemiological evidence (Taylor, 1984). However, many of the high-fibre commodities found on the mass-market have been developed for prophylactic use. Food manufacturers have aimed their products at consumers who are healthy and who believe that they would benefit from increasing their daily intake of fibre.

One of the major problems of incorporating fibre into a food system is the deleterious effects it can have on the functional properties of other components in the food. This can lead to changes in appearance, flavour, texture and mouthfeel, changes that are unacceptable to manufacturers and to many (but not all) consumers (Pomeranz *et al.*, 1977; Shafer & Zabik, 1975; Polizzoto *et al.*, 1983). It is not surprising, therefore, that food scientists have attempted to improve the quality of high-fibre foods.

In the USA and Western Europe the main thrust of research has been in the development of high-fibre cereal based products, particularly breakfast cereals such as the traditional wheat bran foods (see previous section on therapeutic use) (Hamilton, 1983). Most of these cereals contain added sugar and artificial flavourings to improve palatability, but with recommendations on sugar in mind (NACNE, 1979; US Department of Agriculture, 1979) and in response to public demand, manufacturers are now producing sugar-free and 'naturally' flavoured varieties (Moore, 1979; Anon, 1981; Hilliam, 1984). A comparatively recent innovation has been the development of cereal snack bars which are now strongly competing for a share of the snack/confectionary market in the UK. The development of high-fibre cakes (Brockmoles & Zabik, 1976; Zabik, Shafer & Kutorowski, 1977), muffins (Polizzoto *et al.*, 1983) and biscuits (Vratanina &

Zabik, 1978; Goreyzca & Zabik, 1979) has also been investigated, but the commodity that has received most attention from food scientists is bread.

By the time the dietary fibre hypothesis was promulgated by the lay press in the 1970s, the British bread manufacturers were already supplying the public with a variety of high-fibre wheat breads including brown (prepared from flour within the range 85–90 per cent extraction rate), granary (containing cracked or kibbled wheat) and wholemeal breads. It is only recently that British manufacturers have added new high-fibre bread products to the range already available (Anon, 1983a,b). One of these is a white high-fibre bread containing peahull fibre (Anon, 1983b). Bakers and many consumers consider bread made from brown or wholemeal flours to be of an inferior quality compared to white bread. The darker brown and wholemeal breads tend to lack volume and have a coarse, dense crumb texture and shorter shelf life than the white varieties (Collins, Fisher & Knight, 1983). Bakers have endeavoured to widen the appeal of the traditional squat wholemeal loaf by producing an expanded, softer version. This has been achieved by careful manipulation of the ingredients and recipe and by using improving agents such as emulsifiers and vital wheat gluten (Collins et al., 1983). The oxidant ascorbic acid, normally used in the British Chorleywood Bread Process in conjunction with potassium bromate for improving loaf quality, has recently been included on the additives list for making wholemeal bread (MAFF, 1984).

Projected figures for bread consumption in USA indicate that the amount of variety bread consumed is increasing, although white pan bread is still the most popular (Jackel, 1981). The American baking industry provides a wide range of variety breads, including not only brown and wholemeal wheat grain types, but also rye and multigrain breads (containing combinations of wheat, rye, oats, millet, maize, etc.). Breads made from rye or rye and wheat form a significant part of the diet in Eastern Europe and Scandinavia (Kent, 1983). At the time of writing, a number of multigrain breads, based mainly on wheat, rye and barley mixtures, have been launched onto the British market. The therapeutic role of bread made with cereals of high soluble fibre content has yet to be evaluated and proof of its prophylactic benefits would be difficult to obtain. Nevertheless, the British bread industry have not been slow to respond to the nutritional propaganda. The utilization of barley, rye and oats for breadmaking in Britain is not a new idea. Breads made from barley and rye were eaten by poor people in England during the Middle Ages (Kent, 1983). The nutritional advantages (if any) of adding barley, rye and oats to the breadmaking recipe is offset by the loss in bread quality. Wheat, and to a lesser extent rye, contain the gluten-forming proteins that are essential for producing good quality leavened bread, whereas oats and barley lack these functional proteins and are only suitable therefore for making flat breads. This lack of leavening is clearly seen in Fig 1, which shows the poor volume of wholegrain rye and barley breads compared to wheat bread and an expanded gluten-supplemented wheat variety.

American food scientists have used other fibre-rich commodities for incorporation into wheat bread including legumes and other vegetables, fruit and even brewer's spent grain (a by-product of the brewing industry) (Pomeranz, 1977; Toma et al., 1979; Finley & Hanamoto, 1980; Collins, Kalantari & Post, 1982). The deleterious effects of fibre on loaf quality are usually very marked, but can be

Anderson, J. W., Chen, W. L. (1983): Legumes and their soluble fiber: effect on cholesterol-rich lipoproteins. In *Unconventional sources of dietary fiber*, ed I. Furda, pp. 49–59. Washington DC: American Chemical Society.

Anon (1981): Kellogg adds a whole grain cereal line without added sugar. *Food Dev.* **15**, 35–36.

Anon (1983*a*): New image for Hovis. *Fd Mf.* **58**, 25 & 27.

Anon (1983*b*): Windmill gives best of both worlds. *Supermarketing. October 21*, 590.

Apling, E. C., Ellis, P. R. (1982): Guar bread: concept to application. *Chem. Inds, Lond.*, 950–954.

Apling, E. C., Ellis, P. R. (1983): Elevation of 'fibre' in bread by guar addition. In *Dietary fibre*, ed G. G. Birch, K. J. Parker, pp. 61–76. London: Applied Science.

Apling, E. C., Khan, P., Ellis, P. R. (1978): Guar/wheat bread for therapeutic use. *Cereal Fd Wld* **23**, 640–644.

Apling, E. C., Leeds, A. R., Wolever, T. M. S., Jenkins, D. J. A. (1977): How to make guar bread. *Lancet* **1**, 975.

Asp, N-G., Johansson, C-G. (1981): Techniques for measuring dietary fiber. In *The analysis of dietary fiber in foods*, ed W. P. T. James, O. Theander, pp. 173–189. New York: Marcel Dekker.

Asp, N-G., Johansson, C-G., Hallmer, H., Siljeström, M. (1983): Rapid enzymatic assay of insoluble and soluble dietary fiber. *J. Agric. Fd Chem.* **31**, 476–482.

Beareboom, J. J. (1979): Low calorie bulking agents. *Crit. Rev. Fd Sci. Nutr.* **11**, 401–413.

Behall, K. M., Lee, K. H., Moser, P. B. (1984): Blood lipids and lipoproteins in adult men fed four refined fibers. *Am. J. Clin. Nutr.* **39**, 209–214.

Bingham, S., Cummings, J. H. (1980): Sources and intakes of dietary fiber in man. In *Medical aspects of dietary fiber*, ed G. A. Spiller, R. M. Kay, pp. 261–284. New York: Plenum Press.

Bingham, S., Cummings, J. H., McNeil, N. I. (1979): Intakes and sources of dietary fibre in the British population. *Am. J. Clin. Nutr.* **32**, 1313–1319.

Björck, I., Asp, N-G., Birkhed, D., Eliassons, A-C., Sjöberg, L-B., Lundquist, I. (1984*a*): Effects of processing on starch availability *in vitro* and *in vivo*. II. Drum-drying of wheat flour. *J. Cereal Sci.* **2**, 165–178.

Björck, I., Asp, N-G., Birkhed, D., Lundquist, I. (1984*b*): Effects of processing on availability of starch for digestion *in vitro* and *in vivo*. I. Extension cooking of wheat flours and starch. *J. Cereal Sci.* **2**, 91–103.

Black, A. E., Ravenscroft, C., Sims, A. J. (1984): The NACNE Report: are the dietary goals realistic? Comparisons with the dietary patterns of dietitians. *Hum Nutr.: Appl. Nutr. 38A*, 165–179.

Brodribb, A. J. M. (1983): Dietary fibre as a tool of the clinician. In *Dietary fibre*, ed G. G. Birch, K. J. Parker, pp. 195–203. London: Applied Science.

Brockmoles, C. L., Zabik, M. E. (1976): Wheat bran and middlings in white layer cakes. *J. Fd Sci.* **41**, 357–360.

Bryson, E., Dore, C., Garrow, J. S. (1980): Wholemeal bread and satiety. *J. Hum. Nutr.* **34**, 113–116.

Burkitt, D. P., Trowell, H. C. eds (1975): *Refined carbohydrate foods and disease. Some implications of dietary fibre*. London: Academic Press.

Burley, V., Leeds, A. R., Ellis, P. R., Peterson, D. B. (1983): Wholemeal guar bread: acceptability combined. A study of blood glucose, plasma insulin and palatability in normal subjects. *Proc. Nutr. Soc.* **43**, 48A.

Cann, P. A., Read, N. W., Holdsworth, C. D. (1984): What is the benefit of coarse wheat bran in patients with irritable bowel syndrome? *Gut* **25**, 168–173.

Chen, W-J. L., Anderson, J. W., Gould, M. R. (1981): Cholesterol-lowering effects of oat bran and oat gum. *Fed. Proc.* **40**, 853.

Collins, T. H., Fisher, N., Knight, R. A. (1983): Breads brown and wholemeal. *BNF Nutr. Bull.* **8**(38), 105–116.

Collins, J. L., Kalantari, S. M., Post, A. R. (1982): Peanut hull flour as dietary fiber in wheat bread. *J. Food Sci.* **47**, 1899–1902 & 1920.

COMA (Committee on Medical Aspects of Food Policy) (1981): *Nutritional aspects of bread and flour*. London: HMSO.

Cummings, J. H. (1981): Dietary fibre. *Br. Med. Bull.* **37**, 65–70.

Cummings, J. H. (1982): Consequences of the metabolism of fiber in the human large intestine. In *Dietary fibre in health and disease*, ed G. V. Vahouny, R. Kritchevsky, pp. 9–22. New York: Plenum Press.

Cummings, J. H., Englyst, H., Wood, R. (in press): *Determination of dietary fibre in cereals and cereal products*. London: Ministry of Agriculture, Fisheries and Food.

Doi, K., Matsuura, M., Kawara, A., Baba, S. (1979): Treatment of diabetes with glucomannan (Konjac mannan). *Lancet* **1**, 987–988.

Dreese, P. C., Hoseney, R. C. (1982): Baking properties of the bran fractions from brewer's spent grains. *Cereal Chem.* **59**, 89–91.

Eastwood, M. A., Passmore, R. (1983): Dietary fibre. *Lancet* **2**, 202–206.

Ebihara, K., Kiriyama, S. (1982): Comparative effects of water-soluble and water-insoluble dietary fibres on various parameters relating to glucose tolerance in rats. *Nutr. Rep. Int.* **26**, 193–201.

Ebihara, K., Masuhara, R., Kiriyama, S. (1981): Effect of Konjac mannan, a water-soluble dietary fiber on plasma glucose and insulin responses in young men undergone glucose tolerance test. *Nutr. Rep. Int.* **23**, 577–583.

Economist Intelligence Unit (1982): Baked beans. *Retail Business No. 298. December*, 30–33.

Englyst, H., Anderson, V., Cummings, J. H. (1983): Starch and non-starch polysaccharides in some cereal foods. *J. Fd Agric.* **34**, 1434–1440.

Englyst, H. N., Cummings, J. H. (1984): Simplified method for the measurement of total non-starch polysaccharides by gas-liquid chromatography of constituent sugars as alditol acetates. *Analyst* **109**, 937–942.

Englyst, H., Wiggins, H. S., Cummings, J. H. (1982): Determination of the non-starch polysaccharides in plant foods by gas-liquid chromatography of constituent sugars as alditol acetates. *Analyst* **107**, 307–318.

Ellis, P. R. (1984): The development and testing of guar bread for use in the treatment of diabetes mellitus. PhD Thesis, Reading University, UK.

Ellis, P. R., Apling, E. C. (1983): The development and acceptability of guar-bran bread. In *Proceedings of 7th World Cereal and Bread Congress*, Prague, 1982, ed J. Holas, J. Kratochvil, pp. 1121–1126. Amsterdam: Elsevier.

Ellis, P. R. Apling, E. C., Leeds, A. R., Bolster, N. R. (1981): Guar bread: acceptability and efficacy combined. Studies on blood glucose, serum insulin and satiety in normal subjects. *Br. J. Nutr.* **46**, 267–276.

Ellis, P. R., Apling, E. C., Leeds, A. R., Peterson, D., Jepson, E. M. (1985): Guar bread and satiety: effect of an acceptable new product in overweight diabetic patients and normal subjects. *J. Plant Foods*, **6** (3), in press.

Evans, E., Miller, D. S. (1975): Bulking agents in the treatment of obesity. *Nutr. Metab.* **18**, 199–203.

Evans, E., Miller, D. S. (1978): Slimming aids. *J. Hum. Nutr.* **32**, 433–438

Finley, J. W., Hanamoto, M. M. (1980): Milling and baking properties of dried brewer's spent grains. *Cereal Chem.* **59**, 89–91.

Furda, I. (1981): Simultaneous analysis of soluble and insoluble dietary fiber. In *The analysis of dietary fiber in food*, ed W. P. T. James, O. Theander, pp. 163–172. New York: Marcel Dekker.

Gatti, E., Catenazzo, G., Camisasca, E., Torri, A., Denegri, E., Sirtori, C. R. (1984): Effects of guar-enriched pasta in the treatment of diabetes and hyperlipidaemia. *Ann. Nutr. Metab.* **28**, 1–10.

Gear, J. S. S., Ware, A-, Furdson, P., Mann, J. I., Nolan, D. J., Brodribb, A. J. M., Vessey, M. P. (1979): Symptomless diverticular disease and intake of dietary fibre. *Lancet* **1**, 511–514.

Glicksman, M. (1979): Gelling hydrocolloids in food product applications. In *Polysaccharides in food*, ed J. M. V. Blanchard, J. R. Mitchell, pp. 185–204. London: Butterworths.

Goreyzca, C. G., Zabik, M. E. (1979): High fiber sugar snap-cookies containing cellulose and coated cellulose products. *Cereal Chem.* **56**, 537–540.

Greenberg, C. J. (1976): Studies on the fibre in human diets and its effect on digestion and absorption of other nutrients. PhD Thesis, University of Cambridge, UK.

Grimes, D. S., Gordon, C. (1978): Satiety value of wholemeal and white bread. *Lancet* **2**, 106.

Hagander, B., Björck, I., Asp, N-G., Lundquist, I., Nilsson-Ehle, P., Schrezenmeir, J., Scherstén, B. (1985): Hormonal and metabolic responses to breakfast meals in NIDDM: comparison of white and whole-grain wheat bread and corresponding extruded products. *Hum. Nutr.: Appl. Nutr.* **39A**, 114–123.

Hamilton, W. D. B. (1983): The role of dietary fibre in food product formulation. In *Dietary fibre*, ed G. G. Birch, K. J. Parker, pp. 29–36. London: Applied Science.

Heaton. K. W. (1983): Dietary fibre: concepts and definitions. In *Fibre in human and animal nutrition*, eds G. Wallace, L. Bell, pp. 19–21. New Zealand: Royal Society of New Zealand.

Heinonen, L., Korpela, R., Mantere, S. (1985): The effect of different types of Finnish bread on postprandial glucose response in diabetic patients. *Hum. Nutr.: Appl. Nutr.* **39A**, 108–113.

Hellendoorn, E. W., Nordhoff, M. G., Slagman, J., (1975): Enzymatic determination of the indigestible residue (dietary fibre) content of human food. *J. Sci. Fd Agric.* **26**, 1461–1468.

Heller, S. N., Hackler, L. R., Rivers, J. M., Van Soest, P. J., Roe, D. A., Lewis, B. A., Robertson, J. (1980): Dietary fiber: the effect of particle size of wheat bran on colonic function in young adult men. *Am. J. Clin. Nutr.* **33**, 1734–1744.

Hill, M. A., French, S. J., Sunman, M. L., Sutton, C. M. (1984): The preparation and use of guar bread in diet therapy. *Hum. Nutr.: Appl. Nutr.* **38A**, 227–228.

Hill, M. A., Leeds, A. R. (1979): High-fibre foods: a feasibility study using guar gum. *J. Hum. Nutr.* **33**, 253–258.

Hilliam, M. A. (1984): Health foods in the UK. *Food market updates (No. 5)*, Information Group Services, Leatherhead Food RA, UK.

Hipsley, E. A. (1953): Dietary fibre and pregnancy toxaemia. *Br. Med. J.* **2**, 420–422.

Hudson, G. J., Bailey, B. S. (1980): Mutual interference effects in the colorimetric methods used to determine the sugar composition of dietary fibre. *Food Chem.* **5**, 201–206.

Iwasaki, Y., Aono, M., Aoki, N., Uchino, H. (1982): Guar jelly for the treatment of diabetes mellitus in humans. *Nutr. Rep. Int.* **26**, 203–207.

Jackel, S. S. (1981): Established variety breads in the United States. In *Variety breads in the United States*, ed B. S. Miller, pp. 3–8. St Paul, MN: AACC.

James, W. P. T., Theander, O., eds (1981): *The analysis of dietary fibre in food.* New York: Marcel Dekker.

Jenkins, D. J. A. (1980): Dietary fiber and carbohydrate metabolism. In *Medical aspects of dietary fiber*, ed G. A. Spiller, R. M. Kay, pp. 175–192. New York: Plenum Press.

Jenkins, D. J. A., Leeds, A. R., Gassull, M. A., Cochet, B., Alberti, K. G. M. M. (1977a): Decrease in postprandial insulin and glucose concentrations by guar and pectin. *Ann. Intern. Med.* **86**, 20–23.

Jenkins, D. J. A., Leeds, A. R., Slavin, B., Mann, J., Jepson, E. M. (1979): Dietary fibre and blood lipids: reduction of serum cholesterol in type II hyperlipidaemia by guar gum. *Am. J. Clin. Nutr.* **32**, 16–18.

Jenkins, D. J. A., Reynolds, D., Slavin, B., Leeds, A. R., Jenkins, A. L., Jepson, E. M. (1980a): Dietary fiber and blood lipids: treatment of hypercholesterolemia with guar crispbread. *Am. J. Clin. Nutr.* **33**, 575–581.

Jenkins, D. J. A., Taylor, R. H., Wolever, T. M. S. (1982): The diabetic diet, dietary differences in digestibility. *Diabetologia* **23**, 477–484.

Jenkins, D. J. A., Wolever, T. M. S., Bacon, S., Nineham, R., Lees, R., Rowden, R., Love, M., Hockaday, T. D. R. (1980b): Diabetic diets: high carbohydrate combined with high fiber. *Am. J. Clin. Nutr.* **33**, 1729–1733.

Jenkins, D. J. A., Wolever, T. M. S., Hockaday, T. D. R., Leeds, A. R., Howarth, R., Bacon, S., Apling, E. C., Dilawari, J. (1977b): Treatment of diabetes with guar gum. Reduction of urinary glucose loss in diabetics. *Lancet* **2**, 779–780.

Jenkins, D. J. A., Wolever, T. M. S., Jenkins, A. L., Lee, R., Wong, G. S., Josse, R. (1983): Glycaemic response to wheat products: reduced response to pasta but no effect of fiber. *Diabetes Care* **6**, 155–159.

Jenkins, D. J. A., Wolever, T. M. S., Leeds, A. R., Gassull, M. A., Haisman, P., Dilawari, J., Goff, D. V., Metz, G. L., Alberti, K. G. M. M. (1978a): Dietary fibres, fibre analogues and glucose tolerance: importance of viscosity. *Br. Med. J.* **1**, 1392–1394.

Jenkins, D. J. A., Wolever, T. M. S., Nineham, R., Taylor, R., Metz, G. L., Bacon, S., Hockaday, T. D. R. (1978b): Guar crispbread in the diabetic diet. *Br. Med. J.* **2**, 1744–1746.

Jenkins, D. J. A., Wolever, T. M. S., Taylor, R. H., Barker, H. M., Fielden, H., Gassull, M. A. (1981): Lack of effect of refining on the glycaemic response to cereals. *Diabetes Care* **4**, 509–513.

Kay, R. M., Truswell, A. S. (1980): Dietary fiber: effects on plasma and biliary lipids in man. In *Medical aspects of dietary fiber*, ed G. A. Spiller, R. M. Kay, pp. 153–173. New York: Plenum Press.

Kent, N. L. (1983): *Technology of cereals*, 3rd edn, p. 175. Oxford: Pergamon.

Khan, M. N., Hagenmaier, R. D., Rooney, L. W., Mattil, K. F. (1976): High fiber coconut products for baking systems. *Bakers' Dig.* **50**, 19–23 & 50.

Kirwan, W. O., Smith, A. N., McConnell, A. A., Mitchell, W. D., Eastwood, M. A. (1974): Action of different bran preparations on colonic function. *Br. Med. J.* **4**, 187–189.

Krotkiewski, M. (1984): Effect of guar gum on body-weight, hunger ratings and metabolism in obese subjects. *Br. J. Nutr.* **52**, 97–105.

Leeds, A. R. (1982): Modification of intestinal absorption by dietary fiber and fiber components. In *Dietary fiber in health and disease*, eds G. V. Vahouny, D. Kritchevsky, pp. 53–71. New York: Plenum

Lithell, H., Selinus, I., Vessby, B. (1984): Lack of effect of a purified bran preparation in men with low HDL cholesterol. *Hum. Nutr.: Clin. Nutr.* **38C**, 309–313.

Mann, J. (1984): Dietary fibre and diabetes. In *Dietary fibre in the management of the diabetic* , pp. 7–13. Oxford: Medical Education Services.

McCance, R. A., Widdowson, E. M., Shackleton, L. R. B. (1936): *The nutritive value of fruits, vegetables and nuts*. Spec. Rep. Ser. Med. Res. Coun. Lond. 213. London: HMSO.

McIvor, M. E., Cummings, C. C., Leo, T. A., Mendeloff, A. I. (1984): Acute and chronic effects of high carbohydrate, high fiber food supplements in patients with NIDDM. *Diabetes* **33**(Suppl. 1), 191A.

Micklesen, O., Makdani, D. D., Cotton, R. H., Titcomb, S. T., Colmey, J. C., Gatty, R. (1979): Effects of a high fiber bread diet on weight loss in college-age males. *Am. J. Clin. Nutr.* **32**, 1703–1709.

Miettinen, T. A. (1983): Effects of dietary fibre on cholesterol metabolism in man. In *Fibre in human and animal nutrition*, ed G. Wallace, G. Bell, pp. 173–177. New Zealand: Royal Society of New Zealand.

MAFF (Ministry of Agriculture, Fisheries and Food) (1956–1982): *Household food consumption and expenditure*. Annual Reports of the National Food Survey Committee. London: HMSO.

MAFF (Ministry of Agriculture, Fisheries and Food) (1984): *The Bread and Flour Regulations, Statutory Instruments No. 1304*. London: HMSO.

MAFF (Ministry of Agriculture, Fisheries and Food) (1985): *Food Facts*. London: MAFF.

Mintel, (1984): Breakfast Cereals. *Mark. Intell. April*, 13–25.

Moore, K. (1979): Bran nuggets provide 'golden' method for fiber incorporation — naturally. *Food Prod. Dev.* **13**, 38.

NACNE (National Advisory Committee on Nutrition Education) (1983): *Proposals for nutritional guidelines for health education in Britain*. London: Health Education Council.

Nygren, C., Hallmans, G., Lithner, F. (1984): Effects of high-bran bread on blood glucose control in insulin-dependent diabetic patients. *Diabete Metab.* **10**, 39–43.

O'Connor, N., Tredger, J., Morgan, L. (1981): Viscosity differences between various guar gums. *Diabetologia* **20**, 612–615.

Paul, A. A., Southgate, D. A. T. (1978): *McCance and Widdowson's The composition of foods*, 4th edn. Spec. Rep. Med. Res. Council, No. 297. London:HMSO.

Peterson, D. (1984): Guar in the management of non-insulin dependent diabetic patients. In *Dietary fibre in the management of the diabetic*, pp. 33–38. Oxford: Medical Education Series.

Peterson, D., Ellis, P. R., Baylis, J. M., Frost, P. G., Leeds, A. R., Jepson, E. M. (1984): Effects of guar on diabetes and lipids — food and pharmacology compared. *Diabetologia* **27**, 319A.

Pikaar, N. A., Wedel, M., Van Dokkum, W., Hernius, R. J. J. (1985): The influence of the type of starch and of the incorporation of soluble dietary fibre in breakfast and lunch on the levels of glucose, insulin and C-peptide in plasma. *Proc. Nutr. Soc.* **44**, in press.

Polizzoto, L. M., Tinsley, A. M., Webber, C. W., Berry, J. W. (1983): Dietary fibers in muffins. *J. Food Sci.* **48**, 111–118.

Pomeranz, Y. (1977): Fiber in breadmaking — a review of recent findings. *Bakers' Dig.* **51**, 94–96 & 142.

Pomeranz, Y., Shogren, M. D., Finney, K. F., Bechtel, D. B. (1977): Fiber in breadmaking — effects on functional properties. *Cereal Chem.* **54**, 25–41.

Prosky, L., Asp, N-G., Furda, I., DeVries, J. W., Schweizer, T. F., Harland, B. F. (1984): Determination of total dietary fiber in foods, food products and ingredients. *Jnl Ass. Off. Analyt. Chem.* **67**, 1044–1052.

Rajchel, C. L., Zabik, M. E., Everson, E. (1975): Wheat bran and middlings as a source of dietary fiber in banana, chocolate nut and spice cakes. *Bakers' Digest* **49**, 27–30.

Rivellese, A., Riccardi, G., Giacco, A., Pacioni, D., Genovene, S., Mattioli, P. L., Mancini, M. (1980): Effect of dietary fibre on glucose control and serum lipoproteins in diabetic patients. *Lancet* **2**, 447–450.

Robertson, J. B., Van Soest, P. J. (1977): Dietary fiber estimation in concentrate feed stuffs. *J. Anim. Sci.* **45**(Suppl. 1), 254.

Royal College of Physicians of London (1980): *Medical aspects of dietary fibre*. London: Pitman Medical.

Sartor, G., Carlström, S., Scherstén, B. (1981): Dietary supplementation of fibre (Lunelax[R]) as a means to reduce postprandial glucose in diabetics. *Acta Med. Scand.* **665**, 51–53.

Satin, M. (1980): *High fiber white bread*, U.S. Patent 4,237,170.

Schaller, D. R. (1977): Analysis of dietary fiber. *Food Prod. Dev.* **11**, 70–72.

Schweizer, T. F., Würsch, P. (1979): Analysis of dietary fibre. *J. Sci. Fd Agric.* **30**, 613–619.

Selvendran, R. R. (1983): The plant cell wall as a source of dietary fiber chemistry and structure. *Am. J. Clin. Nutr.* **39**, 320–337.

Selvendran, R. R. (1984): The chemistry of plant cell walls. In *Dietary fibre*, eds G. G. Birch, K. J. Parker, pp. 95–147. London: Applied Science.

Selvendran, R. R., March, J. F., Ring, S. G. (1979*b*): Determination of aldoses and uronic acid content of vegetable fibre. *Analyt. Biochem.* **96**, 282–292.

Selvendran, R. R., Ring, S. G., Du Pont, M. S. (1979*a*): Assessment of procedures used for analysing dietary fibre. *Chem. Inds.* Lond.: 225–230.

Shafer, M. A. M., Zabik, M. E. (1975): Dietary fiber sources for baked products: Comparison of wheat brans and other cereal brans in layer cakes. *J. Food Sci.* **43**, 375–379.

Shogren, M. D., Pomeranz, Y., Finney, K. F. (1981): Counteracting the deleterious effects of fiber in breadmaking. *Cereal Chem.* **58**, 142–144.

Smith, A. N., Drummond, E., Eastwood, M. A. (1981): The effect of coarse and fine Canadian red spring wheat and French soft wheat on colonic motility in patients with diverticular disease. *Am. J. Clin. Nutr.* **34**, 2460–2463.

Smith, C. J., Rosman, M. S., Levitt, N. S., Jackson, W. P. U. (1982): Guar biscuits in the diabetic diet. *S. Afr. Med. J.* **61**, 196–198.

Southgate, D. A. T. (1969): Determination of carbohydrates in foods. II. Unavailable carbohydrates. *J. Sci. Fd Agric.* **20**, 331–335.

Southgate, D. A. T. (1976*a*): The chemistry of dietary fiber. In *Fiber in human nutrition*, eds G. A. Spiller, R. J. Amen, pp. 31–72. New York: Plenum Press.

Southgate, D. A. T. (1976*b*): The analysis of dietary fiber. In *Fiber in human nutrition*, ed G. A. Spiller, R. J. Amen, pp. 73–107. New York: Plenum Press.

Southgate, D. A. T. (1976*c*): *Determination of food carbohydrates*. London: Applied Science.

Southgate, D. A. T. (1978): Dietary fiber: analysis and food sources. *Am. J. Clin. Nutr.* **31**, S106–S110.

Southgate, D. A. T. (1982): Definitions and terminology of dietary fiber. In *Dietary fiber in health and disease*, ed G. V. Vahouny, D. Kritchevsky, pp. 1–7. New York: Plenum Press.

Southgate, D. A. T., Bailey, B., Collinson, E., Walker, A. F. (1976): A guide to calculating intakes of dietary fibre. *J. Hum. Nutr.* **30**, 303–313.

Southgate, D. A. T., Hudson, G. J., Englyst, H. (1978): The analysis of dietary fibre — the choices for the analyst. *J. Sci. Fd Agric.* **29**, 979–988.

Southgate, D. A. T., White, M. A. (1981): Commentary on results obtained by the different laboratories using the Southgate method. In *The analysis of dietary fiber in food*, ed W. P. T. James, O. Theander, pp. 37–50. New York: Marcel Dekker.

Springsteen, E., Zabik, M. E., Shafer, M. A. M. (1977): Note on layer cakes containing 30 to 70% wheat bran. *Cereal Chem.* **54**, 193–198.

Taylor, R. H. (1984): Bran yesterday … bran tomorrow? *Br. Med. J.* **289**, 69–70.

Theander, O. (1981): Review of the different analytical methods and remaining problems. In *The analysis of dietary fiber in food*, ed W. P. T. James, O. Theander, pp. 263–276. New York: Marcel Dekker.

Theander, O., Åman, P. (1979): Studies on dietary fibres. 1. Analysis and chemical characterization of water-soluble and water-insoluble dietary fibres. *Swed. J. Agric. Res.* **9**, 97–106.

Theander, O., Åman, P. (1982): Studies on dietary fibre. A method for the analysis and chemical characterization of total dietary fibre. *J. Sci. Fd Agric.* **33**, 340–344.

Thomas, B., Elchazly, M. (1976): Funktionelle wirkungen und veränderungen der ballaststoffe des weizens während des verdauungsablaufes. *Qual. Plant.-Pl. Fds Hum. Nutr.* **26**, 211–226.

Thorne, M. J., Thompson, L. U., Jenkins, D. J. A. (1983): Factors affecting starch digestibility and the glycaemic response with special reference to legumes. *Am. J. Clin. Nutr.* **38**, 481–488.

Toma, R. B., Orr, P. H., D'Appolonia, B., Dintzis, F. R., Tabekhia, M. M. (1979): Physical and chemical properties of potato peel as a source of dietary fiber in bread. *J. Fd Sci.* **44**, 1403–1407 & 1417.

Tredger, J., Ransley, J. (1978): Guar gum — its acceptability to diabetic patients when incorporated into baked food products. *J. Hum. Nutr.* **32**, 427–432.

Trowell, H. C. (1972): Crude fibre, dietary fibre and atherosclerosis. *Atherosclerosis* **16**, 138–140.

Trowell, H. C. (1978): The development of the concept of dietary fiber in human nutrition. *Am. J. Clin Nutr.* **31**, S3–S11.

Trowell, H., Southgate, D. A. T., Wolever, T. M. S., Leeds, A. R., Gassull, M. A., Jenkins, D. J. A. (1976): Dietary fibre redefined. *Lancet* **1**, 967.

Tuomilehto, J., Voutilainen, E., Huttunen, J., Vinni, S., Homan, K. (1980): Effect of guar gum on body weight and serum lipids in hypercholesterolaemic females. *Acta Med. Scand.* **208**, 45–48.

US Department of Agriculture. (1979): *Food.* Home and Garden Bull. No. 228. Washington DC: US Department of Agriculture.

Vaaler, S., Hanssen, K. F., Dahl-Jorgensen, K., Frolich, W., Aaseth, J., Odegaard, B., Aagenaes, O. (1983): Improvement in long-term diabetic control after high fibre (bran and guar) diets. *Diabetologia* **25**, 200.

Vahouny, G. V., Kritchevsky, D. eds (1982): *Dietary fiber in health and disease.* New York: Plenum Press.

Valle-Jones, J. C. (1980): The evaluation of a new appetite-reducing agent (Prefil) in the management of obesity. *Br. J. Clin. Pract.* **34**, 72–74.

Van Soest, P. (1967): Development of a comprehensive system of feed analyses and its application to forages. *J. Anim. Sci.* **26**, 119–128.

Van Soest, P. J. (1978): Dietary fibers: their definition and nutritional properties. *Am. J. Clin. Nutr.* **31**, S12–S20.

Volpe, T., Lehmann, T. (1977): Production and evaluation of a high-fiber bread. *Bakers' Dig.* **51**, 24–26.

Vratanina, D. L., Zabik, M. E. (1978): Dietary fiber sources for baked products: Bran in sugar-snap cookies. *J. Fd Sci.* **43**, 1590–1594.

Walker, C. L. (1984): The national diet. *Postgrad. Med. J.* **60**, 26–33.

Walsh, D. E., Yaghoubian, V., Behforooz, A. (1984): Effect of glucomannan on obese patients: a clinical study. *Int. J. Obesity* **8**, 289–293.

Wenlock, R. W., Buss, D. H., Agater, I. B. (1984): New estimates of fibre in the diet in Britain. *Br. Med. J.* **288**, 1873.

Wenlock, R. W., Sivell, L. M., Agater, I. B. (1985): Dietary fibre fractions in cereal and cereal-containing products in Britain. *J. Sci. Fd Agric.* **36**, 113–121.

Wolever, T. M. S., Jenkins, D. J. A., Nineham, R., Alberti, K. G. M. M. (1979): Guar gum and reduction of post-prandial glycaemia: effect of incorporation into solid food, liquid, and both. *Br. J. Nutr.* **41**, 505–510.

Wyman, J. B., Heaton, K. W., Manning, A. P., Wicks, A. C. B. (1976): The effect on intestinal transit and the feces of raw and cooked bran in different doses. *Am. J. Clin. Nutr.* **29**, 1474–1479.

Zabik, M. E., Shafer, M. A. M., Kutorowski, B. W. (1977): Dietary fiber sources for baked products. Comparison of cellulose types and coated-cellulose products in layer cakes. *J. Fd Sci.* **42**, 1428–1431.

Zavoral, J. H., Hannan, P., Fields, D. J., Hanson, M. N., Franz, I. D., Kuba, K., Elmer, P., Jacobs, D. R. (1983): The hypolipidemic effect of locust bean gum food products in familial hypercholesterolemic adults and children. *Am. J. Clin. Nutr.* **38**, 285–294.

Dietary fibre in human nutrition: a bibliography

HUGH C. TROWELL

This bibliography, which covers the years up to and including 1977, was first published in 1979 for The Kellogg Company of Great Britain.

FOREWORD

By K. W. Heaton, MA, MD, FRCP, Consultant Senior Lecturer in Medicine, University Department of Medicine, Bristol Royal Infirmary, Bristol.

If there was ever a case of a new concept really being an old one rediscovered, then dietary fibre is surely it. The older literature on fibre is surprisingly extensive (and rewarding) and since 1970 there has been a wave of new papers and books. Literature searches are always time-consuming and, perhaps because of this, they are all too often skimped by the modern research worker. With dietary fibre, even the conscientious worker finds it difficult to do a good literature search because there are so many synonyms for fibre and its various sub-classes, and the nomenclature keeps changing. In addition, there are many papers and books which are relevant to dietary fibre and its role in health and disease but which do not mention fibre or any of its synonyms in the title.

Everyone interested in dietary fibre will therefore be deeply indebted to Dr Trowell for compiling this massive bibliography. It is a major achievement by any standards, but for a man well past retirement age it is a veritable *tour de force*. Actually, Dr Trowell is probably the only person alive who could have brought it off. His deep involvement in the fibre field since 1970 has been almost a second professional career. As an indefatigable letter writer and an intrepid traveller he has established personal contacts with almost every research worker and writer in this field, and these he has grafted on to his already wide acquaintance with the world of nutrition. He must be a familiar figure in many great medical libraries.

Dr Trowell has plenty of other distinguished achievements behind him, but I suspect that few of his earlier writings will be as widely used as this bibliography. On behalf of all workers in the field of diet and human disease, I should like to say 'Thank you, Hugh'.

PREFACE

Dietary fibre has been defined as the substances present in the residue of the plant foods of man that are resistant to digestion by human digestive enzymes. The main components are cellulose, non-cellulosic polysaccharides (hemicelluloses) and lignin.

In 1977 the Cumulated Index Medicus began to publish citations concerning 'DIETARY FIBER — see under CELLULOSE', listing about 50 citations concerning dietary fibre in human nutrition for the year 1977. The present bibliography contains 182 citations concerning dietary fibre for 1977. The difference in the number of citations is due to various factors. This bibliography includes, as far as possible, citations from all medical and scientific journals and books published during 1977, and in previous years. The Index Medicus compiles citations from its list of the major medical and scientific journals.

Uncertainties surround the preparation of any medical bibliography of dietary fibre. For instance, it is apparent that dietary fibre cannot concern itself exclusively with cellulose: citations concerning hemicelluloses and lignin should not be excluded. Other uncertainties have been discussed in a joint letter to the Editor of the American Journal of Clinical Nutrition entitled 'Fiber Bibliographies and Terminology' (H. Trowell, E. Godding, G. Spiller and G. Briggs, 1978 31, 1480 00). This letter made four points. The bibliography should be restricted to 1) dietary fibre and 2) its main components — cellulose, hemicelluloses and lignin — derived from 3) plant foods of man 4) with respect to human nutrition and animal experiments planned to throw light on human disease. This medical bibliography of dietary fibre in human nutrition has been prepared in conformity with these four principles. Some citations in the 1977 Index Medicus list have therefore been omitted, such as those on 'Analogues, Biosynthesis and Pharmacodynamics'. All these subjects, however, may be relevant to the action of dietary fibre in human nutrition. This bibliography is therefore a restricted bibliography.

The joint letter discussed also wider issues. It suggested that a new term 'Edible fibre' is required and would include four groups of substances: a) undigested dietary fibre from the plant foods of man; b) undigested partially synthetic polysaccharides such as methyl cellulose; c) undigested animal polysaccharides such as aminopolysaccharides present in connective tissues and eaten by certain ethnic groups; d) undigested pharmaceutical preparations from plants not eaten as foodstuffs by man, such as those from ispaghula bark. This medical bibliography is concerned only with dietary fibre; it does not include citations concerning b), c) and d).

This dietary fibre bibliography is clinically oriented and is retrospective for the years 1977, 1976, 1975 and so on. This will enable readers to consult the latest publications. The Yearly Index is preceded by the Subject Index. The latter will enable readers to consult the latest citations of a certain subject. The more informative citations are marked by an asterisk. The main subjects are grouped into seven sections: 1) Gastrointestinal, including gallstones and bile-salt metabolism. 2) Cardiovascular, including lipid metabolism and thrombosis. 3) Metabolic, including diabetes mellitus and obesity. 4) Fibre and food. 5) Miscellaneous. 6) General hypotheses. 7) Books, reviews and symposia.

An attempt has been made to include a few citations concerning the early history of fibre, such as the laxative action of bran, and early studies concerning the cellulose, hemicelluloses and lignin of plant foods of man. There was also a long controversy concerning the alleged merits of wholemeal versus white bread. This has been reviewed by R.A. McCance and E.M. Widdowson: *Breads, White and Brown* (1956) and included 720 references. No fibre bibliography would be complete without citations concerning dietary changes in Britain and other countries during the last two centuries. Other changes occurred during the World War (1939 - 1945); then high-fibre flour was milled in many countries. Efforts were made to keep the fibre content of wartime flour as low as possible, for roughage was considered to be a gastro-intestinal irritant. This view is reflected in citations from medical journals 1919-1940, a few of which are included in this bibliography.

The citations have been presented as far as possible in the style of the Index Medicus of the year concerned. Thus in recent years initials of an author have been restricted to two. Square brackets denote translation. Checking, whenever possible, has been through this invaluable Index.

The inadequacy of the citations in foreign medical journals, except in recent years, is regretted. Their inclusion can be accomplished only be someone familiar with their languages.

1 November, 1978

Hugh C. Trowell
Woodgreen
Nr. Fordingbridge, Hants
SP6 2AZ

ACKNOWLEDGEMENTS

This literature search has been assisted by a grant from the Pharmaceutical Division, Reckitt and Colman. Mr M.T. Wheeler of their staff has provided the references for 1977. Mr F.M. Sutherland, Librarian of the Nuffield Library, British Medical Association, kindly checked the early references for 1935 and all previous years. Professor B. Thomas provided the German citations. All these I thank and also Dr K.W. Heaton, who made many valuable suggestions.

This bibliography was prepared for the Kellogg Nutrition Symposium at the Royal Society of Medicine, December 1977*. It proved impossible to complete the bibliography for this conference: fortunately the delay allowed the 1977 citations to be completed.

Mrs Priscilla Tippett and Mrs Sheila King have both rendered careful secretarial assistance. Finally it remains to thank the Kellogg Company of Great Britain, Stretford, Manchester, whose generous help made publication possible.

Sources of citations

Two literature searches of US National Library of Medicine Jan 1973 to Mar 1977[1]	200
Commonwealth Bureau of Nutrition compilation 1951-1976[2]	95
Cumulated Index Medicus for 1977	50
German[3]	19
Literature search (H.C.T.) 1976 retrospectively and in collaboration with Mr M. Wheeler for 1977	674
Total	1038

[1]Published in Citation 1977, No. 151, pp. 214-239   [2]Compiled from Nutrition Abstracts and Reviews
[3]Courtesy of Professor Dr B. Thomas

* *Journal of Plant Foods* (1978) **3**, issue number 1 & 2. Book: *Dietary fibre: current developments of importance to health*, ed K.W. Heaton, 1978, London: Newman.

Contents

Subject Index

1. Gastrointestinal

An asterisk (*) marks some of the more important citations

1.1. Colonic function, faecal weight, transit time, constipation
1977: 6*, 31*, 34, 44, 51, 55, 65*, 79*, 94, 100*, 117, 123*, 132*, 134, 142, 158*, 162*,
    168, 171, 180
1976: 5*, 18, 25, 28*, 29*, 30*, 36, 39*, 43*, 45*, 52, 54, 58, 96*, 111, 137*, 161, 162*, 163
1975: 27, 28, 40*, 51, 81, 96*, 120*, 124, 125   *1974:* 24, 25, 26, 33, 40*, 41, 46*, 53
1973: 12, 14*, 16, 18, 19*, 24, 25, 38, 41, 42   *1972:* 7, 12, 14, 16*   *1971:* 5, 9, 19
1970: 6, 7, 14*, 15, 17   *1969:* 3   *1962:* 2, 8   *1961:* 6*   *1959:* 3   *1953:* 2
1947: 3*   *1945:* 2*   *1943:* 2*, 3, 5   *1942:* 2   *1941:* 2, 4*, 5*, 7, 15, 16
1940: 2, 3*   *1938:* 2   *1937:* 1*, 3*   *1936:* 1*, 3*, 9*, 10, 11*, 12*
1935: 1*, 3, 5*, 8*   *1934:* 3*, 4, 5   *1933:* 1*, 2*, 3   *1932:* 1*, 4   *1930:* 3, 4
1928: 3   *1927:* 2   *1919:* 1   *1912:* 1*   *1610:* 1   *BC 430:* 1, 2

1.2. Diverticular disease
1977: 13*, 27*, 35, 43, 54, 62*, 79*, 91*, 94*, 101, 111*, 125*, 126*, 137, 170*, 171, 175, 179
1976: 10*, 11*, 12*, 53*, 65, 66, 114, 127*, 133   *1975:* 6*, 75*, 77, 78*, 79, 80
1974: 2, 16, 17, 23, 24*, 25, 32*, 54, 55, 64*, 80*   *1973:* 3*, 5, 32, 36*, 39, 43
1972: 1, 9, 18, 19, 21*, 25   *1971:* 12, 13*, 17   *1969:* 7*   *1968:* 7*   *1967:* 7
1964: 8, 13   *1962:* 7*   *1949:* 1*, 8

1.3. Irritable bowel syndrome
1977: 4, 39*, 50*, 79*, 93*, 159*, 171, 174, 177*
1976: 24, 53*, 89, 90*, 99, 100, 101, 102, 115*, 116*, 159   *1975:* 89*, 97
1974: 57, 71, 77   *1972:* 20

1.4. Large bowel cancer, colonic and faecal bacteria
1977: 6*, 55*, 60, 65*, 92, 160*, 161*, 164
1976: 1, 34, 35*, 45, 93*, 106, 126*, 154*, 157*, 164
1975: 6*, 7, 8*, 49*, 50*, 65, 69*, 70*   *1974:* 7, 18, 26*, 30, 47, 60*
1973: 13, 15, 31, 46, 65*   *1972:* 2*, 3*   *1971:* 2*, 3, 14, 19, 20   *1970:* 16
1969: 11   *1964:* 12   *1960:* 4*   *1936:* 2

1.5. Appendicitis
1977: 19, 142   *1975:* 6*, 26   *1973:* 64*   *1971:* 1*   *1926:* 3   *1920:* 2*

1.6. Ulcerative colitis, Crohn's disease
1975: 29, 114*

1.7. The group of large bowel disorders (see also *2.3. Haemorrhoids*)
1977: 115*, 142*   1976: 38*, 155*   1975: 2, 12, 84, 85*, 112
1973: 14*, 16*, 17, 40   *1972:* 11, 15   *1971:* 11   *1964:* 3   *1962:* 8
1960: 4   *1936:* 3

1.8. Dental caries
1975: 1*   *1974:* 9*

1.9. Hiatus hernia
1975: 6*, 9*, 10   *1974:* 9   *1973:* 10   *1964:* 8*

1.10. Stomach, gastric ulcer, small intestine, duodenal ulcer
1977: 10, 57*, 122, 134, 173   *1976:* 57   *1975:* 100*, 101*, 102*   *1974:* 9, 72*
1973: 59*   *1972:* 27, 28*, 33   *1962:* 4

1.11. Digestibility, absorption of nutrients, minerals and drugs
1977: 8, 14, 15, 32*, 36*, 37*, 46*, 53*, 66*, 67*, 100*, 109, 118*, 119, 152, 155, 156*, 162*
1976: 22*, 40*, 62, 69*, 98, 103, 108*, 110, 123*, 160
1975: 4, 28*, 45*, 56, 63, 86*, 87, 95, 120*   *1974:* 3, 6*, 29   *1973:* 2, 60
1972: 8   *1970:* 4, 12, 13*   *1969:* 3, 5   *1966:* 8*   *1961:* 2*, 5*
1960: 6   *1958:* 7   *1957:* 6   *1956:* 11   *1954:* 4   *1949:* 7   *1948:* 1, 2*, 3
1947: 1, 2   *1946:* 3*   *1945:* 2   *1942:* 4, 5, 6, 8, 9, 10   *1941:* 12*, 14*, 17
1940: 3   *1936:* 4   *1935:* 4   *1934:* 1, 3, 4, 7   *1932:* 3   *1930:* 1, 2, 5
1929: 3   *1926:* 2   *1917:* 3   *1912:* 2   *1911:* 1, 2, 3, 5, 6   *1888-89:* 2

1.12. Gallstones, bile salt metabolism (see also *2.1. Cholesterol metabolism*)
1977: 5*, 6*, 41*, 61, 105*, 165, 181*   *1976:* 23*, 37, 40, 81, 104*, 123, 129*, 131*
1975: 20*, 41*, 43, 45*, 59, 64*   *1974:* 5*, 9*, 22, 25, 39, 44*, 58*
1973: 2, 26*. 44, 51*   *1972:* 13*   *1971:* 6*   *1968:* 1, 2*, 3*   *1967:* 1

2. Cardiovascular
2.1. Lipid metabolism, cholesterol, triglyceride
1977: 1, 3, 5*, 24, 33, 65, 74, 76*, 77, 81, 83*, 84, 85, 86*, 90, 96*, 97, 105*, 107*, 114*,
     133, 135, 143, 158, 159, 162*, 163
1976: 12*, 23*, 36*, 56, 60, 62*, 64*, 72, 73, 75, 80*, 86, 88, 95*, 103, 105*, 123*, 130*,
     131*, 145*, 146, 147, 162*
1975: 1, 3, 5, 21, 22, 32, 38*, 44, 46, 54, 55, 56*, 57, 60, 74, 82, 109, 116, 123
1974: 3, 10, 27, 29, 38, 43, 50, 52*, 60*   *1973:* 13, 30, 35, 45*, 48*, 52, 62*, 63*
1972: 35, 36   *1971:* 10, 15, 16   *1969:* 4*, 6*   *1968:* 4, 6*   *1967;* 2*, 6*, 8
1966: 2, 3, 5, 7, 9, 10   *1965:* 1, 2, 3, 4, 5, 8*   *1964:* 10, 14   *1963:* 2
1962: 1*, 2*, 5, 6*   *1961:* 3*   *1960:* 2   *1958:* 1   *1957:* 7   *1956:* 7

2.2. Atherosclerosis, ischaemic heart disease
1977: 85*, 86*, 87, 88, 107*, 124*, 140, 143, 148*   *1976:* 6, 60, 79, 80*, 87, 97*
1975: 44, 110, 114*, 121*   *1974:* 1*, 9, 12, 42*, 65, 78, 80, 83*   *1973:* 48*, 55*
1972: 29, 30, 31, 32*   *1971:* 8, 17   *1970:* 2*   *1969:* 9, 10   *1968:* 5*, 8*
1967: 4, 5*, 6   *1964:* 15   *1957:* 1   *1956:* 1   *1954:* 1, 3

2.3. Venous thrombosis, varicose veins, haemorrhoids, fibrinolysis
1977: 38, 116*, 148*, 172   *1976:* 14*, 15*, 20*, 44, 67, 83, 92*, 139*
1975: 6*, 9*, 10, 11, 12, 15*, 16*, 35, 58, 73, 99, 105, 107, 122   *1974:* 51, 85
1973: 4*, 32, 47   *1972:* 4*, 5   *1971:* 18   *1968:* 5*   *1964:* 2*, 5
1960: 1*   *1959:* 1*

2.4. Phleboliths
1977: 21*, 80*

2.5. Pregnancy toxaemia, eclampsia
1974: 31   *1957:* 4*   *1953:* 1*   *1949:* 5

3. Metabolic

3.1. Diabetes mellitus, carbohydrate metabolism
1977: 2*, 29, 59*, 68, 69*, 70*, 71*, 72, 73, 106*, 146*
1976: 4*, 12*, 33, 47, 48, 71*, 74, 77*, 84, 109*   *1975:* 31*, 53*, 103*, 114*
1974: 9*, 34, 36*, 48, 73*, 74, 78   *1973:* 54, 55*, 57, 66   *1972:* 34*, 38*   *1969:* 2*

3.2. Obesity (see also *1.11 Absorption of nutrients*)
1977: 11, 59*   *1976:* 61, 112*, 113*   *1975:* 106*, 114*   *1974:* 9*, 28, 35, 63, 75
1973: 27*, 28, 50*, 54   *1970:* 13*   *1969:* 2   *1966:* 8*   *1961:* 2*, 5*
1958: 7

4. Fibre and food

4.1. Fibre: definition, terminology, composition, analysis
1977: 12*, 42*, 63, 89, 120*, 121*, 127*, 139*, 141*, 153*
1976: 27*, 41*, 51*, 68*, 117*, 118*, 119*, 120*, 121, 125*, 134*, 144*, 151*, 152*, 153*
1975: 47, 52, 88*, 117, 119   *1974:* 4, 9*, 37, 45*, 66*, 76*
1973: 20, 22, 23*, 33, 34, 37, 50*, 53*, 61*   *1972:* 26*   *1971:* 14*   *1970:* 1*, 9*
1969: 4, 8*   *1965:* 6, 9   *1963:* 3*, 4*, 5*   *1959:* 2*   *1958:* 7
1957: 3*, 4, 5*   *1956:* 5, 6, 11   *1953:* 1*, 5*   *1943:* 1   *1940:* 6   *1936:* 8
1935: 7, 8*   *1930:* 5   *1929:* 1*

4.2. Fibre in the diet and food, except cereals
1977: 51, 182   *1976:* 32*, 122*, 155*   *1975:* 72, 114, 117   *1974:* 49
1973: 1   *1972:* 17, 22*, 24   *1971:* 7*   *1970:* 5, 10, 11   *1964:* 6, 7, 9
1963: 5*   *1960:* 3   *1956:* 15   *1953:* 5*, 7   *1943:* 3   *1940:* 6

4.3. Fibre in cereals, bran, breads brown and white
1977: 113, 169   *1976:* 42, 70, 122*   *1975:* 23, 76, 111, 114
1974: 4, 68   *1973:* 22*, 33, 34, 37   *1972:* 22*   *1971:* 7   *1970:* 8*, 10, 11*
1967: 3   *1966:* 6*   *1965:* 7   *1964:* 11   *1963:* 1*   *1962:* 3   *1961:* 1
1960: 5   *1959:* 2*, 4   *1958:* 2, 3*, 4, 5, 6, 8, 9, 10   *1957:* 3*, 5*
1956: 3, 4, 6, 8*, 9, 10, 11, 12, 13, 14*   *1955:* 1, 2*, 3   *1954:* 2*, 4
1953: 3, 4, 6, 7   *1952:* 1   *1951:* 2*, 3   *1950:* 1, 2, 3
1949: 3   *1946:* 1, 2, 4, 5, 6   *1945:* 1, 3, 4, 5   *1944:* 1, 2, 3, 4, 5
1943: 4, 6, 7   *1942:* 1, 3, 7   *1941:* 1, 3, 6, 8, 9, 10, 11, 13, 18   *1940:* 1, 5
1939: 2, 3   *1937:* 2*   *1929:* 1*   *1928:* 1   *1925:* 1   *1924:* 3   *1923:* 1
1920: 1*   *1919:* 3   *1917:* 2, 3   *1911:* 1, 2, 3, 5, 6   *1900-05:* 1
1898-1900: 1   *1892:* 1   *1889:* 1, 2   *1849:* 1   *1847:* 1   *1837:* 1
1821: 1   *1610:* 1   *1542:* 1   *BC 430:* 1, 2

4.4. Modern dietary change
1977: 150*   *1976:* 49   *1975:* 114*   *1974:* 49   *1973:* 56   *1972:* 22*
1971: 7   *1966:* 4*, 11   *1964:* 1*   *1957:* 2*   *1951:* 1*   *1949:* 1, 4*, 6
1947: 3   *1939:* 1*   *1938:* 1*   *1928:* 1*   *1917:* 1*   *1911:* 4*
1871: 1   *1856:* 1   *1830:* 1

Yearly Index

1977

1   Ahuja MM: Hypolipidaemic drugs of indigenous origin. J Indian Med Assoc 68: 214-215 (77)

2   Anderson JW: polysaccharide diet studies in patients with diabetes and vascular disease. Cereal Foods World 22: 12-14, 22 (77)

3   Arvanitakis C, Staınnes CL, Folscroft J, et al: Failure of bran to alter diet-induced hyperlipidemia in the rat. Proc Soc Exp Biol Med 154: 550-552 (77)

4   Austad WI: The irritable bowel syndrome. N Z Med J 86: 291-293 (77)

5   Avgerinos GC, Fuchs HM, Floch MH: Increased cholesterol and bile acid excretion during a high fiber diet. Gastroenterology 72: A-3/1026 (77)

6   Baird IM, Walters RL, Davies PS, et al: The effects of two dietary fibre supplements on gastrointestinal transit, stool weight and frequency, and bacterial flora and fecal bile acids in normal subjects. Metabolism 26: 117-128 (77)

7   Barness LA: Pediatrics, pp 441-462. In: Schneider HA et al, ed. *Nutritional Support Of Medical Practice.* London, Harper and Row (77)

8   Beshgetoor D, Keis C, Fox HM: Zinc utilisation as affected by dietary pectin, cellulose and hemicellulose. Fed Proc 36: 1118 (77)

9   Bine R. Jr: Cardiology, pp 236-262. In: Schneider HA et al, ed. *Nutritional Support of Medical Practice.* London, Harper and Row (77)

10   Bingham S, McNeil NI, Cummings JH: Diet for the ileostomist. J Hum Nutr 31: 365-366 (77)

11   Bray GA: Current status of intestinal bypass surgery in the treatment of obesity Diabetes 26: 1072-1079 (77)

12   Briggs GM, Spiller GA: 'Dietary fibre' or 'Plantix' (letter). Lancet 2: 563 (77)

13   Brodribb AJ: Treatment of symptomatic diverticular disease with a high-fibre diet. Lancet 1: 664-666 (77)

14   Brown RC, Kelleher J, Walker BE, et al: Dietary fibre and drug absorption: the effect of pectin and bran on paracetamol absorption in the rat. Gut 18: A964 (77)

15   Budhiraja RD, Bala S, Garg KN: Effects of dietary factors on drug action. Clinician 41: 257-264 (77)

16   Burkitt DP: Are our commonest diseases preventable? (Editorial). Prev Med 6: 556-559 (77)

17   Burkitt DP: Diet and diseases of affluence. Qual Plant-P1 Fds Hum Nutr 27, 3-4: 227-238 (77)

18   Burkitt DP: Food fiber: benefits from a surgeon's perspective. Cereal Foods World 22: 6-9 (77)

19   Burkitt DP: Appendicitis and diabetes (letter). Br Med J 1: 1413-1414 (77)

20   Burkitt DP: The Burkitt hypothesis (letter). Am J Dig Dis 22: 75 (77)

21   Burkitt DP, Latto C, Janvrin SB, et al: Pelvic phleboliths: epidemiology and postulated etiology. New Engl J Med 296: 1387-1389 (77)

22   Burkitt DP: Relationships between diseases and their etiological significance. Am J Clin Nutr 30: 262-267 (77)

23 Burkitt DP, Trowell, HC: Dietary fibre and western diseases. Ir Med J 70: 272-277 (77)
24 Chang ML, Johnson MA: Influence of dietary fiber (from soybean flour) on
    lipid metabolism in rats. Nutr Rep Internat 16: 573-577 (77)
25 Cleave TL: Fibre pathfinder. General Practitioner: 44, 9 Sep (77)
26 Cleave TL: Over-consumption: now the most dangerous cause of disease in
    westernized countries. Public Health 91: 127-131, (77)
27 Connell AM: Pathogenesis of diverticular disease of the colon, pp 377-395. In:
    Stollerman GH ed. *Advances in Internal Medicine* 22: Chicago Year Book Medical
    Publishers (77)
28 Connell AM: Wheat bran as an etiological factor in certain diseases. Some second
    thoughts. J Am Diet Assoc 71: 235-239 (77)
29 Corridan JP, O'Regan JP, O'Sullivan DJ: Diabetes and appendectomy: testing a
    hypothesis. Br Med J 1: 1135 (77)
30 Cummings JH: Treatment of diarrhoea in adults. Prescribers J 17: 27-39 (77)
31 Cummings JH, Branch WJ, Houston H, et al: Effect of dietary protein with and
    without added dietary fibre on faecal ammonia and on colonic function. Gut 18:
    A411-412 (77)
32 Davies NT, Hristic V, Flett AA: Phytate rather than fibre in bran as the major
    determinant of zinc availability in rats. Nutr Rep Internat 15: 207-214 (77)
33 Delbarre F, Rondier J, De Géry A: Lack of effect of two pectins on idiopathic or
    gout-associated hyperdyslipidemia hypercholesterolemia (letter). Am J Clin Nutr 30:
    463-465 (77)
34 Devereux DF, Baker AR: The effect of dietary fiber on stool bulk and gut transit
    time. Gastroenterology 72: A-25/1048 (77)
35 Devroede G, Vobecky IS, Vobecky JM, et al: Medical management of diverticular
    disease: a random trial. Gastroenterology 72: A-134/1157 (77)
36 Dilawari JB, Leeds AR, Gassull MA, et al: The effect of dietary fiber (guar gum)
    on carbohydrate absorption. Gastroenterology 72: A-26/1049 (77)
37 Dobbs RJ, Baird IM: Effect of wholemeal and white bread on iron absorption in
    normal people. Br Med J 1: 1641-1642 (77)
38 Dolman W, Southcott D: For piles, surgery is not always the answer. Mod Medicine
    22: 66-71 (77)
39 Drossman DA, Powell DW, Sessions JT Jr: Clinical gastroenterology conference.
    The irritable bowel syndrome. Gastroenterology 73: 811-822 (77)
40 Eastwood MA: Statement at hearings on fiber, pp 75-87. In: *Dietary Fiber and
    Health,* US Senate Select Committee on Nutrition and Human Needs, Washington,
    US Government Printing Office (77)
41 Eastwood MA: Fibre and enterohepatic circulation. Nutr Rev 35: 42-44 (77)
42 Eastwood MA, Smith AN: Nomenclature and definition of dietary fiber (letter).
    Am J Clin Nutr 30: 658-659 (77)
43 Eastwood MA, Sanderson J, Pocock SJ, et al: Variation in the incidence of diverticular
    disease within the city of Edinburgh. Gut 18: 571-574 (77)
44 Eastwood MA, Smith AN, Mitchell WD, et al: Physical characteristics of fiber
    influencing the bowel. Cereal Foods World 22: 10-11 (77)
45 Editorial: Food and Fibre. Br Med J 2: 418 (77)
46 Editorial: Effect of wholemeal and white bread on iron absorption. Br Med J 2:
    771-772 (77)
47 Editorial: Dietary fibre. Lancet 2: 337-338 (77)
48 Editorial: Dietary fibre in perspective. N Z Med J 85: 17-18 (77)

49 Ershoff BH: The virtues of dietary fibre. Fd Cosmet Toxicol 15: 358-359 (77)
50 Fielding JF: The irritable bowel syndrome. 1. Clinical spectrum. Clin. Gastroenterol
    6: 607-620 (77)
51 Flynn JF, O'Beirne SF, Burkitt DP: The potato as a source of fibre in the diet.
    Ir J Med Sci 146: 285-288 (77)
52 Forrester JM: Small-bowel volvulus (letter). Lancet 2: 349-350 (77)
53 Förster H, Hoos I: Influence of gums on intestinal absorption. Nutr Metab 21:
    262-264 (77)
54 Gear JS, Ware AC, Nolan DJ, et al: Dietary fibre and asymptomatic diverticular
    disease of the colon. Proc Nutr Soc 37: 13A (77)
55 Glober GA, Nomura A, Kamiyama S, et al: Bowel transit-time and stool weight in
    populations with different colon-cancer risks. Lancet 2: 110-111 (77)
56 Goldsmith HS, Gross SD: The Burkitt hypothesis (letter). Am J Dig Dis 22: 73 (77)
57 Grimes DS, Goddard J: Gastric emptying of wholemeal and white bread. Gut 18:
    725-729 (77)
58 Gunby P, Fiber catches fancy of nutrition congress. J Am Med Assoc 238: 1715-1716
    (77)
59 Haber GB, Heaton KW, Murphy D, et al: Depletion and disruption of dietary fibre.
    Effects on satiety, plasma-glucose and serum insulin. Lancet 2: 679-682 (77)
60 Heaton KW: Dietary fibre in Scandinavia (letter). Lancet 2: 407-408 (77)
61 Heaton KW, Wicks AC: Bran and bile: time-course of changes in normal young
    men given a standard dose. Gut 18: A951 (77)
62 Hodgson JW: The placebo effect, is it important in diverticular disease? Am J
    Gastroenterol 67: 157-162 (77)
63 Holloway WD, Tasman-Jones C, Maher K: Towards an accurate measurement of
    dietary fibre. N Z Med J 85: 420-423 (77)
64 Hunter BT: Dietary fibre: a panacea? A cure for our various ills as some are
    suggesting? Consumers Research Magazine: 32-33, Jul (77)
65 International Agency for Research on Cancer Intestinal Microecology Group:
    Dietary fibre, transit-time, faecal bacteria, steroids and colon cancer in two
    Scandinavian populations. Lancet 2: 207-211 (77)
66 Ismail-Beigi F, Reinhold JG, Faraji B, et al: Effects of cellulose added to diets of
    low and high fiber content upon the metabolism of calcium, magnesium, zinc and
    phosphorus by man. J Nutr 107: 510-518 (77)
67 Ismail-Beigi F, Faradji B, Reinhold JG, et al: Binding of zinc and iron to wheat bread,
    wheat bran and their components. Am J Clin Nutr 30: 1721-1725 (77)
68 Jenkins DJ, Gassull MA, Leeds AR, et al: Pectin and post-gastric surgery: prevention
    of postprandial hypoglycaemia. Gut 18: A412-A413 (77)
69 Jenkins DJ, Gassull MA, Leeds AR: Effect of dietary fiber on complications of
    gastric surgery: prevention of postprandial hypoglycemia by pectin. Gastroenterology
    73: 215-217 (77)
70 Jenkins DJ, Hockaday TD, Howarth R, et al: Treatment of diabetes with guar gum:
    reduction of urinary glucose loss in diabetics. Lancet 2: 779-780 (77)
71 Jenkins DJ, Leeds AR, Gassull MA, et al: Decrease in postprandial insulin and
    glucose concentrations by guar and pectin. Ann Intern Med 86: 20-23 (77)
72 Jenkins DJ, Leeds AR, Gassull MA, et al: Viscosity and the action of unavailable
    carbohydrate in reducing postprandial glucose and insulin levels. Proc Nutr Soc 36:
    44A (77)
73 Jenkins DJ, Leeds AR, Houston H, et al: Carbohydrate tolerance in man after

six weeks of pectin administration. Proc Nutr Soc 36: 62A (77)

74 Jenkins DJ, Leeds AR, Slavin B, et al: Reduction of serum cholesterol in type II hyperlipidaemia by guar gum. Proc Nutr Soc 36: 94A (77)

75 Jones JM: Trace elements in human nutrition. Cereal Foods World 22: 573-574, 576-578 (77)

76 Kay RM, Truswell AS: The effect of wheat fibre on plasma lipids and faecal steroid excretion in man. Br J Nutr 37: 227-235 (77)

77 Kay RM, Truswell AS: The effect of citrus pectin on blood lipids and fecal steroid excretion in man. Am J Clin Nutr 30: 171-175 (77)

78 Kimura KK: High fiber diet – who needs it? Cereal Foods World 22: 16-19 (77)

79 Kirwan WO, Smith AN: Colonic propulsion in diverticular disease, idiopathic constipation and irritable colon syndrome. Scand J Gastroenterol 12: 331-335 (77)

80 Kloppers PJ, Fehrsen GS: Western diseases in developing peoples: in search of a 'marker'. S Afr Med J 51: 745-746 (77)

81 Kritchevsky D: Diet and cholesterolemia. Lipids 12: 49-52 (77)

82 Kritchevsky D: Modification by fiber of toxic dietary effects. Fed Proc 36: 1692-1695 (77)

83 Kritchevsky D: Dietary fiber and other dietary factors in hypercholesterolemia. Am J Clin Nutr 30: 979-984 (77)

84 Kritchevsky D: Diet and atherosclerosis, pp 93-106. In: *Dietary Fiber and Health,* US Senate Select Committee on Nutrition and Human Needs, Washington, US Government Printing Office (77)

85 Kritchevsky D: Atherosclerosis and dietary fiber, pp 179-185. In: *Atherosclerosis Reviews* vol 2: ed. Paoletti R and Gotto AM Jr. New York, Raven Press (77)

86 Kritchevsky D: Dietary fiber: what it is and what it does. Ann NY Acad Sci 300: 283-289 (77)

87 Kritchevsky D, Davidson LM, Kim HK, et al: Influence of semi-purified diets on atherosclerosis in African green monkeys. Exp Mol Pathol 26: 28-51 (77)

88 Kritchevsky D, Tepper SA, Williams DE, et al: Experimental atherosclerosis in rabbits fed cholesterol-free diets. Part 7. Interaction of animal or vegetable protein with fiber. Atherosclerosis 26: 397-403 (77)

89 Kuroda N, Ohnishi M, Fuyino Y: Sterol lipids in rice bran. Cereal Chem 54: 997-1006 (77)

90 Langley NJ, Thye FW: The effect of wheat bran and/or citrus pectin on serum cholesterol and triglycerides in middle-aged men. Fed Proc 36: 1118 (77)

91 Levy N, Luboshitzki R, Shiratzki Y, et al: Diverticulosis of the colon in Israel. Dis Colon Rectum 20: 477-481 (77)

92 Malhotra SL: Dietary factors in a study of cancer colon from Cancer Registry, with special reference to the role of saliva, milk and fermented milk products and vegetable fibre. Med Hypotheses 3: 122-126 (77)

93 Manning AP, Heaton KW, Harvey RF, et al: Wheat fibre and irritable bowel syndrome. A controlled trial. Lancet 2: 417-418 (77)

94 Manousos ON, Nicolaou A, Trichopoulos D: Bowel transit, stool weight, and diverticular disease (letter). Lancet 2: 360 (77)

95 *Marabou Symposium: Food and Fibre.* Nutr Rev 35: 6-54 (77)

96 Mathé D, Lutton C, Routureau J, et al: Effects of dietary fiber and salt mixtures on the cholesterol metabolism of rats. J Nutr 107: 466-474 (77)

97 Mathur MS, Singh F, Chadda VS: Effect of bran on blood lipids. J Assoc Physicians India 25: 275-278 (77)

98 Mattha AG: Rheological studies of Plantago Albicans (Psyllium) seed gum dispersions. General flow characteristics. Pharm Acta Helv 52: 210-213 (77)

99 Mattha AG: Rheological studies of Plantago Albicans (Psyllium) seed gum dispersions. II. Effect of some pharmaceutical additives. Pharm Acta Helv 52: 214-217 (77)

100 McNeil NI, Cummings JH, James WP: Short chain fatty acid absorption in the human large bowel. Gut 18: A425-A426 (77)

101 Mehta A: When the complaint is abdominal pain, consider diverticular disease. Mod Geriatrics 7: 64-67 (77)

102 Mendeloff AI: The Burkitt hypothesis (letter). Am J Dig Dis 22: 73-76 (77)

103 Mendeloff AI: Dietary fiber and human health. New Engl J Med 297: 811-814 (77)

104 Mendeloff AI: Statement at hearings on fiber, pp 72-75. In: *Dietary Fiber and Health,* US Senate Select Committee on Nutrition and Human Needs, Washington, US Government Printing Office (77)

105 Miettinen TA, Tarpila S: Effect of pectin on serum cholesterol, faecal bile acids and biliary lipids in normolipidaemic and hyperlipidaemic individuals. Clin Chim Acta 79: 471-477 (77)

106 Miranda PM, Horowitz DL: The effect of dietary fiber on plasma glucose levels in diabetes. Diabetes 26 (Suppl 1): 356 (77)

107 Morris JN, Marr JW, Clayton DG: Diet and heart: a postscript. Br Med J 2: 1307-1314 (77)

108 Moynahan EJ: Nutritional hazards of high-fibre diet (letter). Lancet 1: 654-655 (77)

109 Omori M, Muto Y: Effects of dietary protein, calcium, phosphorus and fibre on renal accumulation of exogenous cadmium in young rats. J Nutr Sci Vitaminol 23: 361-373 (77)

110 Painter NS: The Burkitt Hypothesis (letter). Am J Dig Dis 22: 74 (77)

111 Painter NS: The epidemiology, history and pathogenesis of diverticulosis coli – basis for its treatment with unprocessed bran. Schweiz Med Wochenschr 107: 486-493 (77)

112 Pomare EW: Dietary fibre: when is it worth a trial. Drugs 14: 213-219 (77)

113 Prentice N, D'Appolonia BL: High fiber bread containing brewer's spent grain. Cereal Chem 54: 1084-1095 (77)

114 Raymond TL, Connor WE, Lin DS, et al: The interaction of dietary fibers and cholesterol upon the plasma lipids and lipoproteins, sterol balance and bowel function in human subjects. J Clin Invest 60: 1429-1437 (77)

115 Reilly RW, Kirsner JB: Dietary fiber and the colon, pp 521-524. In: Glass GB, ed. *Progress in Gastroenterology,* Vol 3. New York, Grune and Stratton (77)

116 Richardson JB, Dixon M: Varicose veins in tropical Africa. Lancet 1: 791-792 (77)

117 Salter RH: Idiopathic slow transit constipation. Practitioner 218: 623 (77)

118 Sanders TA, Ellis FR, Baird IM, et al: Effect of wholemeal and white bread on iron absorption (letter). Br Med J 2: 236-237 (77)

119 Sandstead HH, Klevay L, Munoz J, et al: Zinc and copper balance in humans fed fiber. Fed Proc 36: 1118 (77)

120 Schaller D: Analysis of dietary fiber. Food Proc Dev 11: 70-72 (77)

121 Schaller D: Fiber content and structure in foods, pp 112-116. In: *Dietary Fiber and Health,* US Senate Select Committee on Nutrition and Human Needs, Washington, US Government Printing Office (77)

122 Schneeman BO: The effect of plant fiber on trypsin and chymotrypsin activity in vitro. Fed Proc 36: 1118 (77)

123 Schuster MM: Constipation and anorectal disorders. Clin Gastroenterol 6: 643-658 (77)

124   Schwartz K: Silicon, fibre, and atherosclerosis. Lancet 1: 454-457 (77)
125   Segal I, Soloman A, Hunt JA: Emergence of diverticular disease in the urban South African Black. Gastroenterology 72: 215-219 (77)
126   Smith AN: Fibre, intra-colonic pressure and diverticular disease. Health Bull (Edinb) 35: 49-54 (77)
127   Southgate DA: The definition and analysis of dietary fibre. Nutr Rev 35: 31-37 (77)
128   Southgate DA: Non-assimilable components of food, pp 199-204. In: Hollingsworth D, Russell M, ed *Nutritional Problems in a Changing World,* Barking, Applied Science (77)
129   Spiller GA: 'Fibre' in the vocabulary of nutrition (letter). Lancet 1: 198 (77)
130   Spiller GA, Shipley EA: Perspectives in dietary fiber in human nutrition. World Rev Nutr Diet 27: 105-131 (77)
131   Spiller GA, Shipley EA: Observation on dietary fiber terminology and possible requirement in human nutrition, pp 107-111. In: *Dietary Fiber and Human Needs,* US Senate Select Committee on Nutrition and Human Needs, Washington, US Government Printing Office (77)
132   Spiller GA, Chernoff MC, Shipley EA, et al: Can fecal weight be used to establish a recommended intake of dietary fiber (plantix)? (letter). Am J Clin Nutr 30: 659-661 (77)
133   Story JA, Czarnecki SK, Baldino A, et al: Effect of components of fiber on dietary cholesterol in rats. Fed Proc 36: 1134 (77)
134   Tadesse K, Eastwood MA: Metabolism of dietary fibre components in man, as assessed by breath hydrogen and methane. Gut 18: A944 (77)
135   Tarpila S, Miettinen TA: Effects of plantago fibre on serum lipids and faecal composition in hypercholesterolaemic patients. Scand J Gastroenterol (Suppl) 45: 105 (77)
136   Taylor KB: Gastroenterology, pp 332-340. In: Schneider HA et al. ed. *Nutritional Support of Medical Practice,* London, Harper and Row (77)
137   Thompson WG: Diet and diverticula (Editorial). Can Med Assoc J 116: 468 (77)
138   Trowell H: Food and dietary fibre. Nutr Rev 35: 6-11 (77)
139   Trowell H: Dietary fibre versus plantix (letter). Lancet 1: 655 (77)
140   Trowell H: Diet and coronary heart disease (letter). Br Med J 1: 1283-1284 (77)
141   Trowell H: Why a new term for dietary fiber? (letter). Am J Clin Nutr 30: 1003-1004 (77)
142   Trowell HC: Dietary fibre and diseases of the large bowel. Practitioner 219: 350-354 (77)
143   Trowell H: Cardiovascular diseases and fibre. Chest Heart and Stroke J 2: 1-7 (77)
144   Trowell HC: Western diseases, starchy foods and fibre. Medicine Digest 3: 6-14 (77)
145   Trowell HC: Statement at fibre hearings, pp 50-57. In: *Dietary Fiber and Health,* US Senate Select Committee on Nutrition and Human Needs, Washington, US Government Printing Office (77)
146   Trowell HC: Diabetes mellitus and the dietary fiber of the starchy foods, pp 116-121. In: *Dietary Fiber and Health.* US Senate Select Committee on Nutrition and Human Needs, Washington, US Government Printing Office (77)
147   Trowell HC: Pathological growth and maturation in infants and children associated with modern methods of feeding, pp 181-188. In: *Dietary Fiber and Health,* US Senate Select Committee on Nutrition and Human Needs, Washington, US Government Printing Office (77)

148 Trowell HC, Burkitt DP: Dietary fiber and cardiovascular disease. Artery 3: 107-119 (77)

149 Tudge C: Bread in the head. New Scientist 76: 812-813 (77)

150 United States Senate Select Committee on Nutrition and Human Needs: *Dietary Goals for the United States,* Washington, US Government Printing Office (77)

151 United States Senate Select Committee on Nutrition and Human Needs: *Diet Related to Killer Diseases. 4. Dietary Fiber and Health,* Washington, US Government Printing Office (77)

152 Uwaifo AO, Bassir O: The effect of functional groups on the interaction of aflatoxins B1 and G1 with starch, cellulose and seven cellulose derivatives. Biochem Pharmacol 26: 863-866 (77)

153 Van Soest PJ: Statement at Fiber Hearings, pp 60-72. In: *Dietary Fiber and Health,* US Senate Select Committee on Nutrition and Human Needs, Washington, US Government Printing Office (77)

154 Vickery K: Dietary fiber in perspective (letter). Lancet 2: 408 (77)

155 Walan A, Bergdahl B, Skoog ML, et al: Study of digoxin bioavailability during treatment with a bulk forming laxative (Metamucil). Scand J Gastroenterol (Suppl) 45: 111 (77)

156 Walker AR, Walker BF: Effect of wholemeal and white bread on iron absorption (letter). Br Med J 2: 771-772 (77)

157 Walker AR: Health implications of fibre-depleted diets. S Afr Med J 52: 767-770 (77)

158 Walker AR, Gajjar D: Gastro-intestinal transit times and serum lipid levels in Black schoolchildren. S Afr Med J 52: 677-679 (77)

159 Watson WC, Corke M, Pomare EW, et al: A double blind study on the effect of dietary fibre on stool frequency and appearance, abdominal symptoms and serum lipid levels in patients with the irritable bowel syndrome (IBS). Gastroenterology 72: A-123/1146 (77)

160 Weisburger JH, Reddy BS, Wynder EL: Colon cancer: its epidemiology and experimental production. Cancer 40: 2414-2420 (77)

161 Wilson RB, Hutchinson DP, Wideman L: Dimethylhydrazine-induced colon tumors in rats fed diets containing beef fat or corn oil with or without wheat bran. Am J Clin Nutr 30: 176-181 (77)

162 Weinreich J, Pedersen O, Dinesen K: Role of bran in normals. Serum levels of cholesterols, triglyceride, calcium and total 3-alpha-hydroxy-cholanic acid and intestinal transit time. Acta Med Scand 202: 125-130 (77)

163 Woolfe JA: The effects of okra mucilage (Hibiscus Esculentus L) on the plasma cholesterol level in rats. Proc Nutr Soc 36: 59A (77)

164 Wynder EL, Reddy BS, McCoy DG, et al: Diet and cancer of the gastrointestinal tract, pp 397-419. In: Stollerman GH ed. *Advances in Internal Medicine,* Chicago, Year Book Medical Publishers, Vol 22 (77)

Foreign Language Citations 1977

French:

165 Capron JP: Essais therapeutiques de la lithiase biliar en dehors l'acide chenodeoxycholique (Therapy of gallstones excluding the use of chenodeoxycholic acid). Therapie 32: 409-416 (77)

166 Claude R: Regimes riches en fibres (Regimens rich in fibre). Gaz Med France 84: 4087-4090 (77)

167   Frexinos J, Escourrau J: Du bon usage de son de blé (Proper use of dietary fibre).
      Nouv Presse Med 6: 3328-3329 (77)
168   Lambert R, Audiger J-C: Laxatifs ou fibres alimentaires. Plaidoyer pour un trait-
      ment rationnel de la constipation (Laxatives or dietary fibre. A plea for a rational
      treatment for constipation). Nouv Presse Med 6: 2219-2221 (77)
169   Bure J, Guinet R: Le pain de demain? (The bread of tomorrow?). Ind Aliment Agric
      94: 999-1006 (77)

German:
170   Filippini L: Die Divertelkrankheit des Sigmas (Diverticular disease of the sigmoid
      colon). Praxis 66: 295-302 (77)
171   Gnauck R: Die bedentung fasserreicher Kost bie der Therapie von Divertikulose,
      Obstipation und Colon irritable (Dietary measures in the therapy of diverticulosis,
      chronic constipation and irritable colon). Therapiewoche 27: 6411-6412 (77)
172   Hansen HH; Pathomorphology und Therapie des Haemorrhoidalleidens (Pathomor-
      phology and therapy of haemorrhoids). Hautarzt 28: 364-367 (77)
173   Knick B: Ernaehrung bei funktionallen margen Darmstoerungen (Treatment of
      functional gastric disorders). Therapiewoche 27: 6404-6406, 6409-6410 (77)
174   Linhart P: Colon irritable (Irritable colon). Therapiewoche 27: 6396-6400, 6403 (77)
175   Philip J, Fuchs HF: Divertikulosis und Divertikulitis. Pathogenese, Diagnose und
      Therapie (Diverticulosis and diverticulitis. Pathogenesis, diagnosis and therapy). Med
      Welt 28: 1744-1747 (77)
176   Schardt F: Wechselwirkungen von Antirheumatika (Interactions of antirheumatics).
      Therapiewoche 27: 8805-8808 (77)

Dutch:
177   Bartelink A: Het irritable bowel syndroom (The irritable bowel syndrome). Ned
      Tijdschr Geneesk 121: 1462-1465 (77)

Italian:
178   Bassello O, Ostuzzi R, Armellini F: Il ruolo della fibra grezza nella pathologia
      metabolica (The role of dietary fibre in metabolic pathology). Recent Prog Med
      (Roma) 63: 1-12 (77)
179   Feruglio FS: Terapia della malatta diverticulare del colon (Therapy of diverticular
      disease of the colon). Minerva Med 68: 3724-3726 (77)
180   Romanelli R, Romoli R, Cini F, et al: Dieta alto contenato fibroso e patologia gastro-
      enterica dell anziano (Fibre content of diet and gastrointestinal pathology in the
      elderly). G Gerontol 25: 1040 (77)

Spanish:
181   Villalonga EF, Benitez JH, Ramos EF: Encuesta sobre la alimentacion que han lecho
      los enfermos de litiasis biliar (Dietary survey among gallstone patients). Rev Clin
      Esp 147: 61-66 (77)

Russian:
182   Surikova VV: Pectin content in some products manufactured by the food industry in
      the BSSR. Zdravokhr Beloruss (12): 42-43 (77)

1976

1   Alcantara EN, Speckmann EW, Graham GG: Diet, nutrition, and cancer. Am J Clin Nutr 29: 1035-1047 (76)

2   Almy TP: The role of fiber in the diet. Curr Concepts Nutr 4: 155-169 (76)

3   Ammann R: [Is chronic constipation harmless? From cellulose to arteriosclerosis, colonic carcinoma and other 'western diseases']. Schweiz Med Wochenschr 106: 697-699 (76)

4   Anderson JW: Influence of type of carbohydrate on the triglyceride response to high carbohydrate diets in diabetic men (abstract). Am J Clin Nutr 29: 471 (76)

5   Balasegaram M, Burkitt DP: Stool characteristics and western diseases (letter). Lancet 1: 152 (76)

6   Bassler TJ, Cardello FP: Fiber-feeding and atherosclerosis (letter). J Am Med Assoc 235: 1841-1842 (76)

7   Bing FC: Dietary fiber — in historical perspective. J Am Diet Assoc 69: 498-505 (76)

8   Bonnevie-Nielson V: [Dietary fibre: a protective factor in the diet]. Ugeskr Laeger 138: 199-203 (76)

9   Brasher C: Dietary fibre: search for the facts (letter). Br Med J 1: 94-95 (76)

10   Brodribb AJ, Humphreys DM: Diverticular disease: three studies. Part I Relation to other disorders and fibre intake. Br Med J 1: 424-425 (76)

11   Brodribb AJ, Humphreys DM: Diverticular disease: three studies. Part II Treatment with bran. Ibid 425-428 (76)

12   Brodribb AJ, Humphreys DM: Diverticular disease: three studies. Part III Metabolic effect of bran in patients with diverticular disease. Ibid 428-430 (76)

13   Brown KL: Dietary fiber — what is it? J Arkansas Med Soc 73: 275-277 (76)

14   Burkitt DP: Varicose veins: facts and fantasy. Arch Surg 111: 1327-1332 (76)

15   Burkitt DP: Varicose veins in developing countries (letter). Lancet 2: 472 (76)

16   Burkitt DP: The role of fibre in the human diet. Finska Läkar Hand Arg 120: 123-127 (76)

17   Burkitt DP: A deficiency of dietary fiber may be one cause of certain colonic and venous disorders. Am J Dig Dis 21: 104-108 (76)

18   Burkitt DP: Stool weights in western children (letter). Lancet 2: 633 (76)

19   Burkitt DP: Some mechanical effects of fibre-depleted diets. In: *Dietary Fibre,* Miles Symposium, editor W W Hawkins, 5-12. Halifax Canada (76)

20   Burkitt DP, Townsend AJ, Patel K, et al: Varicose veins in developing countries (letter). Lancet 2: 202-203 (76)

21   Burkitt DP, Walker AR: Saint's triad: confirmation and explanation. S Afr Med J 50: 2136-2138 (76)

22   Campbell BJ, Reinhold JG, Cannell JS, et al: The effects of prolonged consumption of wholemeal bread upon metabolism of calcium, magnesium, zinc and phosphorus of two young American adults. Pahlavi Med J 7: 1-17 (76)

23   Chang ML, Johnson MA: Influence of fat level and type of carbohydrate on the capacity of pectin in lowering serum and liver lipids of young rats. J Nutr 106: 1562-1568 (76)

24   Cleave TL: Bran and the irritable bowel (letter). Lancet 1: 540 (76)

25   Connell AM: Natural fiber and bowel dysfunction. Am J Clin Nutr 29: 1427-1431 (76)

26   Coste T et al: [Current concepts on dietary fibres. Their role in human pathology]. Med Chir Dig 5: 287-291 (76)

27   Cummings JH: What is fiber? In: *Fiber in Human Nutrition,* editors GA Spiller, RJ Amen 1-30. Plenum Press New York and London (76)

28   Cummings JH, Hill MJ, Jenkins DJ, et al: Changes in fecal composition and colonic function due to cereal fiber. Am J Clin Nutr 29: 1468-1473 (76)

29   Cummings JH, Jenkins DJ, Wiggins HS: Measurement of the mean transit time of dietary residue through the human gut. Gut 17: 210-218 (76)

30   Cummings JH, Wiggins HS: Transit through the gut measured by analysis of a single stool. Gut 17: 219-223 (76)

31   Donefer E: The importance of fibre for herbivorous animals. In: *Dietary Fibre,* editor WW Hawkins, 51-56 Miles Symposium, Halifax Canada (76)

32   Dorfman, SH, Ali M, Floch MH: Low fiber content of Connecticut diets. Am J Clin Nutr 29:87-89 (76)

33   Douglass J, Rasgon I: Diet and diabetes (letter). Lancet 2: 1306-1307 (76)

34   Drasar BS, Jenkins DJ: Bacteria, diet and large bowel cancer. Am J. Clin Nutr 29: 1410-1416 (76)

35   Drasar BS, Jenkins DJ, Cummings JH: The influence of a diet rich in wheat fibre on the human faecal flora. J Med Microbiol 9: 423-431 (76)

36   Durrington PN, Manning AP, Bolton CH, et al: Effect of pectin on serum lipids and lipoproteins, whole-gut transit-time and stool weight. Lancet 2: 394-396 (76)

37   Eastwood MA: Fibre and enterohepatic circulation. In: *Food and Fibre.* Marabou Symposium 42-44. Sundbyberg Sweden (76)

38   Eastwood MA, Eastwood J, Ward M: Epidemiology of bowel disease. In: *Fiber in Human Nutrition,* editors GA Spiller, RJ Amen 207-240. Plenum Press New York and London (76)

39   Eastwood MA, Mitchell WD: Physical properties of fiber: a biological evaluation. In: *Fiber in Human Nutrition,* editors GA Spiller, RJ Amen 109-129. Plenum Press New York and London (76)

40   Eastwood M, Mowbray L: The binding of the components of mixed micelle to dietary fiber. Am J Clin Nutr 29: 1461-1467 (76)

41   Elchazly M, Thomas B: [A simple biochemical method for the determination of dietary fibre in plant foods.] Z Lebensm Unters-Forsch 162: 329-340 (76)

42   Fisher N: Bran content of wholemeal bread (letter). Br Med J 1: 647 (76)

43   Floch MH editor: Symposium on diet, bacteria, and the colon. Am J Clin Nutr 29: 1405-1484 (76)

44   Frohn MJ: Left-leg varicose veins and deep-vein thrombosis (letter). Lancet 2: 1019-1020 (76)

45   Fuchs H-M, Dorfman S, Floch MH: The effect of dietary fiber supplementation in man. II, Alterations in fecal physiology and bacterial flora. Am J Clin Nutr 29: 1443-1447 (76)

46   Galton L: *The Truth About Fiber in Your Food.* Crown Publishers New York (76)

47   Gassull MA, Goff DV, Haisman P, et al: The effect of unavailable carbohydrate gelling agents in reducing the post-prandial glycaemia in normal volunteers and diabetics. J Physiol 256: 52P-53P (76)

48   Gassull MA, Leeds A, Jenkins DJ: Glucose absorption and diabetes (letter). Br Med J 1: 1279-1280 (76)

49   Gelfand M: The pattern of disease in Africa and the Western way of life. Trop Doctor 6: 173-179 (76)

50   Glasby M: Pityrophagous gingivitis or bran-gum? (letter). Lancet 2: 1087 (76)

51   Godding EW: Dietary fibre redefined (letter). Lancet 1: 1129 (76)

52   Godding EW: What are healthy bowels? (letter). Lancet 1: 1294-1295 (76)

53   Goy JA, Eastwood MA, Mitchell WD, et al: Fecal characteristics contrasted in the irritable bowel syndrome and diverticular disease. Am J Clin Nutr 29: 1480-1484 (76)

54   Grimes DS: Refined carbohydrate, smooth-muscle spasm and disease of the colon. Lancet 1: 395-397 (76)

55   Hall RC: The bran-wagon (letter). Br Med J 1: 1076 (76)

56   Hamilton RM, Carroll KK: Plasma cholesterol levels in rabbits fed low fat, low cholesterol diets: effects of dietary proteins, carbohydrates and fibre from different sources. Atherosclerosis 24: 47-62 (76)

57   Hansen OH, Pederson T, Larsen JK: Cell proliferation kinetics in normal human gastric mucosa. Studies on diurnal fluctuations and effect of food ingestion. Gastroenterology 70: 1051-1054 (76)

58   Hart GR, Gunnin BE: The effect of fiber on intestinal transit time in mice (abstract). Am J Clin Nutr 29: 478 (76)

59   Hawkins WW (editor): *Dietary Fibre,* Miles Symposium, Nutrition Society of Canada Halifax Canda (76)

60   Heaton KW: Fiber, blood lipids, and heart disease (letter). Am J Clin Nutr 29: 125-126 (76)

61   Heaton KW, Low-Beer TS: Unrefined carbohydrate diet and weight (letter). New Eng J Med 294: 177 (76)

62   Heaton KW, Manning AP, Hartog M: Lack of effect on blood lipid and calcium concentrations of young men on changing from white to wholemeal bread. Br J Nutr 35: 55-60 (76)

63   Hegsted DM: Food and fibre: evidence from experimental animals. In: *Food and Fibre,* Marabou Symposium, Syndbyberg Sweden 45-50 (76)

64   Hellendoorn EW: Beneficial physiologic action of beans. J Am Diet Assoc 69: 248-253 (76)

65   Herrera AF: Medical treatment of diverticular disease. Postgrad Med 60: 107-109 (76)

66   Herxheimer A: Bran tablets and diverticular disease (letter). Br Med J 1: 1341 (76)

67   Hobbs JT: Varicose veins in developing countries (letter). Lancet 2: 259 (76)

68   Hudson GJ, John PM, Bailey BS, et al: The automated determination of carbohydrate. Development of a method for available carbohydrates and its application to foodstuffs. J Sci Food Agric 27: 681-687 (76)

69   Hungate RE: Microbial activities related to mammalian digestion and absorption of food. In: *Fiber in Human Nutrition,* editors GA Spiller and RJ Amen 131-149. Plenum Press New York and London (76)

70   Hunt T: Dr Allinson and the wholemeal load. World Med 11: 58-60 (76)

71   Jenkins DJ, Leeds AR, Gassull MA, et al: Unabsorbable carbohydrates and diabetes: decreased post-prandial hyperglycaemia. Lancet 2: 172-174 (76)

72   Jenkins DJ, Goff DV, Leeds AR, et al: The cholesterol lowering properties of guar and pectin. Clin Sci Mol Med 51: 8p-9p (76)

73   Jenkins DJ, Leeds AR, Slavin B, et al: Guar gum in hyperlipidaemia (letter). Lancet 2: 1351 (76)

74   Jenkins DJ, Wolever TM, Haworth R, et al: Guar gum in diabetes (letter). Lancet 2: 1086-1087 (76)

75   Judd PA, Kay RM, Truswell AS: Cholesterol-lowering effect of lignin in rats (abstract). Proc Nutr Soc 35: 73A (76)

76   Kahaner N, Fuchs H-M, Floch MH: The effect of dietary fiber supplementation in man. 1. Modification of eating habits. Am J Clin Nutr 29: 1437-1442 (76)

77   Kiehm TG, Anderson JW, Ward K: Beneficial effects of a high carbohydrate, high fiber diet on hyperglycemic diabetic men. Am J Clin Nutr 29: 895-899 (76)

78   Kimura KK: Refined carbohydrates, dietary fiber, and gastrointestinal abnormality (letter). J Am Med Assoc 235: 375 (76)

79   Klevay LM: Ischemic heart disease: the fiber hypothesis. In: *Dietary Fibre,* editor WW Hawkins 33-39. Miles Symposium Halifax Canada (76)

80   Kritchevsky D: Diet and atherosclerosis. Am J Pathol 84: 615-632 (76)

81   Kritchevsky D, Story JA, Walker AR: Binding of sodium taurocholate by cereal products. S Afr Med J 50: 1831 (76)

82   Lang JA, Briggs GM: The use and function of fiber in diets of monogastric animals. In: *Fiber in Human Nutrition,* editors GA Spiller, RJ Amen 151-169. Plenum Press New York and London (76)

83   Latto C: Postoperative deep-vein thrombosis, pulmonary embolism, and high-fibre diet (letter). Lancet 2: 1197 (76)

84   Leeds A, Gassull MA, Jenkins DJ, et al: Metabolic effects of bran (letter). Br Med J 1: 900-901 (76)

85   Macdonald I: The effects of dietary fiber: are they all good? In: *Fiber in Human Nutrition,* editors GA Spiller and RJ Amen 263-269. Plenum Press New York and London (76)

86   MacLean WC Jr, De Romana GL, Graham GG: Short-term effect of wheat based diets on serum lipids in children (abstract). Am J Clin Nutr 29: 480 (76)

87   Malhotra SL: Protective role of dietary factors in coronary heart disease. Practitioner 217: 929-934 (76)

88   Malinow MR, McLaughlin P, Papworth L, et al: Effect of bran and cholestyramine on plasma lipids in monkeys. Am J Clin Nutr 29: 905-911 (76)

89   Manning AP, Heaton KW: Bran and the irritable bowel (letter). Lancet 1: 588 (76)

90   Manning AP, Heaton KW, Harvey RF, et al: Cereal fibre and irritable bowel – a controlled trial. Gut 17: 822-823 (76)

91   Marabou Symposium: *Food and Fibre,* editor not stated. Sundbyberg Sweden Sept (76)

92   Martin A, Olding-Smee W: Pressure changes in varicose veins. Lancet 1: 768-700 (76)

93   Mastromarino A, Reddy BS, Wynder EL: Metabolic epidemiology of colon cancer: enzymic activity of fecal flora. Am J Clin Nutr 29: 1455-1460 (76)

94   Mendeloff AI: A critique of 'fiber deficiency'. Am J Dig Dis 21: 109-122 (76)

95   Menon PV, Kurup PA: Dietary fibre and cholesterol metabolism: effect of fibre rich polysaccharide from Blackgram (Phaseolus Mungo) on cholesterol metabolism in rats fed normal and atherogenic diet. Biomedicine 24: 248-253 (76)

96   Mitchell WD, Eastwood MA: Dietary fiber and colon function. In: *Fiber in human Nutrition,* editors GA Spiller and RJ Amen 185-206. Plenum Press New York and London (76)

97   Moore MC, Guzman MA, Schilling PE, et al: Dietary-atherosclerosis study on deceased persons. Relation of selected dietary components to raised coronary lesions. J Am Diet Assoc 68: 216-223 (76)

98   Morris ER, Ellis R: Isolation of monoferric phytate from wheat bran and its biological value as an iron source in the rat. J Nutr 106: 753-760 (76)

99   Painter NS: Bran and the irritable bowel (letter). Lancet 1: 540 (76)

100   Painter NS: Diverticular disease of the colon: a bane of the elderly. Geriatrics 31: 89-94 (76)

101   Painter NS: The bran-wagon (letter). Brit Med J 1: 1400 (76)

102   Painter NS: Diverticular disease of the colon and dietary fiber. In: *Gastrointestinal*

Emergencies, editors HR Clearfield and VP Dinoso Jr. 143-152. Grune and Stratton New York (76)

103 Persson I, Raby K, Fønns-Bech P, et al: Effect of prolonged bran administration on serum levels of cholesterol, ionised calcium and iron in the elderly. J Am Ger Soc 24: 334-335 (76)

104 Pomare EW, Heaton KW, Low-Beer TS, et al: The effect of wheat bran upon bile salt metabolism and upon lipid composition of bile in gallstone patients. Am J Digest Dis 21: 521-526 (76)

105 Pore MS, Magar NG: Effect of ragi feeding on serum cholesterol level. Ind J Med Res 64: 909-914 (76)

106 Reddy BS: Dietary factors and cancer of the large bowel. Semin Oncol 3: 351-359 (76)

107 Reinhold JG: Rickets in Asian immigrants (letter). Lancet 2: 1132-1133 (76)

108 Reinhold JG, Faradji B, Abadi P, et al: Decreased absorption of calcium, magnesium, zinc and phosphorus by humans due to increased fiber and phosphorus consumption of wheat bread. J Nutr 106: 493-503 (76)

109 Ricketts HT: Fiber and diabetes (editorial). J Am Med Assoc 236: 2321-2322 (76)

110 Russell RM, Ismail-Beigi F, Reinhold JG: Folate content of Iranian breads and the effect of their fiber content on the intestinal absorption of folic acid. Am J Clin Nutr 29: 799-802 (76)

111 Rutter K, Maxwell D: Diseases of the alimentary system. Constipation and laxative abuse. Br Med J 2: 997-1000 (76)

112 Savory CJ et al: Effects of dietary dilution with fibre on the food intake and gut dimensions of Japanese quail. Br Poult Sci 17: 561-570 (76)

113 Savory CJ et al: Changes in food intake and gut size in Japanese quail in response to manipulation of dietary fibre content. Br Poult Sci 17: 571-580 (76)

114 Sethbhakdi S: Pathogenesis of colonic diverticulitis and diverticulosis. Postgrad Med 60: 76-81 (76)

115 Søltoft J, Gudmand-Høyer E, Krag B, et al: [Bran in the treatment of irritable colon. A double-blind controlled investigation]. Ugeskr Laeger 138: 3316-3318 (76)

116 Søltoft J, Gudmand-Høyer E, Krag B, et al: A double-blind trial of the effect of wheat bran on symptoms of irritable bowel syndrome. Lancet 1: 270-272 (76)

117 Southgate DA: *Determination of Food Carbohydrates.* Applied Science Publishers London (76)

118 Southgate DA: The definition and analysis of dietary fibre. In: *Food and Dietary Fibre,* editor not stated, 31-37. Marabou Symposium Sundbyberg Sweden (76)

119 Southgate DA: The chemistry of dietary fiber. In: *Fiber in Human Nutrition,* editors GA Spiller and RJ Amen 31-72. Plenum Press New York and London (76)

120 Southgate DA: The analysis of fiber. Ibid 73-107 (76)

121 Southgate DA: Dietary fibre (letter). Br Med J 2: 236 (76)

122 Southgate DA, Bailey B, Collinson E, et al: A guide to calculating intakes of dietary fibre. J Hum Nutr 30: 303-313 (76)

123 Southgate DA, Branch WJ, Hill MJ, et al: Metabolic responses to dietary supplements of bran. Metabolism 25: 1129-1135 (76)

124 Spiller GA, Amen RJ (editors): *Fiber in Human Nutrition.* Plenum Press New York and London (76)

125 Spiller GA, Fassett-Cornelius G, Briggs GM: A new term for plant fibers in nutrition (letter). Am J Clin Nutr 29: 934-935 (76)

126 Spiller GA, Sorensen SG: Dietary fiber and human intestinal microflora. In: *Dietary Fibre,* editor WW Hawkins 41-49. Miles Symposium Halifax Canada (76)

127 Srivastava GR, Smith AN, Painter NS: Sterculia bulk-forming agent with smooth-muscle relaxant versus bran in diverticular disease. Br Med J 1: 315-318 (76)

128 Stanway A: *Taking the Routh With The Smooth. Dietary Fibre and Your Health — a new medical breakthrough.* Souvenir Press London (76)

129 Story JA, Kritchevsky D: Comparison of the binding of various bile acids and bile salts *in vitro* by various types of fiber. J Nutr 106: 1292-1294 (76)

130 Story JA, Kritchevsky D: Dietary fiber and lipid metabolism. In: *Fiber in Human Nutrition,* editors GA Spiller and RJ Amen 171-184. Plenum Press New York and London (76)

131 Story JA, Tepper SA, Kritchevsky D: Influence of fibre on intestinal function: involvement in cholesterol and bile acid metabolism. In: *Dietary Fibre,* editor WW Hawkins 27-31. Miles Symposium Halifax Canada (76)

132 Tasman-Jones C: Does dietary fibre deficiency kill? N Z Med J 83: 275-278 (76)

133 Taylor I, Duthie HL: Bran tablets and diverticular disease. Br Med J 1: 988-990 (76)

134 Theander O: The chemistry of dietary fibres. In: *Food and Fibre,* Marabou Symposium 23-30. Sundbyberg Sweden (76)

135 Thomas B: [Fiber-rich food as a diet form]. Dtsch Krankempenflegez 29: 425-429 (76)

136 Thomas B, Riewermann U: *Veränderungen de Rohfasergehalts der Kostder letzen 100 Jahre in Deütschland.* Berlin (76)

137 Thomas B, Elchazly M: [The physiological effects and changes of the dietary-fibre of wheat in the digestive tract]. Qual Plant Fds Hum Nutr 26: 211-226 (76)

138 Trowell H: Definition of dietary fiber and hypotheses that it is a protective factor in certain diseases. Am J Clin Nutr 29: 417-427 (76)

139 Trowell H: Fibre inadequately replaced by cellulose or other forms of roughage in animal experimental diets (letter). Thromb Haemostasis (Stuttg) 36: 489-492 (76)

140 Trowell H: Food and dietary fibre. In: *Food and Fibre,* Marabou Symposium 6-11. Sundbyberg Sweden (76)

141 Trowell H: Difficulties surround fiber (letter). J Am Med Assoc 236: 252 (76)

142 Trowell HC: The effects of dietary fibre on the alimentary tract and its possible role in the causation of disease. Voeding 37: 205-207 (76)

143 Trowell HC: *Dietary Fibre: Metabolic And Vascular Diseases.* Norgine London (76)

144 Trowell H, Southgate DA, Wolever TM, et al: Dietary fibre redefined (letter). Lancet 1: 967 (76)

145 Truswell AS, Kay RM: Bran and blood-lipids (letter). Lancet 1 367 (76)

146 Truswell AS: Food Fibre and blood lipids. In: *Food and Fibre,* Marabou Symposium 51-54. Sundbyberg Sweden (76)

147 Tsai AC, Elias J, Kelley JJ, et al: Influence of certain dietary fibers on serum and tissue cholesterol levels in rats. J Nutr 106: 118-123 (76)

148 Tudge C: Fibre revisited. Wld Med 11: 47-66 (76)

149 Vaisrub S: Fiber feeding — fad or finger of fate? (editorial). J Am Med Assoc 235: 182 (76)

150 van Soest PJ: Food and Fibre. Närings-forskning 20: Suppl 14 61-62 (76)

151 van Soest PJ, Robertson JB: What is fibre and fibre in food? In: *Food and Fibre,* Marabou Symposium 12-22. Sundbyberg Sweden (76)

152 van Soest PJ, Robertson JB: Chemical and physical properties of dietary fibre. In: *Dietary Fibre,* Miles Symposium, editor WW Hawkins 13-25. Hamilton Canada (76)

153 van Soest PJ, Robertson JB: Analytical problems of fiber. Symposium on

Carbohydrate Metabolism , Institute of Food Technologists. Anaheim California (76)

154 Walker AR: Colon cancer and diet, with special reference to intakes of fat and fiber. Am J Clin Nutr 29: 1417-1426 (76)

155 Walker AR: Gastrointestinal diseases and fiber intakes with special reference to South African populations. In: *Fiber in human Nutrition,* editors GA Spiller and RJ Amen 241-261. Plenum Press New York and London (76)

156 Walker AR, Burkitt DP: Colon cancer: epidemiology. Semin Oncol 3: 341-350 (76)

157 Walker AR, Burkitt DP: Colonic cancer – hypotheses of causation, dietary prophylaxis and future research. Am J Dig Dis 21: 910-917 (76)

158 Weill JP: [Dietetic fibre] (letter). Nouv Presse Med 5: 2633-2634 (76)

159 Weinreich J: Bran and the irritable bowel (letter). Lancet 1: 810-811 (76)

160 Weinreich J, Pederson O, Dinesen K: [The effect of wheat bran on serum cholesterol, serum triglyceride, serum calcium and serum total 3 alpha-hydroxy-cholic acid and the duration of food transit time]. Ugeskr Laeger 138: 3112-3115 (76)

161 Wiggins HS, Cummings JH: Evidence for the mixing of residue in the human gut. Gut 17: 1007-1011 (76)

162 Wyman JB, Heaton KW, Manning AP, et al: The effect on intestinal transit and the feces of raw and cooked bran in different doses. Am J Clin Nutr 29: 1474-1479 (76)

163 Wyman JB, Heaton KW, Manning AP, et al: Laxative effect of All-Bran (letter). Br Med J 2: 944 (76)

164 Zald'ivar R, Watterstrand WH: High-fibre, low-saturated-fat diet and the aetiology of colo-rectal carcinomata in a low-risk population. Z Krebsforsch 87: 41-45 (76)

165 Anon: What is the most effective source of fibre in the diet and how much should be taken? Br Med J 1: 1461 (76)

1975

1 Adatia AK: Dental caries and periodontal disease. In: *Refined Carbohydrate Foods and Disease,* editors DP Burkitt, HC Trowell 251-277. Academic Press London and New York (75)

2 Arvidson J: [Fibre poor diet causes intestinal diseases]. Tidskr Sver Sjukskot 42: 47-49 (75)

3 Berenson LM, Bhandaru RR, Radhakrishnamurthy B et al: The effect of dietary pectin on serum lipoprotein cholesterol in rabbits. Life Sci 16: 1533-1543 (75)

4 Branch WJ, Southgate DA, James WP: Binding of calcium by dietary fibre: its relationship to unsubstituted uronic acids. Proc Nutr Soc 34: 120A (75)

5 Bremner WF, Brooks PM, Third JL et al: Bran in hypertriglyceridaemia: a failure of response. Br Med J 3: 574 (75)

6 Burkitt DP: In: *Refined Carbohydrate Foods and Disease,* editors DP Burkitt, HC Trowell. Appendicitis 87-97, diverticular disease 99-116, benign and malignant tumours of large bowel 117-133, varicose veins, deep vein thrombosis and haemorrhoids 143-160, hiatus hernia 161-169. Academic Press London and New York (75)

7 Burkitt DP: Cancer of the GI tract: colon, rectum and anus. Epidemiology and etiology. J Am Med Assoc 231: 517-518 (75)

8 Burkitt DP: (editorial): Large bowel cancer: an epidemiologic jigsaw puzzle. J Natl Cancer Inst 54: 3-6 (75)

9 Burkitt DP: Dietary fibre and 'pressure diseases'. J Roy Coll Phycns Lond 9: 138-147 (75)

10 Burkitt DP: Diet and Disease: Dietary Fibre (a) Diet-determined pressure phenomena.

R Soc Health J 95: 186-188 (75)

11 Burkitt DP: Hemorrhoids, varicose veins and deep vein thrombosis: epidemiologic features and suggested causative factors. Can J Surg 18: 483-488 (75)

12 Burkitt DP: A deficiency of dietary fiber may be one cause of certain colonic and venous disorders. Am J Dig Dis 21: 104-108 (75)

13 Burkitt DP: Fibre-depleted carbohydrates and disease. Community Health (Bristol) 6: 190-194 (75)

14 Burkitt DP: Some diseases related to fibre-depleted diets. In: *The Man/Food Equation*. Editors F Steele and A Bourne 247-256 Academic Press London (75)

15 Burkitt DP, Graham-Stewart CW: Haemorrhoids – postulated pathogenesis and proposed prevention. Postgrad Med J 51: 631-636 (75)

16 Burkitt DP, Jansen HK, Mategaonker DW et al: Varicose veins in India (letter). Lancet 2: 765 (75)

17 Burkitt DP, Trowell HC (editors): *Refined Carbohydrate Foods and Disease. Some Implications of Dietary Fibre*. Academic Press London and New York (75)

18 Burkitt DP: Food fiber and disease prevention. Compr Ther 1: 19-22 (75)

19 Burkitt DP, Tunstall M: Common geography as a clue to causation. Trop Geogr Med 27: 117-124 (75)

20 Burkitt DP, Tunstall M: Gall-stones: geographical and chronological features. J Trop Med Hyg 78: 140-144 (75)

21 Cleave TL: Bran and blood-lipids (letter). Lancet 1: 857 (75)

22 Connell AM, Smith CL, Somsel M: Absence of effect of bran on blood-lipids. Lancet 1: 496-497 (75)

23 Copeland CL: Fibre content of bread (letter). Br Med J 2: 503 (75)

24 Copeland CL: Dietary fibre. search for the facts (letter). Br Med J 4: 404-405 (75)

25 Coste T, Routureau J, Gouffier E: ['Dietary fibres', their role in pathology]. Nouv Presse Med 4: 2551-2554 (75)

26 Cove-Smith JR, Langman MJ: Proceedings: appendicitis and dietary fibre. Gut 16: 409 (75)

27 Crofts TJ: Bowel-transit times and diet (letter). Lancet 1: 801 (75)

28 Cummings JH: Absorption and secretion by the colon. Gut 16: 323-329 (75)

29 de Klerk WA, du Bruyn DB: Chronic typhlitis in baboons fed a semi-synthetic low-fibre diet. S Afr Med J 49: 2233-2234 (75)

30 de Moraes Filho JP, Bettarello A: [Fibre diet]. Rev Assoc Med Bras 21: 303-306 (75)

31 Douglass JM: Raw diet and insulin requirements (letter). Ann Int Med 82: 61-63 (75)

32 Durrington P, Wicks AC, Heaton KW: Effect of bran on blood-lipids (letter). Lancet 2: 133 (75)

33 Eastwood MA: Diet and Disease (b) Vegetable dietary fibre – potent pith. R Soc Health J 95: 188-190 (75)

34 Eastwood MA: The role of vegetable dietary fibre in human nutrition. Med Hypotheses 1: 46-53 (75)

35 Eastwood M, Mitchell WD, Smith AN: Straining, sitting, and squatting at stool (letter). Lancet 2: 560 (75)

36 Editorial: Faecal fibre fortunes. Br Med J 2: 580-581 (75)

37 Editorial: Idea Exchange: Fiber in the diet. J Am Diet Assoc 66: 50-53 (75)

38 Editorial: Dietary fibre and plasma-lipids. Lancet 2: 353-354 (75)

39 Ershoff BH, Marshall WE: Protective effects of dietary fiber in rats fed toxic doses of sodium cyclamate and polyoxyethylene sorbitan monostearate (Tween 60). J Food Sci 40: 357-361 (75)

40 Goldsmith HS, Burkitt DP: Stool characteristics of black and white Americans (letter). Lancet 2: 407 (75)

41 Hall RC, Klauda HC, Waite VM et al: Improved lithogenicity of fasting hepatic bile by dietary fiber and cholestyramine: studies in mice and humans. Surg Forum 26: 435-437 (75)

42 Heaton KW: Diet fibre and disease. Trans Med Soc Lond 91: 55-62 (75)

43 Heaton KW: [Effects of a cellulose fibre based diet on the bile salt metabolism and on the composition of bile]. Med Chir Dig 4: Suppl 1 27-29 (75)

44 Heaton KW: Fibre, blood-lipids, and heart-disease (letter). Lancet 2: 927 (75)

45 Heaton KW: The effects of carbohydrate refining on food ingestion, digestion and absorption 59-67. Gallstones and cholecystitis 173-194. In: *Refined Carbohydrate Foods and Disease,* editors DP Burkitt, HC Trowell. Academic Press London and New York (75)

46 Heaton KW, Pomare EW: Bran and blood-lipids (letter). Lancet 1: 800-801 (75)

47 Hellendoorn EW, Noordhoff MG, Slagman J: Enzymatic determination of the indigestible residue (dietary fibre) content of human food. J Sci Fd Agric 26: 1461-1468 (75)

48 Heywood PF: Nutrition 13. Fibre. Med J Aust 2: 179-182 (75)

49 Hill MJ: Metabolic epidemiology of dietary factors in large bowel cancer. Cancer Res 35: 3398-3402 (75)

50 Hill MJ, Drasar BS: The normal colonic bacterial flora. Gut 16: 318-323 (75)

51 Holm CN, Hansen LP: [Plant fibre and gastrointestinal transit time]. Ugeskr Laeg 137: 561-565 (75)

52 Holst DO, Gehrke CW: Crude fiber analysis without asbestos. J Assoc Offic Anal Chem 58: 474-476 (75)

53 Horwitz DL, Slowie L: Raw diet in diabetes mellitus. Ann Int Med 82: 853-854 (75)

54 Huth K, Fettel M: Bran and blood-lipids (letter). Lancet 2: 456 (75)

55 James WP, Southgate DA: Bran and blood-lipids (letter). Lancet 1: 800 (75)

56 Jenkins DJ, Hill MS, Cummings JH: Effect of wheat fiber on blood lipids, fecal steroid excretion and serum iron. Am J Clin Nutr 28: 1408-1411 (75)

57 Jenkins DJ, Leeds AR, Newton C et al: Effect of pectin, guar gum and wheat fibre on serum-cholesterol (letter). Lancet 1: 1116-1117 (75)

58 Kataria MS: Straining, sitting, and squatting at stool (letter). Lancet 2: 407 (75)

59 Kritchevsky D, Story JA: In vitro binding of bile acids and bile salts (letter). Am J Clin Nutr 28: 305-306 (75)

60 Kritchevsky D, Tepper SA, Story JA: Nonnutritive fiber and lipid metabolism. J Food Sci 40: 8-11 (75)

61 Le Quintrec M, Le Quintrec Y: [Fibre and residue free diets]. Rev Prat 25: 4403-4408 (75)

62 Leader RW, Hayden DW: Some diseases characteristic of western civilization prevalent in wild and domestic animals. In: *Refined Carbohydrate Foods and Disease,* editors DP Burkitt, HC Trowell 311-317. Academic Press London and New York (75)

63 Leeds AR, Gassull MA, Metz GL et al: Food: influence of form on absorption (letter). Lancet 2: 1213 (75)

64 Low-Beer TS, Pomare EW: Can colonic bacterial metabolites predispose to cholesterol gallstones? Br Med J 1: 438-440 (75)

65 Maclennan R: [Epidemiology of colorectal cancer]. Bull Cancer (Paris) 62: 411-418 (75)

66 Mendeloff AI: A critique of 'fiber deficiency'. Am J Dig Dis 21: 109-112 (75)

68   Merrington HN: Nutrition 14: Fact and Fancy in food and feeding. The application of nutrition science on primary care. Med J Aust 2: 261-262 (75)

69   Modan B, Barell V, Lubin F et al: Low-fiber intake as an etiological factor in cancer of the colon. J Natl Cancer Inst 55: 15-18 (75)

70   Modan B, Barell V, Lubin F et al: Dietary factors and cancer in Israel. Cancer Res 35: 3503-3506 (75)

71   Mokhobo KP: Saccharine diseases and profiles of possibly related diseases (letter). S Afr Med J 49: 1906 (75)

72   O'Beirne SF, Flynn JR: The potato as a source of dietary fibre. Ir J Med Sci 144: 76-77 (75)

73   Osman AA: Etiology of venous disorders. Int Surg 60: 540-543 (75)

74   Owen DE, Munday KA, Taylor TG et al: Hypocholesterolaemic action of wheat bran and a mould (Fusarium) in rats and hamsters. Proc Nutr Soc 34: 16A-17A (75)

75   Painter NS: *Diverticular Disease of the Colon. A Deficiency Disease of Western Civilisation.* Heinemann London (75)

76   Painter NS: Brown bread. Practitioner 215: 93 (75)

77   Painter NS: Diet and disease: dietary fibre. (d) Diverticular disease of the colon: the effect of the high-fibre diet. R Soc Health J 95: 194-198 (75)

78   Painter NS, Burkitt DP: Diverticular disease of the colon. In: *Refined Carbohydrate Foods and Disease,* editors DP Burkitt, HC Trowell 99-116. Academic Press London and New York (75)

79   Painter NS, Burkitt DP: Diverticular disease of the colon, a 20th century problem. Clin Gastroenterol 4: 3-21 (75)

80   Parks AG: [Etiology and pathogenesis of diverticulosis]. Schweiz Med Wochenschr 103: 825-827 (75)

81   Payler DK, Pomare EW, Heaton KW et al: The effect of wheat bran on intestinal transit. Gut 16: 209-213 (75)

82   Persson I, Raby K, Fønns-Bech P et al: Bran and blood-lipids (letter). Lancet 2: 1208 (75)

83   Plumley P: Faecal fibre fortunes (letter). Br Med J 3: 305 (75)

84   Reilly RW, Kirsner JB: Fiber deficiency and colonic disorders. Am J Clin Nutr 28: 293-294 (75)

85   Reilly RW, Kirsner JB (editors): *Fiber Deficiency and Colonic Disorders.* Plenum Medical Book Co New York and London (75)

86   Reinhold JG, Ismail-Beigi F, Faradji B: Fibre vs. phytate as determinant of the availability of calcium, zinc and iron of breadstuffs. Nutr Rep Internat 12: 75-85 (75)

87   Reinhold JG: Phytate destruction by yeast fermentation in whole wheatmeals. J Am Diet Assoc 66: 38-41 (75)

88   Schaller D: Plant fibers in nutrition: need for better nomenclature (letter). Am J Clin Nutr 28: 1347 (75)

89   Segal I, Hunt JA: The irritable bowel syndrome in the urban South African Negro. S Afr Med J 49: 1645-1646 (75)

90   Sorokin M: Hospital morbidity in the Fiji Islands with special reference to the saccharine disease. S Afr Med J 49: 1481-1485 (75)

91   Southgate DA: Diet and disease: dietary fibre (c) dietary fibre – its nature and role in the diet. R Soc Health J 95: 191-194 (75)

92   Southgate DA: Fibre in nutrition. Bibl Nutr Dieta 22: 109-124 (75)

93   Spiller GA, Amen RJ: Dietary fiber in human nutrition. Crit Rev Fd Sci 7: 39-70 (75)

94   Spiller GA, Amen RJ: Plant fibers in nutrition: need for better nomenclature (letter).

Am J Clin Nutr 28: 675-676 (75)

95   Spiller GA, Saperstein S, Beigler MA et al: Effect on fecal output of various dietary nitrogen sources in pig-tailed monkeys (Macaca nemestrina) fed fiber-free semi-synthetic diets. Am J Clin Nutr 28: 502-506 (75)

96   Tandon RK, Tandon BN: Stool weights in North Indians (letter). Lancet 2: 560-561 (75)

97   Texter EC Jr, Butler RC: The irritable bowel syndrome. Am Fam Physician 11: 169-173 (75)

98   Thaler H: [Stomach carcinoma and nutrition] (letter). Dtsch Med Wochenschr 100: 1515 (75)

99   Thomson H: Piles: and their nature and management. Lancet 2: 494-495 (75)

100 Tovey FI: Duodenal ulcer and diet. In: *Refined Carbohydrate Foods and Disease,* editors DP Burkitt, HC Trowell 279-309. Academic Press London and New York (75)

101 Tovey, FI, Jayaraj AP, Clarke C: The possibility of dietary protective factors in duodenal ulcer. Postgrad Med J 51: 366-372 (75)

102 Tovey FI, Tunstall M: Progress Report. Duodenal ulcer in black populations in Africa south of the Sahara. Gut 16: 564-576 (75)

103 Trowell HC: Dietary-fiber hypothesis of the etiology of diabetes mellitus. Diabetes 24: 762-765 (75)

104 Trowell H: Pathological growth and maturation in infants and children associated with modern methods of feeding. Envir Child Health 21: 192-198 (75)

105 Trowell H: Straining, sitting and squatting at stool (letter). Lancet 2: 456 (75)

106 Trowell H: Obesity in the western world. Plant Foods for Man 1: 157-168 (75)

107 Trowell H: Prevalence of haemorrhoids (letter). Lancet 2: 821 (75)

108 Trowell HC: Dietary fibre hypothesis (letter). Br Med J 4: 649 (75)

109 Trowell H: Bran and blood-lipids (letter). Lancet 1: 801 (75)

110 Trowell H: Coronary heart disease and dietary fiber (letter). Am J Clin Nutr 28: 798-800 (75)

111 Trowell H: Fibre content of bread (letter). Br Med J 3: 101 (75)

112 Trowell HC: *Dietary Fibre and Colonic Diseases.* Norgine London (75)

113 Trowell HC: The importance of fibre. Chemist Drug 204: 692-694 (75)

114 Trowell HC: In: *Refined Carbohydrate Foods and Disease. Some Implications of Dietary Fibre,* editors DP Burkitt, HC Trowell. Historical aspects of milling cereals and refining sugar 43-46. Dietary changes in modern times 47-56. Ulcerative colitis and Crohn's disease 135-140. Ischaemic heart disease, atheroma and fibrinolysis 195-226. Diabetes mellitus and obesity 227-249. Disorders of unknown aetiology showing certain environmental associations 319-331. Academic Press London and New York (75)

115 Trowell H, Burkitt DP: Faecal fibre fortunes (letter). Br Med J 3: 305 (75)

116 Truswell AS, Kay RM: Absence of effect of bran on blood-lipids (letter). Lancet 1: 922-923 (75)

117 Tyler C: Albrecht Thaer's hay equivalents: fact or fiction? Nutr Astr Rev 45: 1-11 (75)

118 Tytgat GN, Dekker W: [Is the fibre content of the diet of pathological significance?] Ned Tijdschr Geneeskd 119: 750-755 (75)

119 van Soest PJ: Physico-chemical aspects of fibre digestion. Proceedings 4th International Symposium Ruminant Physiology, Sydney, Australia 351-365 (75)

120 Walker AR: Effect of high crude fiber intake on transit time and the absorption of nutriments in South African Negro schoolchildren. Am J Clin Nutr 28: 1161-1169 (75)

121 Walker AR: The epidemiological emergence of ischaemic arterial diseases. Am Heart
     J 89: 133-136 (75)
122 Walker AR: Plumbing and bowel habit (letter). Lancet 2: 456 (75)
123 Walters RL, Baird IM, Davies PS et al: Effects of two types of dietary fibre on
     faecal steroid and lipid excretion. Br Med J 2: 536-538 (75)
124 Anon: Laxatives and dietary fiber (letter). Med Lett Drugs Ther 15: 98-100 (75)
125 Anon: Dietary fiber and colonic function – an effect of particle size? Nutr Rev 33:
     70-72 (75)

1974

  1 Advisory Panel of the Committee on Medical Aspects of Food Policy (Nutrition)
     on Diet in relation to Cardiovascular and Cerebrovascular Disease. *Diet and Coronary
     Heart Disease* 18, 21. H.M. Stationery Office London (74)
  2 Antia FP, Desai HG: Colonic diverticular and dietary fibre (letter). Lancet 1: 814 (74)
  3 Balmer J, Zilversmit DB: Effects of dietary roughage on cholesterol absorption,
     cholesterol turnover and steroid excretion in the rat. J. Nutr 104: 1319-1328 (74)
  4 Bing FC: Indigestible carbohydrates (letter). Am J Clin Nutr 27: 1201-1202 (74)
  5 Birkner HJ, Kern F Jr: In vitro absorption of bile salts to food residues, salicyla-
     zosulfapyride, and hemicellulose. Gastroenterology 67: 237-244 (74)
  6 Björn-Rasmussen E: Iron absorption from wheat bread. Influence of various
     amounts of bran. Nutr Metab 16: 101-110 (74)
  7 Bryant MP: Nutritional features and ecology of predominant anerobic organisms of
     the intestinal tract. Am J Clin Nutr 27: 1313-1319 (74)
  8 Burkitt DP, Walker AR, Painter NS: Dietary fiber and disease. J Am Med Ass
     229: 1068-1074 (74)
  9 Cleave TL: *The Saccharine Disease. Conditions Caused by the Taking of Refined
     Carbohydrates, such as Sugar and White Flour.* John Wright Bristol (74)
 10 Cleave TL: Effect of bran on blood lipids and calcium (letter). Lancet 1: 137 (74)
 11 Cleave TL: The bran hypothesis (letter). Lancet 1: 1173 (74)
 12 Cleave TL: Sugar, heart disease and diabetes (letter). Lancet 1: 515 (74)
 13 Eastwood MA: Dietary fibre in human nutrition. J Sci Fd Agric 25: 1523-1527 (74)
 14 Eastwood MA, Fisher N, Greenwood CT et al: Perspectives on the bran hypothesis.
     Lancet 1: 1029-1033 (74)
 15 Eastwood MA, Mitchell WD: The place of vegetable fibre in the diet. Br J Hosp Med
     11: 123-126 (74)
 16 Eastwood MA, Mitchell WD, McConnell AA et al: Diverticular disease and fibre.
     Nutr Food Sci 35: 2-4 (74)
 17 Eggleston FC: Colonic diverticula and dietary fibre (letter). Lancet 2: 1324 (74)
 18 Ellis FR, Sanders TA: Diet and colonic cancer (letter). Br Med J 2: 505 (74)
 19 Ershoff BH: Nutritional effects of dietary fibers. J Appl Nutr 26: 22-26 (74)
 20 Ershoff BH: Antitoxic effects of plant fiber. Am J Clin Nutr 27: 1395-1398 (74)
 21 Ershoff BH, Thurston EW: Effects of diet on Amaranth (FD and C Red No 2)
     toxicity in the rat. J Nutr 104: 937-942 (74)
 22 Falaiye JM: Bile-salt patterns in Nigerians on a high-fibre diet (letter). Lancet 1: 1002 (74)
 23 Findlay JM, Mitchell WD, Eastwood MA et al: Intestinal streaming patterns in
     cholerrhoeic enteropathy and diverticular disease. Gut 15: 207-212 (74)
 24 Findlay JM, Smith AN, Mitchell WD et al: Effects of unprocessed bran on colon
     function in normal subjects and in diverticular disease. Lancet 1: 146-149 (74)
 25 Findlay JM, Smith AN, Shariff S et al: The effect of bran on transit time, bile acid

134

concentration and motility in colonic diverticular disease. Br J Surg 61: 323 (74)

26 Glober GA, Klein KL, Moore JO et al: Bowel transit-times in two populations experiencing similar colon-cancer rates. Lancet 2: 80-81 (74)

27 Hart JT, Scott I: Bran and blood-lipids (letter). Lancet 1: 175 (74)

28 Heaton KW: Dietary fibre and energy intake (letter). Lancet 1: 368-369 (74)

29 Heaton KW, Pomare EW: Effect of bran on blood lipids and calcium. Lancet 1: 49-50 (74)

30 Hill MJ: Colon cancer: a disease of fibre depletion or dietary excess? Digestion 11: 289-306 (74)

31 Hipsley EH: Dietary 'fibre' and pregnancy toxaemia (letter). Med J Aust 2: 341-342 (74)

32 Hodgson J: Diverticular disease. Possible correlation between low residue diet and intracolonic pressures in the rabbit model. Am J Gastroenterol 62: 116-123 (74)

33 Hyams DE: Gastrointestinal problems in the old – 1: Br Med J 1: 107-110 (74)

34 James WP: Food and death-rates from diabetes (letter). Lancet 2: 1201-1202 (74)

35 James WP, Cummings JH: Dietary fibre and energy regulation (letter). Lancet 1: 61-62 (74)

36 Jeffreys DB: The effect of dietary fibre on the response to orally administered glucose. Proc Nutr Soc 33: 11A-12A (74)

37 Kato M, Hiromi K, Morita Y: Purification and kinetic studies of wheat bran beta-amylase. Evaluation of subsite affinities. J Biochem (Tokyo) 75: 563-576 (74)

38 Kay RM, Truswell AS: The effect of wheat fibre on the plasma cholesterol in rats. Proc Nutr Soc 34: 17A-18A (74)

39 Kiriyama S, Enishi A, Yura K: Inhibitory effect of Konjac mannan on bile acid transport in the everted sacs from rat ileum. J. Nutr 104: 69-78 (74)

40 Kirwan WO, Smith AN, McConnell AA et al: Action of different bran preparations on colonic function. Br Med J 4: 187-189 (74)

41 Kirwan WO, Smith AN, McConnell AA et al: Proceedings: Action of bran on colonic motility related to its physical properties. Gut 15: 828 (74)

42 Klevay LM: Coronary heart disease and dietary fiber (letter). Am J Clin Nutr 27: 1202-1203 (74)

43 Kritchevsky D, Davidson LM, Shapiro IL et al: Lipid metabolism and experimental atherosclerosis in baboons: influence of cholesterol-free semisynthetic diets. Am J Clin Nutr 27: 29-50 (74)

44 Kritchevsky D, Story JA: Binding of bile salts in vitro by non-nutritive fiber. J Nutr 104: 458-462 (74)

45 McConnell AA, Eastwood MA: A comparison of methods of measuring 'fibre' in vegetable material. J Sci Fd Agric 25: 1451-1456 (74)

46 McConnell AA, Eastwood MA, Mitchell WD: Physical characteristics of vegetable foodstuffs that could influence bowel function. J. Sci Fd Agric 25: 1457-1464 (74)

47 Malhotra SL: Diet and colonic cancer (letter). Br Med J 4: 532 (74)

48 Malins JM: Food and death-rates from diabetes (letter). Lancet 2: 1201 (74)

49 Manning EB, Mann JI, Sophangisa E et al: Dietary patterns in urbanised Blacks. A study in Guguletu, Cape Town, 1971. S Afr Med J 48: 485-498 (74)

50 Menon PV, Kurup PA: Hypolipidaemic action of the polysaccharide from Phaseolus mungo (Black gram). Effect on glycosaminoglycans, lipids and lipoprotein lipase activity in normal rats. Atherosclerosis 19: 315-316 (74)

51 Milton-Thompson DG: Varicose veins in tropical Africa (letter). Lancet 1: 1174 (74)

52 Morgan B, Heald M, Atkin SD et al: Dietary fibre and sterol metabolism in the rat.

Br J. Nutr 32: 447-455 (74)

53   Nielsen JA: Behandling af kronisk obstipation hosimmobile plejehjemspatienter med hoedeklid og methylcellolosesuspension. Ugeskr Laeg 136: 967-971 (74)

54   Painter NS: The high fibre diet in the treatment of diverticular disease of the colon. Postgrad Med J 50: 629-635 (74)

55   Painter NS: Diverticular disease of the colon – a disease caused by fibre deficiency. Plant Foods for Man 1: 67-79 (74)

56   Phillpotts JS: The bran hypothesis (letter). Lancet 2: 102 (74)

57   Piepmeyer JL: Use of unprocessed bran in the treatment of irritable bowel syndrome (letter). Am J Clin Nutr 27: 106-107 (74)

58   Pomare EW, Heaton KW, Low-Beer TS: Proceedings: Effect of wheat bran on bile salt metabolism and bile composition. Gut 15: 824-825 (74)

59   Preston RD: *The Physical Biology of Plant Cell Walls.* Chapman and Hall London (74)

60   Rose G, Blackburn H, Keys A et al: Bowell cancer and blood-cholesterol. Lancet 1: 181-183 (74)

61   Scala J: Physiological effects of dietary fiber. In: *Physiological Effects of Food Carbohydrates,* editors A Jeanes, J Hodge 325-335. American Chemical Society Washington (74)

62   Schreiber G: Ingested dyed cellulose in the blood and urine of man. Arch Environ Health 29: 39-42 (74)

63   Sittwer SH: Food, fiber and energy. Am J Dis Child 128: 13-15 (74)

64   Smith AN, Kirwan WO, Shariff S: Motility effects of operations performed for diverticular disease. Proc Roy Soc Med 67: 1041-1043 (74)

65   Sorokin M: Controlling heart disease (letter). Med J Aust 1: 1047 (74)

66   Southgate DA: Problem on the analysis of the polysaccharides in foods. J Assoc Pub Analysts 12: 114-118 (74)

67   Spiller GA, Amen RJ: Research on dietary fibre (letter). Lancet 2: 1259 (74)

68   Technology Assessment Consumption Centre (TACC): *Bread: TACC Report* 40-48. Intermediate Publishing London (74)

69   *Thickening Agents A: Celluloses.* In: *Toxicological Evaluation of Some Food Additives including anticaking agents, antimicrobials, antioxidants, emulsifiers and thickening agents.* World Health Organisation, Geneva (74)

70   Thomas B: Zur Bewertung der Ballaststoffkomponenten des Brotes. Internationale Zeischrift für Vitamin und Ernährungsforschung. Beiheft Nr 14, Qualitätskriterien der Nahrung 53-62. Verlag Hans Huber Bern Stuttgart Wein (74)

71   Thompson WG: The irritable colon. Can Med Assoc J 111: 1241-1244 (74)

72   Tovey FI: Aetiology of duodenal ulcer: an investigation into the buffering action and effect on pepsin of bran and unrefined carbohydrate foods. Postgrad Med J 50: 683-688 (74)

73   Trowell H: Diabetes mellitus death-rates in England and Wales 1920-70 and food supplies. Lancet 2: 998-1002 (74)

74   Trowell H: Incidence of diabetes in children (letter). Lancet 2: 1510 (74)

75   Trowell H: Fibre and obesity (letter). Lancet 1: 95 (74)

76   Trowell H: Definitions of fibre (letter). Lancet 1: 503 (74)

77   Trowell H: Fibre and irritable bowels (letter). Br Med J 3: 44 (74)

78   Trowell HC: Dietary fibre, coronary heart disease and diabetes mellitus. Part 2. Coronary heart disease and diabetes mellitus. Plant Foods for Man 1: 91-97 (74)

79   Trowell H: Bran hypothesis. Lancet 2: 54 (74)

80   Trowell H, Painter N, Burkitt D: Aspects of the epidemiology of diverticular disease

and ischemic heart disease. Am J Dig Dis 19: 864-873 (74)

81 Voinchet C, Mouchat A: Obstruction of the oesophagus by mucilage. Nouv Presse Med 3: 1223-1225 (74)

82 Walker AR: Dietary fiber and the pattern of disease (editorial). Ann Int Med 80: 663-664 (74)

83 Walker AR: Survival rate at middle age in developing and western populations. Postgrad Med J 50: 29-32 (74)

84 Walker AR: The bran hypothesis (letter). Lancet 2: 341 (74)

85 Williams EH: Varicose veins in tropical Africa (letter). Lancet 1: 1291 (74)

86 Yellowlees WW: The bran hypothesis (letter). Lancet 1: 1282-1283 (74)

87 Anon: Fibre and moral fibre (editorial). Br Med J 2: 457-458 (74)

1973

1 Adamson CJ, Brown AM, Truswell AS: Survey of high and low residue (fibre) diets in British hospitals. Nutrition Lond 27: 159-169 (73)

2 Barnard DL, Heaton KW: Bile acids and vitamin A absorption in man: the effects of two bile acid-binding agents cholestryamine and lignin. Gut 14: 316-318 (73)

3 Berman PM, Kirsner JB: Diverticular disease of the colon – the possible role of 'roughage' in both food and life. Am J Dig Dis 18: 506-507 (73)

4 Burkitt DP: Varicose veins, deep vein thrombosis and hemorrhoids. Am Heart J 85: 572-573 (73)

5 Burkitt DP: Diverticular disease of the colon and epidemiological evidence relating it to fibre-depleted diets. Trans Med Soc Lond 89: 81-84 (73

6 Burkitt DP: Some diseases characteristic of modern Western civilization. Br Med J 1: 274-278 (73)

7 Burkitt DP: Epidemiology of large bowel diseases: the role of fibre. Proc Nutr Soc 32: 145-149 (73)

8 Burkitt DP: Some diseases characteristic of modern western civilization. A possible common causative factor. Clin Radiol 24: 271-280 (73)

9 Burkitt DP: Diseases of the alimentary tract and western diets. Proceedings 11th Conference International Society of Geographical Pathology. Path Microbiol (Basel) 39: 177-186 (73)

10 Burkitt DP, James PA: Low residue diets and hiatus hernia. Lancet 2: 128-130 (73)

11 Cleave TL: Diseases of western civilization (letter). Br Med J 1: 678-679 (73)

12 Cleave TL: Effects of dietary fibre on intestinal transit (letter). Lancet 1: 1443 (73)

13 Crowther JS, Drasar BS, Goddard P et al: The effect of a chemically defined diet on the faecal flora and faecal steroid concentration. Gut 14: 790-793 (73)

14 Cummings JH: Progress report: Dietary fibre. Gut 14: 69-81 (73)

15 Drasar BS, Irving D: Environmental factors and cancer of colon and breast. Br J Cancer 27: 167-172 (73)

16 Eastwood MA: Vegetable fibre: its physical properties. Proc Nutr Soc 32: 137-143 (73) •

17 Eastwood MA: Dietary fibre and gastroenterology. Digestion 8: 368-371 (73)

18 Eastwood MA, Hamilton T, Kirkpatrick JR et al: The effects of dietary supplements of wheat bran and cellulose on faeces. Proc Nutr Soc 32: 22A (73)

19 Eastwood MA, Kirkpatrick JR, Mitchell WD et al: Effects of dietary supplements of wheat bran and cellulose on faeces and bowel function. Br Med J 4: 392-394 (73)

20 Edwards CS: Determination of lignin and cellulose in forages by extraction with triethylene glycol. J Sci Fd Agric 24: 381-386 (73)

21 Field AC (editor): *Fibre in human nutrition*. Proc Symp Nutr Soc Edinburgh 1973.

Proc Nutr Soc 32: 123-167 (73)

22   Fisher N: Indigestible constituents of cereals and other foodstuffs. In: *Molecular Structure and Function of Food Carbohydrate,* editors AG Birch, LF Green. Applied Science Publishers London (73)

23   Goering HK, van Soest PJ: Forage fiber analysis (apparatus) reagents, procedures and some applications. US Department Agriculture Handbook No 379 Washington (73)

24   Harvey RF, Pomare EW, Heaton KW: Effects of increased dietary fibre on intestinal transit. Lancet 1: 1278-1280 (73)

25   Harvey RF, Pomare EW, Heaton KW: Effect of bran on bowel function (letter). Br Med J 4: 614 (73)

26   Heaton KW: The epidemiology of gallstones and suggested aetiology. Clin Gastroenterol 2: 67-83 (73)

27   Heaton KW: Food fibre as an obstacle to energy intake. Lancet 2: 1418-1421 (73)

28   Heaton KW: Are we getting too much out of food? Nutrition Lond 27: 170-183 (73)

29   Hellendoorn EW: Physiological importance of indigestible carbohydrates in human nutrition. Voeding 34: 618-636 (73)

30   Huth K, Lück M, Stiehl A et al: Pulverisierte Cellulose als Füllstoff, insebesondere ihre Wirkung auf das Serumcholesterin. Verh Dtsch Ges Inn Med 79: 1270-1272 (73)

31   Irving D, Drasar BS: Fibre and cancer of the colon. Br J Cancer 28: 462-463 (73)

32   Latto C, Wilkinson RW, Gilmore OJ: Diverticular disease and varicose veins. Lancet 1: 1089-1090 (73)

33   Lee JW, Stenvert NL: Conditioning studies on Australian wheat. IV. Compositional variations in the bran layers of wheat and their relation to milling. J Sci Fd Agric 24: 1565-1569 (73)

34   Lim PE, Tate ME: The phytases. II. Properties of phytase fractions F1 and F2 from wheat bran and the myoinositol phosphates produced by fraction F2. Biochim Biophys Acta 302: 316-328 (73)

35   Lindner P, Moller B: Lignin: a cholesterol-lowering agent? (letter). Lancet 2: 1259-1260 (73)

36   Manousos ON, Vrachliotis G, Papaevangelou G et al: Relation of diverticulosis of the colon to environmental factors. Am J Dig Dis 18: 174-176 (73)

37   Mason JB, Gibson N, Kodicek E: The chemical nature of the bound nicotinic acid of wheat bran: studies of nicotinic acid-containing macromolecules. Br J Nutr 30: 297-311 (73)

38   Painter NS: Food fibre and bowel behaviour (letter). Lancet 1: 1508-1509 (73)

39   Painter NS: A disease of Western civilisation caused by a deficiency of dietary fibre. Trans Med Soc Lond 89: 85-91 (73)

40   Parks TG: The role of dietary fibre in the prevention and treatment of diseases of the colon. Proc R Soc Med 66: 681-683 (73)

41   Parsons DS: Dietary fibre, stool output and transit time (letter). Lancet 1: 152 (73)

42   Payler DF: Food fibre and bowel behaviour (letter). Lancet 1: 1394 (73)

43   Plumley PF, Francis B: Dietary management of diverticular disease. J Am Diet Assoc 63: 527-530 (73)

44   Pomare EW, Heaton KW: Alteration of bile salt metabolism by dietary fibre (bran). Br Med J 4: 262-264 (73)

45   Ranhotra GS: Effect of cellulose and wheat mill fractions on plasma and liver cholesterol levels in cholesterol-fed rats. Cereal Chem 50: 358-363 (73)

46   Reddy BS, Wynder EL: Large bowel carcinogenesis: fecal constituents of populations with diverse rates of colon cancer. J Natl Cancer Inst 50: 1437-1442 (73)

47   Rougemont A: Varicose veins in the tropics (letter). Br Med J 2: 547 (73)
48   Sinnett PF, Whyte HM: Epidemiological studies in a total highland population, Tukisenta, New Guinea. Cardiovascular disease and relevant chemical, electrocardiographic, radiological and biochemical findings. J Chronic Dis 26: 265-290 (73)
49   Southgate DA: Dietary fibre. Plant Foods for Man 1:45-47 (73)
50   Southgate DA: Fibre and other unavailable carbohydrates and their effects on the energy value of the diet. Proc Nutr Soc 32: 131-136 (73)
51   Stanley MM, Paul D, Gackle D et al: Effects of cholestyramine, metamucil, and cellulose on fecal bile salt excretion in man. Gastroenterology 65: 889-894 (73)
52   Sundaravalli OE, Shurpalekar KS, Rao MN: Inclusion of cellulose in calorie-restricted diets. Effect on body composition, nitrogen balance, and cholesterol levels in obese rats. J Am Diet Assoc 62: 41-43 (73)
53   Thomas B: [Analysis of whole wheat fibre]. Ernäh Umsch 20: 456 (73)
54   Tikhonova EP, Berdichevski VKH, Palei AA: [Use of methyl cellulose in diets for patients with obesity and diabetes mellitus]. Voprosy Pitaniya 32: 9-13 (73)
55   Trowell H: Dietary fibre, ischaemic heart disease and diabetes mellitus. Proc Nutr Soc 32: 151-157 (73)
56   Trowell H: Dietary fibre, coronary thrombosis and diabetes mellitus. Part 1. Historical aspects of fibre in the food of western man. Plant Foods for Man 1: 11-16 (73)
57   Trowell HC: Diabetes mellitus and refined carbohydrates (letter). Br Med J 1: 365 (73)
58   Trowell HC: Digestive diseases: the changing scene (letter). Br Med J 1: 295 (73)
59   Trowell H: Tropical malabsorption and fiber-depleted starchy carbohydrates (letter). Am J Clin Nutr 26: 477-478 (73)
60   van Soest PJ: The uniformity and nutritive availability of cellulose. Fed Proc 32: 1804-1808 (73)
61   van Soest PJ, McQueen RW: The chemistry and estimation of fibre. Proc Nutr Soc 32: 123-130 (73)
62   Vijayagopal P, Devi KS, Kurup PA: Fibre content of different dietary starches and their effect on lipid levels in high fat-high cholesterol fed rats. Atherosclerosis 17: 158-160 (73)
63   Vijayagopal P, Kurup PA: Hypolipidaemic principle of the husk and bran of paddy. Nature of the substance and its effects on cholesterol absorption and faecal bile salt excretion in rats fed high fat-high cholesterol diet. Atherosclerosis 18: 379-387 (73)
64   Walker AR, Richardson BD, Walker BF et al: Appendicitis, fibre intake and bowel behaviour in ethnic groups in South Africa. Postgrad Med J 49: 243-249 (73)
65   Ward JM, Yamamoto RS, Weisburger J: Cellulose dietary bulk and azomethane-induced intestinal cancer. J Natl Cancer Inst 51: 713-715 (73)
66   Wicks AC, Jones JJ: Insulinopenic diabetes in Africa. Br Med J 1: 773-776 (73)

1972

1   Almy TP: High-residue diet for diverticular disease. J Am Med Assoc 221: 1058 (72)
2   Attebery HR, Sutter VL, Finegold SM: Effect of a partially chemically defined diet on normal human fecal flora. Am J Clin Nutr 25: 1391-1398 (72)
3   Burkitt DP: Cancer of the colon and rectum. Epidemiology and possible causative factors. Minn Med 55: 779-783 (72)
4   Burkitt DP: Varicose veins, deep vein thrombosis and haemorrhoids: epidemiology and suggested aetiology. Br Med J 2: 556-561 (72)

5   Burkitt DP: Aetiology of varicosity (letter). Br Med J 4: 231 (72)

6   Burkitt DP: Geographical pathology related to diet. In: *Medical Annual,* editors RB Scott and RM Walker 5-16. Wright Bristol (72)

7   Burkitt DP, Walker AR, Painter NS: Effect of dietary fibre on stools and transit times, and its role in the causation of disease. Lancet 2: 1408-1412 (72)

8   Butler HS: Dietary fibre and calcium metabolism (letter). Br Med J 4: 363-364 (72)

9   Cleave TL: Bran and diverticular disease (letter). Br Med J 2: 408-409 (72)

10 Dodds C, Fisher N, Greenwood CT et al: Effects of dietary fibre (letter). Br Med J 3: 472-473 (72)

11 Goldstein F: Diet and colonic disease. J Am Diet Assoc 60: 499-503 (72)

12 Hamilton T, Kirkpatrick JR, Mitchell D et al: The effects of dietary supplements of wheat bran and cellulose upon bowel action. Br J Surg 59: 910 (72)

13 Heaton KW: *Bile salts in Health and Disease* 180-195. Churchill Livingstone Edinburgh (72)

14 Holmgreen GO, Mynors JM: The effect of diet on bowel transit times. S Afr Med J 46: 918-920 (72)

15 Hunt T: Digestive diseases: the changing scene. Br Med J 4: 689-694 (72)

16 Jones A, Godding EW, (editors): *Management of Constipation* 27-31 Blackwell Oxford (72)

17 Konlande JE, Robson JR: The nutritive value of cooked cannas as consumed by Flathead Indians. Ecol Fd Nutr 2: 193-195 (72)

18 Painter NS: The importance of dietary fibre, with special reference to diverticular disease of the colon. Nutrition Lond 26: 95-109 (72)

19 Painter NS: High-residue diet for diverticular disease of the colon. J Am Med Ass 221: 1058 (72)

20 Painter NS: Irritable or irritated bowel (letter). Br Med J 2: 46 (72)

21 Painter NS, Almeida AZ, Colebourne KW: Unprocessed bran in the treatment of diverticular disease of the colon. Br Med J 2: 137-140 (72)

22 Robertson J: Changes in the fibre content of the British diet. Nature Lond 238: 290-292 (72)

23 Rukosuev AN, Silant'eva AG: Aminokislotnyi sostav serna rzhl rzhanolselanoi i obdirnol muki i obrubli. Vopr Pitan 31: 42-45 (72)

24 Sinnett PJ: Nutrition in a New Guinea highland community. Hum Biol Oceania 1: 299-305 (72)

25 Stahl WM: High-residue diet for diverticular disease of colon. J Am Med Assoc 221: 1058 (72)

26 Thomas B: Beiträge zur Nomenklator und Analytik pflanzlicher Zellwandsubstanzen. Getreide Mehl und Brot 26: 158-165 168-169 (72)

27 Tovey FI: Duodenal ulcer in Mysore. Characteristics and aetiological factors. Trop Geogr Med 24: 107-117 (72)

28 Tovey FI: A trial of rice bran as a supplement to polished rice in the treatment of duodenal ulcer. J Christian Med Assoc India 47: 312-313 (72)

29 Trowell H: Crude fibre, dietary fibre and atherosclerosis (letter). Atherosclerosis 16: 138-140 (72)

30 Trowell H: Dietary fibre and coronary heart disease. Rev Eur Etud Clin Biol 17: 345-349 (72)

31 Trowell H: Fiber: a natural hypocholesterolemic agent (letter). Am J Clin Nutr 25: 464-465 (72)

32 Trowell H: Ischemic heart disease and dietary fiber. Am J Clin Nutr 25: 926-932 (72)

34   van der Westhuizen J, Mbizvo MT, Jones J: Unrefined carbohydrate and glucose tolerance (letter). Lancet 2: 719 (72)

35   Vijayagopalan, P, Kurup PA: Hypolipidaemic activity of whole paddy in rats fed a high-fat high-cholesterol diet. Isolation of an active fraction from the husk and bran. Atherosclerosis 15: 215-222 (72)

36   Vijayagopalan P, Kurup PA: Effect of dietary starches on the serum, aorta and hepatic lipid levels in high fat high cholesterol-fed rats. 2. Nature of the starch and hypolipidaemic activity. Atherosclerosis 16: 247-256 (72)

37   Walker AR: Biological and disease patterns in South African inter-racial populations as modified by rise in privilege. S Afr Med J 46: 1127-1134 (72)

38   Wapnick S, Wicks AC, Kanengoni E et al: Can diet be responsible for the initial lesion in diabetes? Lancet 2: 300-302 (72)

1971

1   Burkitt DP: The aetiology of appendicitis. Br J Surg 58: 695-699 (71)

2   Burkitt DP: Epidemiology of cancer of the colon and rectum. Cancer 28: 3-13 (71)

3   Burkitt DP: Some neglected leads to cancer causation (editorial). J Natl Cancer Inst 47: 913-919 (71)

4   Burkitt DP: Possible relationships between bowel cancer and dietary habits. Proc R Soc Med 64: 964-965 (71)

5   Davies PJ: Influence of diet on flatus volume in human subjects. Gut 12: 713-716 (71)

6   Heaton KW, Heaton ST, Barry RE: An in vivo comparison of two bile salt binding agents, cholestyramine and lignin. Scand J Gastroenterol 6: 281-286 (71)

7   Lubbe AM: Dietary evaluation. In: A comparative study of rural and urban Venda males, editors A le R van der Merwe, SA Fellingham. S Afr Med J 45: 1289-1297 (71)

8   Malhotra SL: Dietary factors and ischemic heart disease. Am J Clin Nutr: 24: 1195-1198 (71)

9   Milton-Thompson GT, Lewis B: The breakdown of dietary cellulose in man (Abstract). Gut 12: 853-854 (71)

10   Nel A, du Plessis JP, Fellingham SA: Biochemical evaluation. In: A comparative study of rural and urban Venda males, editors A le R van der Merwe and SA Fellingham. S Afr Med J 45: 1315-1317 (71)

11   Painter NS: Below the belt (letter). Lancet 2: 381-382 (71)

12   Painter NS: Treatment of diverticular disease. Br Med J 2: 156 (71)

13   Painter NS, Burkitt DP: Diverticular disease of the colon: a deficiency disease of western civilization. Br Med J 1: 450-454 (71)

14   Sarkanen KV, Ludwig CH (editors): *Lignins, Occurrence, Formation, Structure and Reactions.* Wiley Interscience, New York (71)

15   Shurpalekar KS, Doraiswamy TR, Sundaravalli OE et al: Effect of inclusion of cellulose in an 'atherogenic' diet on the blood lipids of children. Nature Lond 232: 554-555 (71)

16   Sundaravalli OE, Shurpalekar KS, Rao MN: Effects of dietary cellulose supplements on the body composition and cholesterol metabolism of albino rats. J Agric Food Chem 19: 116-118 (71)

17   Trowell H: Atheroma and diverticulitis (letter). Br Med J 2: 707-708 (71)

18   Trowell H: Deep-vein thrombosis (letter). Lancet 2: 928-929 (71)

19   Walker AR: Diet, bowel motility, faeces composition and colonic cancer. S Afr Med J 45: 377-379 (71)

20   Walker AR: Diet and cancer of the colon (letter). Lancet 1: 593 (71)

1970

1 Aspinall GO: *Polysaccharides*. Pergamon Press Oxford, New York (70)

2 Brown J, Bourke GJ, Gearty GF et al: Nutritional and epidemiological factors related to heart disease. Wld Rev Nutr Diet 12: 1-42 (70)

3 Burkitt DP: Relationship as a clue to causation. Lancet 2: 1237-1240 (70)

4 Denbesten L, Connor WE, Kent TH et al: Effect of cellulose in the diet on the recovery of dietary plant sterols from the feces. J Lipid Res 11: 341-345 (70)

5 De Wit JP, Schweigart F: The potential role of pearl millet as a food in South Africa. S Afr Med J 44: 364-366 (70)

6 Eastwood MA, Erikson S: The use of lignin in controlling diarrhoea due to ileal dysfunction. Gut 11: 370 (70)

7 Eastwood MA, Mowbray SL, Thompson RP et al: Dietary fibre and the pruritus of cholestatic jaundice. Br J Nutr 24: 1029-1032 (70)

8 Eheart JF, Mason BS: Nutrient composition of selected wheats and wheat products. V. Carbohydrate. Cereal Chem 47: 715-719 (70)

9 Goering HK, van Soest PJ: Forage Fiber Analysis. Agriculture Handbook 379 Agriculture Research Service Dept of Agriculture Washington (70) (reprinted 75)

10 Hutchinson JB, Martin HF: Nutritive value of wheat bran. I. Effects of fine grinding upon bran and added bran upon the protein quality of white flour. J Sci Food Agric 21: 148-151 (70)

11 Metz J, Lurie A, Konidaris M et al: A note on the folate content of uncooked maize. S Afr Med J 44: 539-541 (70)

12 Phillips WE, Brien RL: Effect of pectin, a hypocholesterolemic polysaccharide on vitamin A utilization in the rat. J Nutr 100: 289-292 (70)

13 Southgate DA, Durnin JV: Caloric conversion factors. An experimental reassessment of the factors used in the calculation of the energy value of human diets. Br J Nutr 24: 517-535 (70)

14 Walker AR, Walker BF, Richardson BD: Bowel transit times in Bantu populations (letter). Br Med J 3: 48-49 (70)

15 Winitz M, Seedman DA, Graff J et al: Studies in metabolic nutrition employing chemically defined diets. I. Extended feeding of normal human adult males. Am J Clin Nutr 23: 525-545 (70)

16 Winitz M, Seedman DA, Graff J: Studies in metabolic nutrition employing chemically defined diets. II. Effects on gut microflora. Ibid. 546-559 (70)

17 Wood TM: Cellulose and cellulolysis. Wld Rev Nutr Diet 12: 227-265 (70)

1969

1 Burkitt DP: Related disease – related cause. Lancet 2: 1229-1231 (69)

2 Cleave TL, Campbell GD, Painter NS: *Diabetes, Coronary Thrombosis, and the Saccharine Disease,* 2nd edition. John Wright Bristol (70)

3 Dreyer JJ: The biological assessment of protein quality: effects of consumption of 'crude' fibre, NaCl and body hair on faecal nitrogen excretion. S Afr Med J 43: 776-786 (69)

4 Eastwood M: Dietary fibre and serum-lipids. Lancet 2: 1222-1225 (69)

5 Kemp JE, Van Soest PJ, Young EP: Comparative study of the digestibility of forage cellulose and hemicellulose in ruminants and non-ruminants. J Am Sci 29: 11-15 (69)

6 Mathur KS: Bengal gram: an effective hypocholesterolemic substance. Ann Ind Acad Med Sci 5: 1-25 (69)

7 Painter NS: Diverticular disease of the colon: a disease of this century. Lancet 2:

586-588 (69)

8   Southgate DA: Determination of carbohydrates in foods. II Unavailable carbohydrates. J Sci Food Agric 20: 331-335 (69)

9   Walker AR: Can expectation of life in western populations be increased by changes in diet? Part 2. S Afr Med J 43: 768-775 (69)

10   Walker AR: What can be done to retard ageing and increase expectation of life? Ann Life Insur Med 4: 176-203 (69)

11   Walker AR, Walker BF: Bowel motility and colonic cancer (letter). Br Med J 3: 238 (69)

12   Wood TM: The relationship between cellulolytic and pseudo-cellulolytic micro-organisms. Biochim Biophys Acta 192: 531-534 (69)

1968

1   Boyd GS, Eastwood MA: Studies on the quantitative distribution of bile salts along the rat small intestine under varying dietary regimes. Biochim Biophys Acta 152: 159-164 (68)

2   Eastwood MA, Girdwood RH: Lignin: a bile-salt sequestrating agent. Lancet 2: 1170-1172 (68)

3   Eastwood MA, Hamilton D: Studies on the adsorption of bile salts in non-absorbed components of the diet. Biochim Biophys Acta 152: 165-173 (68)

4   Lopez SA, Hopson J, Krehl WA: Effect of dietary pectin on plasma and fecal lipids. Fed Proc 27: 485 (68)

5   Malhotra SL: Studies in blood coagulation, diet, and ischaemic heart disease in two population groups in India. Br Heart J 30: 303-308 (68)

6   Mathur KS, Khan MA, Sharma RD: Hypocholesterolaemic effect of Bengal gram: a long-term study in man. Br Med J 1: 30-31 (68)

7   Painter NS: Diverticular disease of the colon. Br Med J 3: 475-479 (68)

8   Walker AR: Can expectation of life in western populations be increased by changes in diet? Part I. S Afr Med J 42: 944-950 (68)

1967

1   Eastwood MA, Boyd GS: The distribution of bile salts along the small intestine of rats. Biochim Biophys Acta 137: 393-396 (67)

2   Fisher H, Griminger P: Cholesterol-lowering effects of certain grains and oat fractions in the chick. Proc Soc Exp Biol Med 126: 108-111 (67)

3   Kent-Jones DW, Amos AJ: *Modern Cereal Chemistry* 6th edition. Food Trade Press London (67)

4   Malhotra SL: Geographical aspects of acute myocardial infarction in India with special reference to patterns of diet and eating. Br Heart J 29: 337-344 (67)

5   Malhotra SL: Epidemiology of ischaemic heart disease in India with special reference to causation. Br Heart J 29: 895-905 (67)

6   Moore JH: The effect of the type of roughage in the diet on plasma cholesterol levels and aortic atherosis in rabbits. Br J Nutr 21: 207-215 (67)

7   Painter NS: Diverticulosis of the colon: fact and speculation. Am J Dig Dis 12: 222-227 (67)

8   Riccardi BA, Fahrenbach MJ: Effect of guar gum and pectin on serum and liver lipids of cholesterol fed rats. Proc Soc Exp Biol Med 124: 749-752 (67)

1966

1   Cleave TL, Campbell GD: *Diabetes, Coronary Thrombosis and the Saccharine*

Disease. Wright Bristol (66)

2   Fahrenbach MJ, Riccardi BA, Grant WC: Hypocholesterolemic activity of mucilaginous polysaccharides in White Leghorn cockerels. Proc Soc Exp Biol Med 123: 321-326 (66)

3   Fisher H, Siller WG, Griminger P: The retardation by pectin of cholesterol-induced atherosclerosis in the fowl. J Atheroscler Res 6: 292-298 (66)

4   Greaves JP, Hollingsworth DF: Trends in food consumption in the United Kingdom. Wrld Rev Nutr Diet 6: 34-89 (66)

5   Griminger P, Fisher H: Antihypercholesterolemic action of scleroglucan and pectin in chickens. Proc Soc Exp Biol Med 122: 551 (66)

6   Kent NL: *Technology of Cereals.* Pergamon Press Oxford (66)

7   Leveille GA, Sauberlich HE: Mechanism of the cholesterol-depressing effect of pectin in the cholesterol-fed rat. J Nutr 88: 209-214 (66)

8   Murthy PS, Belavady B: Faecal loss of calories on Indian diets. Ind J Med Res 54: 1087-1090 (66)

9   Palmer HG, Dixon DG: Effect of pectin on serum cholesterol levels. Am J Clin Nutr 18: 437-442 (66)

10   Riccardi BA, Fahrenbach MJ: Effect of guar gum and pectin NF on serum and liver lipids of cholesterol-fed rats. Proc Soc Exp Biol Med 124: 749-752 (66)

11   Walker AR: Nutritional, biochemical and other studies on African populations. S Afr Med J 40: 814-852 (66)

1965

1   Bruins HW, Potter GC, Hensley GW et al: Factors contributing to the hypocholesterolemic effect of rolled oats. Fed Proc 24: 263 (65)

2   Fisher H, Griminger P, Sostman ER et al: Dietary pectin and plasma cholesterol. J Nutr 86: 113 (65)

3   Garvin JE, Forman DT, Eiseman WR et al: Lowering of human serum cholesterol by an oral hydrophilic colloid. Proc Soc Exp Biol Med 120: 744-746 (65)

4   Grande F, Anderson JT, Keys A: Effect of carbohydrates of leguminous seeds, wheat and potatoes on serum cholesterol concentration in man. J Nutr 86: 313-317 (65)

5   Groen JJ, Balogh M, Yaron E et al: Influence of the nature of the fat in diets high in carbohydrates (mainly derived from bread) on serum cholesterol. Am J Clin Nutr 17: 296-304 (65)

6   Hardinge MG, Swarmer JB, Crooks H: Carbohydrates in foods. J Am Diet Assoc 46: 197-203 (65)

7   Lombard JH, Brandt J, Wehmeyer AS: A study of the nutrient content of the varieties of bread in common use in South Africa. S Afr Med J 39: 488-491 (65)

8   Luyken R, de Wijn JF, Pikaar NA et al: De invloed van havermout op het serumsholeserolgehalte van het bloed. Voeding 26: 229-244 (65)

9   van Soest PJ: Non-nutritive residues: a system of analysis for the replacement of crude fiber. Assoc Off Agr Chem J 49: 546-551 (65)

1964

1   Antar MA, Ohlson MA, Hodges RE: Changes in the retail market food supplies in the United States in the last seventy years in relation to the incidence of coronary heart disease, with special reference to dietary carbohydrates and essential fatty acids. Am J Clin Nutr 14: 169-178 (64)

2   Barker A: Varicose veins (letter). Lancet 2: 970-971 (64)

3   Bremner CG: Ano-rectal disease in the South African Bantu. 1. Bowel habit and physiology. S Afr J Surg 2: 119-123 (64)

4   Dickson JA: Dietary fat and dietary sugar (letter). Lancet 2: 361 (64)

5   Dodd H: The cause, prevention, and arrest of varicose veins. Lancet 2: 809-811 (64)

6   Fox FW: Uncertainties that hinder the accurate determination of the nutritional value of a diet. S Afr Med J 38: 668-673 (64)

7   Groen JJ, Balogh M, Levy M et al: Nutrition of the Bedouins in the Negev desert. Am J Clin Nutr 14: 37-46 (64)

8   Kim EH: Hiatus hernia and diverticulum of the colon. Their low incidence in Korea. New Engl J Med 271: 764-768 (64)

9   Kramer PH: The meaning of high and low residue diets. Gastroenterology 47: 649-652 (64)

10 Mathur KS, Singhai SS, Sharma RD: Effect of Bengal gram on experimentally induced high levels of cholesterol in tissues and serum in albino rats. J Nutr 84: 201-204 (64)

11 Nolte NC: Production and consumption of maize in South Africa. S Afr Med J 38: 642-645 (64)

12 Oettlé AG: Cancer in Africa, especially in regions south of the Sahara. J Natl Cancer Inst 33: 383-439 (64)

13 Painter NS: The aetiology of diverticulosis of the colon with special reference to the action of certain drugs on the behaviour of the colon. Ann Roy Coll Surg Eng 34: 98-119 (64)

14 Prather ES: Effect of cellulose on serum lipids in young women. J Am Diet Assoc 45: 230-233 (64)

15 Walker AR: Coronary heart disease. Limitations of the application to white populations of lessons learned from the underprivileged (editorial). Circulation 29: 1-3 (64)

1963

1   *Bread and Flour Regulations No 1435*. HM Stationery Office London (63)

2   de Groot AP, Luyken R, Pikaar NA: Cholesterol-lowering effect of rolled oats (letter). Lancet 2: 303-304 (63)

3   van Soest PJ: Use of detergents in the analysis of fibrous feeds. 1. Preparation of fiber residues of low nitrogen content. J Ass Off Agric Chem 46: 825-829 (63)

4   van Soest PJ: Use of detergents in the analysis of fibrous feeds. 2. A rapid method for the determination of fiber and lignin. J Ass Off Agric Chem 46: 829-835 (63)

5   Watt BJ, Merrill AL: *Composition of Foods – Raw, Processed, Prepared*. Agriculture Handbook No. 8, United States Department of Agriculture Washington DC (63)

1962

1   Antonis A, Bersohn I: The influence of diet on serum lipids in South African White and Bantu prisoners. Am J Clin Nutr 10: 484-499 (62)

2   Antonis A, Bersohn I: The influence of diet on fecal lipids in South African White and Bantu prisoners. Am J Clin Nutr 11: 142-153 (62)

3   Burgess HJ: Millets and sorghum. E Afr Med J 39: 437-442 (62)

4   Cleave TL: *Peptic Ulcer*. John Wright Bristol (62)

5   Ershoff BH, Wells AF: Effects of gum guar, locust bean gum on liver cholesterol of cholesterol-fed rats. Proc Soc Exp Biol Med 110: 580-582 (62)

6   Luyken R, Pikaar NA, Polman H et al: The influence of legumes on the serum cholesterol level. Voeding 23: 447-453 (62)

7   Painter NS: *Diverticulosis of the Colon*. MS Thesis London University

8   Szczgiel A: [The composition of crude fibre and its influence on some functions

of the digestive tract]. Nahrung 6: 701-707 (62)

1961

1 Carr WR: Observations on the nutritive value of traditionally ground cereals in Southern Rhodesia. Br J Nutr 15: 339-343 (61)
2 Durnin JV: The availability of nutrients in diets containing different quantities of unavailable carbohydrate: a study on young and elderly men and women. 1. General description and proportionate losses of calories (abstract). Proc Nutr Soc 20: ii (61)
3 Keys A, Grande F, Anderson JT: Fiber and pectin in the diet and serum cholesterol concentration in man. Proc Soc Exp Med 106: 555-558 (61)
4 McCarrison R, Sinclair HM: *Nutrition and Health.* Faber and Faber London (61)
5 Southgate DA: The availability of nutrients in diets containing different quantities of unavailable carbohydrates. 2. Nitrogen, fat, carbohydrates and some inorganic constituents (abstract). Proc Nutr Soc 20: iii (61)
6 Walker AR: Crude fibre, bowel motility and pattern of diet. S Afr Med J 35: 114-115 (61)

1960

1 Cleave TL: *On the Causation of Varicose Veins: Their Prevention and Arrest by Natural Means.* Wright Bristol (60)
2 Keys A, Anderson JT, Grande F: Diet-type (fats constant) and blood lipids in man. J Nutr 70: 257-266 (60)
3 McCance RA, Widdowson EM: *The Composition of Foods,* Third impression with minor amendments. Spec Rep Ser Med Res Coun Lond No. 297. HM Stationery Office London (60)
4 Trowell HC: *Non-Infective Disease in Africa* 217-222. Edward Arnold London (60)
5 Whistler RL, Young JR: The role of hemicelluloses in the oat plant. Arch Biochem 89: 1-5 (60)
6 Widdowson EM: A note on the calculation of the calorific value of foods and of diets. In: *The Composition of Foods* editors RA McCance and EM Widdowson, Spec Rep Ser Med Res Coun Lond Third revised edition No 297 171-179. HM Stationery Office London (60)

1959

1 Cleave TL: Varicose veins. Nature's error or man's? Lancet 2: 172-175 (59)
2 Fraser JR, Holmes DC: The proximate analysis of wheat flour carbohydrates. IV. Analysis of wheat flour and some of its fractions. J Sci Fd Agric 10: 506-512 (59)
3 Hughes EW: Low residue diets. Practitioner 182: 374-375 (59)
4 Moran T: Nutritional significance of recent work on wheat, flour and bread. Nutr Abst Reviews 29: 1-16 (59)

1958

1 Aylward F: Excretion of cholesterol (letter). Lancet 2: 852-853 (58)
2 Chick H: Wheat and bread. A historical introduction. Proc Nutr Soc 17: 1-7 (58)
3 Fraser JR: Flour survey 1950-1956. J Sci Fd Agric 9: 125-136 (58)
4 Hardinge MG, Chambers AC, Crooks H et al: Nutritional studies of vegetarians. 3. Dietary levels of fiber. Am J Clin Nutr 6: 523-525 (58)
5 Jones CR: The essentials of flour-milling process. Proc Nutr Soc 17: 7-15 (58)
6 Kent-Jones DW: The case for fortified flour. Proc Nutr Soc 17: 38-43 (58)

146

7 Meyer JH: Interaction of dietary fiber and protein on food intake and body composition of growing rats. Am J Physiol 193: 488-494 (58)

8 Morton RA: The report of the panel on flour. Proc Nutr Soc 17: 20-28 (58)

9 Nicholls JR, Fraser JR: Analytical problems in the determination and control of extraction rates of flour. Proc Nutr Soc 17: 43-49 (58)

10 Sinclair HM: Nutritional aspects of high-extraction flour. Proc Nutr Soc 17: 28-37 (58)

11 Walker AR: Certain biochemical findings in men in relation to diet. Ann New York Acad Sci 69: 989-1008 (58)

1957

1 Cleave TL: *Fat Consumption and Coronary Disease: An Evolutionary Answer to This Problem.* Wright Bristol (57)

2 Drummond JC, Wilbrandon A: *The Englishman's Food: A History of Five Centuries of English Diet.* Cape London (57)

3 Fraser JR, Holmes DC: Proximate analysis of wheat flour. III. Estimation of the hemicellulose fraction. J Sci Fd Agric 8: 715-721 (57)

4 Howeler JF, Hewson AD: Dietary fibre and toxaemia of pregnancy. Med J Aust 1: 761-763 (57)

5 Kent Jones DW, Amos AJ: *Modern Cereal Chemistry,* 5th edition. Northern Publishing Co Liverpool (57)

6 Kowalski J, Piekarska J: [Digestibility of lignin, hemicellulose and cellulose of wheat bread by man]. Rocz Pánslwowego Zakl Hig 8: 557-563 (57)

7 Lin TM, Kim KS, Karvinen E et al: Effect of dietary pectin, protopectin and gum arabic on cholesterol excretion in rats. Am J Physiol 188: 66-70 (57)

1956

1 Bersohn I, Walker AR, Higginson J: Coronary heart disease and dietary fat (letter). S Afr Med J 30: 411-412 (56)

2 Cleave TL: The neglect of natural principles in current medical practice. J R Nav Med Serv 42: 55-83 (56)

3 Editorial: Nutrients in bread. Br Med J 1: 1223-1226 (56)

4 Editorial: End of National flour. Br Med J 1: 1347-1348 (56)

5 Fraser JR, Brendon-Bravo M, Holmes DC: The proximate analysis of wheat flour carbohydrates. 1. Methods and scheme of analysis. J. Sci Fd Agric 7: 577-588 (56)

6 Fraser JR, Holmes DC: 2 The analysis of carbohydrate fractions of different flour types. J Sci Fd Agric 7: 589 (56)

7 Lin TM, Karvinen E, Ivy AC: Effect of indigestible residue (cellulose) on elimination of endogenous and dietary cholesterol. Am J Physiol 187: 170-172 (56)

8 McCance RA, Widdowson EM: *Breads, white and brown.* Pitman Medical London (56) (720 references)

9 Medical Research Council: Nutritional value of flour. Br Med J 1: 1354 (56)

10 Memorandum of a Conference appointed by the Medical Research Council to prepare evidence for submission to the Government Panel on Composition and Nutritive Value of Flour: Flour. Lancet 2: 901-903 (56)

11 Meyer JH: Influence of dietary fiber on metabolic and endogenous nitrogen excretion. J Nutr 58: 407-413 (56)

12 Parliamentary Statement: Nutrients in flour. Br Med J 1: 1246 (56)

13 *Report of the Government Chemist for 1956.* HM Stationery Office London (56)

14 *Report of the Panel on Composition and Nutritive Value of Flour (Cohen Report)*

Cmd 9757. HM Stationery Office London (56)

15 Robinson CH: Fiber in diet. Am J Clin Nutr 4: 288-290 (56)

16 Walker AR: Some aspects of nutritional research in South Africa. Nutr Rev 14: 321-324 (56)

1955

1 National flour committee: Br Med J 1: 1228 (55)

2 McCance RA, Widdowson EM: Old thoughts and new work on breads white and brown. Lancet 2: 205-210 (55)

3 Report of Government Chemist for 1955 18-19. HM Stationery Office London (55)

4 Walker AR: Diet and atherosclerosis (letter). Lancet 1: 565-566 (55)

1954

1 Higginson J, Pepler WJ: Fat intake, serum cholesterol concentration, and atheroma in South African Bantus. II. Atheroma and coronary heart disease. J Clin Invest 33: 1366-1371 (54)

2 Horder (Lord), Dodds C, Moran T: *Bread*. Constable London (54)

3 Walker AR, Arvidsson UB: Fat intake, serum cholesterol concentration, and atherosclerosis in the South African Bantu. I. Low fat intake and the age trend of serum cholesterol concentration in the South African Bantu. J Clin Invest 33: 1358-1365 (54)

4 Widdowson EM, McCance RA: *Nutritive Value of Bread of Various Extraction Rates on Growth of Undernourished Children*. Med Res Coun Spec Rep Ser No 287. HM Stationery Office London (54)

1953

1 Hipsley EH: Dietary 'fibre' and pregnancy toxaemia. Br Med J 2: 420-422 (53)

2 McCance RA, Prior KM, Widdowson EM: A radiological study of the rate of passage of brown and white bread through the digestive tract of man. Br J Nutr 7: 98-104 (53)

3 *Ministry of Food: The Flour Order No. 1282*. HM Stationery Office London (53)

4 *Ministry of Food: The Bread Order No. 1283*. HM Stationery Office London (53)

5 Paloheimo L: Some persistent misconceptions concerning crude fiber and the nitrogen free extract. J Sci Agric Soc Finland 25: 16-22 (53)

6 *Report of Government Chemist for 1953*. HM Stationery Office London (53)

7 Wolf MJ, MacMasters MM, Canon JA et al: Preparation and properties of hemi-celluloses from corn hulls. Cereal Chem 30: 451 (53)

1952

1 *Report of Government Chemist for 1952*. HM Stationery Office London (52)

1951

1 Cruickshank EWH: *Food and Nutrition*. Livingstone Edinburgh (51)

2 Fraser JR: National Flour Survey 1946-50. J Sci Fd Agric 2: 193-198 (51)

3 *Report of Government Chemist for 1951*. HM Stationery Office London (51)

1950

1 British Medical Association Committee on Nutrition (1950). *Report of the Committee on Nutrition*. British Medical Association London (50)

2   Hipsley EH: Should nutritional value of the Australian bread be improved by raising the extraction rate of flour? Med J Aust 1: 720-724 (50)

3   *Report of Government Chemist for 1950.* HM Stationery Office London (50)

1949

1   Carlson AJ, Hoelzel F: Relation of diet to diverticulosis of the colon in rats. Gastroenterology 12: 108-115 (49)

2   Curtis-Bennett N: *The Food of the People.* Faber London (49)

3   Dawbarn MC: The effects of milling upon the nutritive value of wheaten flour and bread. Nutr Abstr Rev 18: 691-706 (49)

4   Deer N: *The History of Sugar.* Chapman and Hall London (49)

5   Hipsley EH: Some aspects of nutrition as related to practice of obstetrics and gynaecology. Med J Aust 1: 775-781 (49)

6   Salaman RN: *The History and Social Influence of the Potato.* Cambridge University (49)

7   Walker AR: Effect of low fat intakes and of crude fibre on the absorption of fat. Nature 164: 825-827 (49)

8   Wells CA: Symposium: diverticula of alimentary tract; diverticula of colon. Br J Radiol 22: 449-458 (49)

1948

1   McCance RA, Glaser EM: The energy value of oatmeal and the digestibility of its proteins, fats and calcium. Br J Nutr 2: 221-228 (48)

2   McCance RA, Walsham CM: The digestibility and absorption of calories, proteins, purines, fat and calcium in wholemeal wheaten bread. Br J Nutr 2: 26-41 (48)

3   Walker AR, Fox FW, Irving JT: Studies in human mineral metabolism. 1. The effect of bread rich in phytate phosphorus on the metabolism of certain mineral salts with special reference to calcium. Biochem J 42: 452-462 (48)

1947

1   Chick H, Cutting ME, Martin CJ et al: Observations on the digestibility and nutritive value of the nitrogenous constituents of wheat bran. Br J Nutr 1: 161-182 (47)

2   McCance RA, Widdowson EM: Digestibility of English and Canadian wheats, with special reference to the digestibility of wheat protein by man. J Hyg Camb 45: 59-64 (47)

3   Walker AR: The effect of recent changes of food habits on bowel motility. S Afr Med J 21: 590-596 (47)

1946

1   Bacharach AL, Rendle T (editors). *The Nation's Food.* Society Chemical Industries London (46)

2   McCance RA: Bread (letter). Lancet 1: 77 (46)

3   McCance RA, Walsham CM: The digestibility and absorption of the calories, proteins, fat, and calcium in wholemeal wheaten breads. Br J Nutr 2: 26-41 (46)

4   MacRae TF, Yudkin S: Palatibility of 85% National wheatmeal bread (letter). Lancet 1: 214 (46)

5   Symposium on Factors Affecting the Nutritive Value of Bread as Human Food. Proc Nutr Soc 4: 1-51 (46)

6   Ministry of Food Scientific Advisers: Eighth Report: National flour (80 per cent

extraction) and bread in Britain. Nature Lond 157: 181 (46).

1945

1 Dunlap FL: *White versus Brown Flour.* Wallace and Tiernan London (45)
2 Hoppert CA, Clark AJ: Digestibility and effect on laxation of crude fiber and cellulose in certain common foods. J Am Diet Assoc 21: 157-160 (45)
3 *Ministry of Food: Report of the Conference on the Post-war Loaf. Cmd 6701.* HM Stationery Office London (45)
4 Ministry of Food Scientific Advisers: Seventh Report. Nature Lond. 155: 717 (45)
5 Moran T, Drummond JC: Scientific basis of 80 per cent extraction flour. Lancet 1: 698-700 (45)

1944

1 Bailey CH: *Constituents of Wheat and Wheat Products.* Reinhold Publishing Co New York (44)
2 Lepkovsky S: The bread problem in war and peace. Physiol Rev 24: 239-276 (44)
3 Ministry of Food Scientific Advisers: Fourth Report. Nature Lond 153: 154 (44)
4 Ministry of Food Scientific Advisers: National flour and bread. Fifth Report. Nature Lond 154: 582 (44)
5 Ministry of Food Scientific Advisers: National flour ($82\frac{1}{2}$ per cent extraction) and bread. Sixth Report.' Nature Lond 154: 788-790 (44)

1943

1 Analytical Methods Committee: Determination of the crude fibre in National flour. Analyst 68: 176-178 (43)
2 Hummel FC, Shepherd M, Macy IG: Disappearance of cellulose and hemicellulose from the digestive tracts of children. J Nutr 25: 59-70 (43)
3 Macy IG, Hummel FC, Shepherd ML: Value of complex carbohydrates in diets of normal children. Am J Dis Child 65: 195-206 (43)
4 Ministry of Food Scientific Advisers: Third Report. Nature Lond 151: 629-630 (43)
5 Streicher MH, Quirk L: Constipation: clinical and roentgenologic evaluation of the use of bran. Am J Digest Dis 10: 179-181 (43)
6 Trémolières J, Erfmann R: Influence sur la digestion de la surcharge cellulosique apportée par le pain actuel. Bull Acad Med 127: 641-646 (43)

1942

1 British Flour Millers Research Association: National bread (First Report). Nature Lond 149: 460-464 (42)
2 Hoppert CA, Clark AJ: Bran muffins and normal laxation. J Am Diet Assoc 18: 524-525 (42)
3 Jenkins GN, McDougall EI, Herbert P: Quality of the national loaf. Lancet 2: 69-70 (42)
4 Krebs HA, Mellanby K: Digestibility of national wheat meal. Lancet 1: 319-321 (42)
5 Macrae TF, Hutchinson JC, Irwin JO et al: Comparative digestibility of wholemeal and white breads and effect of the degree of fineness of grinding on the former. J Hyg 42: 423-435 (42)
6 McCance RA, Widdowson EM: Mineral absorption of healthy adults on white and brown bread dietaries. J. Physiol 101: 44-85 (42)
7 Ministry of Food Scientific Advisers: Second Report: National flour and bread.

Nature Lond 150: 538-539 (42)

8　Moran T, Pace J: Digestibility of high extraction wheat meals. Nature Lond 150: 224 (42)

9　Werch SC, Jung RW, Day AA et al: Decomposition of pectin and galactouronic acid by intestinal bacteria. J Infect Dis 70: 231-242 (42)

10　Widdowson EM, McCance RA: Iron exchanges of adults on white and brown bread diets. Lancet 1: 588-591 (42)

1941

1　Chick H: Nutritive value of bread (letters). Br Med J 2: 790-791 (41)

2　Cleave TL: Natural bran in the treatment of constipation (letter). Br Med J 1: 461 (41)

3　Editorial: Cereals as food. Nature Lond 148: 599 (41)

4　Fantus B, Frank W: The mode of action of bran; effect of bran upon composition of stools. J Lab Clin Med 26: 1774-1777 (41)

5　Fantus B, Hirschberg N, Frankl W: Mode of action of bran: influence of size and shape of bran particles and of crude fiber isolated from bran; preliminary report. Rev Gastroenterology 8: 277-280 (41)

6　Hodder RG: National wheatmeal bread (letter). Br Med J 1: 648 (41)

7　Lampard ME: Bran in the prevention of constipation (letter). Br Med J 1: 390 (41)

8　Medical notes in Parliament: The Nation's bread in wartime. Br Med J 1: 35 (41)

9　Medical notes in Parliament: Fortified bread. Br Med J 1: 180 and 736 (41)

10　Medical Research Council Specification: National flour for Bread. Br Med J 1: 828-829 (41) and Lancet 1: 240 and 703 (41)

11　Mottram JC: Wholemeal bread (letter). Br Med J 2: 244-245 (41)

12　Murlin JR: Marshall ME, Kochakian CD: Digestibility and biological value of whole breads as compared to white breads. J Nutr 22: 573-588 (41)

13　Scott RA: Wholemeal bread (letters). Br Med J 2: 64 and 491 (41)

14　Sealock RR, Basinski DH, Murlin JR: Apparent digestibility of carbohydrates, fats and 'indigestible residue' in whole wheat and white breads. J Nutr 22: 589-506 (41)

15　Weber FP: Prepared bran in the prevention of constipation (letter). Br Med J 1: 252-253 (41)

16　Werch SC, Ivy AC: Study of ingested pectin. Am J Dis Child 62: 499-511 (41)

17　Werch SC, Ivy AC: Is galacturoic acid absorbed by small and large intestine? Proc Soc Exp Biol Med 48: 9-11 (41)

18　Wright MD: The nutritive value of bread. Fortified white flour and national wheatmeal compared. Br Med J 2: 689-692 (41)

1940

1　Anderson JB: Freshly ground whole-wheat bread (letter). Br Med J 2: 72 (40)

2　Fantus B, Kopstein G, Smidt HR: Roentgen study of intestinal motility as influenced by bran. J Am Med Ass 114: 404-408 (40)

3　Hummel FC, Shepherd ML, Macy IG: Effect of changes in food intakes upon the lignin, cellulose and hemicellulose content of diets. J Am Diet Assoc 16: 199-207 (40)

4　McCarrison R: Medical aspects of the use of food. Br Med J 1: 984-987 (40)

5　Medical Research Council: Improved quality of bread: higher extraction flour. Br Med J 2: 164 (40)

6　Williams RD, Wicks L, Bierman HR et al: Carbohydrate values of fruit and vegetables. J Nutr 19: 593-604 (40)

1939

1 Drummond JC: *The Englishman's Food.* Cape London (39)
2 McDougall EJ: Report on Bread in Several European Countries. Bull Hlth Org L o N 4: 498 (39)
3 Taylor G: Virtues of brown bread (letter). Br Med J 2: 1022 (39)

1938

1 Cole GD, Postgate R: *The Common People 1746-1900.* Methuen London (38)
2 Rabinowitch IM, Fowler AF: Variations of weight of dry feces in short period experiments with a low residue – neutral ash diet. J Nutr 16: 565-569 (38)

1937

1 Dimock EM: The prevention of constipation. Br Med J 1: 906-909 (37)
2 Editorial: Brown bread versus white. Br Med J 2: 752-753 (37)
3 Kantor JL, Cooper LF: The dietetic treatment of constipation with special reference to food fiber. Ann Int Med 10: 965-978 (37)

1936

1 American Medical Association Council on Foods: The nutritional significance of bran. J Am Med Ass 107: 874-877 (36)
2 Bergeim O, Hanszen A, Arnold L: The influence of fruit ingestion before meals upon the bacterial flora of stomach and large intestine and on food allergins. Am J Dig Dis Nutr 3: 45-52 (36)
3 Dimock EM: *The Treatment of Habitual Constipation by the Bran Method.* MD Thesis Cambridge (36)
4 Funnell EH, Vahlteich EM, Morris SO et al: Protein utilization as affected by the presence of small amounts of bran or its fiber. J Nutr 11: 37-45 (36)
5 Hardy TL: Spasm of the colon and mucomembranous colitis. Br Med J 1: 487-489 (36)
6 Hutchinson R: Treatment of chronic constipation. Br Med J 1: 374-375 (36)
7 McCarrison R: *Nutrition and National Health* (Cantor Lectures). Faber and Faber London (36)
8 McCance RA, Widdowson EM, Shackleton LR: The nutritive value of fruits, vegetables and nuts. Spec Rep Ser Med Res Coun Lond No 213. HM Stationery Office London (36)
9 Olmsted WH, Williams RD, Bauerlain T: Constipation: the laxative action of bulky foods. Med Clin N Amer 20: 449-459 (36)
10 Parsons LW: Studies on fiber as a factor in intestinal function. J Am Dietet Assoc 12: 11-22 (36)
11 Williams RD, Olmsted WH: The effect of cellulose, hemicellulose and lignin on the weight of the stool: contribution to the study of laxation in men. J Nutr 11: 433-449 (36)
12 Williams RD, Olmsted WH: The manner in which food controls the bulk of the feces. Ann Int Med 10: 717-727 (36)

1935

1 Hay WH: *A New Health Era.* Harrap John Murray London (35)
2 American Medical Association Committee on Food: Accepted Foods. Kellogg's

All-Bran. J Am Med Ass 104: 474 (35)
3   McCance RA, Widdowson EM: Phytin in human nutrition. Biochem J 29:
    2694-2699 (35)
4   Olmsted WH, Curtis G, Timm OK: Stool volatile fatty acids. 4. The influence of
    bran pentosan and fiber to man. J Biol Chem 108: 645-652 (35)
5   Parkes-Weber E: Habitual constipation in old age. Practitioner 135: 229-232 (35)
6   Widdowson EM, McCance RA: The available carbohydrates of fruits. Determination of
    glucose, fructose, sucrose and starch. Biochem J 29: 151-156 (35)
7   Williams RD, Olmsted WH: A biochemical method for determining indigestible
    residue (crude fiber) in feces: lignin, cellulose, non-water soluble hemicelluloses.
    J Biol Chem 108: 653-666 (35)

1934

1   Adolph WH, Wu MY: Influence of roughage on protein digestibility. J Nutr 7:
    381-393 (34)
2   Hurst AF, Holmes G, Burnford J et al: Discussion on the treatment of mucous
    colitis. Proc Roy Soc Med 27: 677-688 (34)
3   Mangold E: The digestion and utilisation of crude fibre. Nutr Abs Rev 3: 647-656 (34)
4   Morgan H: The laxative effect of a regenerated cellulose in the diet, its influence on
    mineral retention. J Am Med Ass 102: 995-997 (34)
5   Olmsted WH, Curtis F, Timm OK: Cause of laxative effect of feeding bran pentosan
    and cellulose to man. Proc Soc Exp Biol Med 32: 141-142 (34)
6   Patterson SW: Diet in diseases of the colon. Practitioner 133: 82-91 (34)
7   Rose MS, Vahlteich EM, MacLeod G: Factors in food influencing hemoglobin
    regeneration. III. Eggs in comparison with whole wheat, prepared bran, oatmeal,
    beef liver and beef muscle. J Biol Chem 104: 217-229 (34)

1933

1   Cowgill GR, Anderson WE, Sullivan AJ: The form of stool as a criterion of laxation.
    J Am Med Assoc 101: 273-275 (33)
2   Cowgill GR, Sullivan AJ: Further studies on the use of wheat bran as a laxative.
    J Am Med Assoc 100: 795-802 (33)
3   Committee on Foods: Whole bran. J Am Med Assoc 100: 1238 (33)

1932

1   Cowgill GR, Anderson WE: Laxative effects of wheat bran and 'washed bran' in
    healthy men. J Am Med Ass 98: 1866-1875 (32)
2   Parsons FB: Constipation and mechanical laxatives. Practitioner 129: 70-83 (32)
3   Rose MS, Vahlteich EM: Factors in food influencing hemoglobin regeneration; whole
    wheat flour, white flour, prepared bran and oatmeal. J Biol Chem 96: 593-608 (32)
4   Rose MS et al: Influence of bran on alimentary tract. J Am Diet Assoc 8: 133-156 (32)

1931

1   Alvarez WC: Opinions of 470 physicians in regard to the advantages and disadvantages
    of using bran and roughage. Minnesota Med 14: 296-300 (31)
2   Cummings R: Chronic constipation. Rational explanation of the symptomatology, with
    suggestions for treatment. Am J Surg 12: 534-536 (31)
3   Davis MB: Intestinal obstruction from eating bran. J Am Med Assoc 97: 24-25 (31)
4   Lichty JA: The present consideration and care of the colon. J Am Med Assoc 96:

649-653 (31)

5   McCarrison R: A lecture on some surgical aspects of faulty nutrition. Br Med J 1: 966-971 (31)

6   McCarrison R: A lecture on the causation of stone in India. Br Med J 1: 1009-1015 (31)

1930

1   Bloom MA: Effect of crude fiber on calcium and phosphorus retention. J Biol Chem 89: 221-233 (30)

2   Childrey JH, Alvarez WC, Mann FC: Digestion: Efficiency with various foods and under various conditions. Archs Int Med 46: 361-374 (30)

3   Falcon-Lesses M: Cause of laxative action of bran. J Nutr 2: 295-310 (30)

4   Mottram JC: The effect of bread on constipation. Practitioner 124: 691-694 (30)

5   Norris FW, Preece IA: Studies on hemicelluloses. I. The hemicelluloses of wheat bran. Biochem J 24: 59-66 (30)

1929

1   McCance RA, Lawrence RD: *The carbohydrate content of Foods*. Med Res Coun Spec Rep Ser No 135 1-73 HM Stationery Office London (29) (340 references)

2   McCarrison R: White and brown bread. Br Med J 2: 913-914 (29)

3   Whitacre J, Willard A, Blunt K: Influence of fiber on nitrogen balance and on fat in feces of human subjects. J Nutr 2: 187-195 (29)

1928

1   Ashley WJ: *The Bread of Our Forefathers: An Inquiry in Economic History*. Clarendon Press Oxford (28)

2   Egglestone EL: Colitis – the spastic type. J Am Med Assoc. 91: 2049-2053 (28)

3   Frey JW et al: Dietetic investigations of edible pure cellulose. Med J Rec 127: 585-589 (28)

4   Hosoi K, Alvarez WC, Mann FC: Intestinal absorption. A search for a low residue diet. Archs Int Med 41: 112-126 (28)

5   Mallory WJ: Medical aspects of colitis J Am Med Assoc 90: 601-603 (28)

6   Ryle JA: Chronic spasmodic affections of the colon and the diseases which they simulate. Lancet 2: 1115-1119 (28)

1927

1   McCarrison R: A good diet and a bad one: an experimental contrast. Ind J Med Res 14: 649-654 (27)

2   Williams GA: A study of the laxative action of wheat bran. Am J Physiol 83: 1-14 (27)

1926

1   McCarrison R: A good diet and a bad one: an experimental contrast. Br Med J 2: 730-732 (26)

2   Murphy JC, Jones DB: Proteins of wheat bran; nutritive properties of proteins of wheat bran. J Biol Chem 69: 85-99 (26)

3   Williamson H: Appendicitis and vegetarianism. Br Med J 2: 714 (26)

1925

1   Moore CV, Brodie JL: The comparative nutritional value of white and whole wheat flour. Archs Pediat 42: 572-577 (25)

2   Weber FP: The clinical significance of constipation. Lancet 1: 53-54 (25)

1924
1   Alvarez WC: Intestinal toxaemia. Physiol Rev 4: 352-393 (24)
2   Halliday H: Intestinal stasis and cancer in Indians. Ind Med Gaz 59: 403-404 (24)
3   Hartwell GA: An experimental study of brown and white bread in the diet of the rat. Biochem J 18: 1323-1326 (24)

1923
1   Kellogg JH: *The New Dietetics: A Guide to the Scientific Feeding in Health and Disease.* Rev. Ed. Modern Medicine Publishing Battle Creek Michigan (23)

1921
1   Dawson (Lord): The colon and colitis. Br Med J 2: 31-35 (21)
2   McCarrison R: *Studies in Deficiency Disease.* Henry Frowde and Hodder and Stoughton London (21)

1920
1   Hindhede M: The effect of food restriction during war on mortality in Copenhagen. J Am Med Assoc 74: 381-382 (20)
2   Short AR: The causation of appendicitis. Br J Surg 8: 171-188 (20)

1919
1   Austen RF: Cellulose and chronic constipation. Ind Med Gaz 54: 56-60 (19)
2   Hurst AF: *Constipation and Allied Intestinal Disorders.* 2nd Ed. Henry Frowde and Hodder and Stoughton London (19)
3   Snyder H: The US Food Administration war flour. Science 50: 130-132 (19)

1917
1   Hammond JL, Hammond LB: *The Town Labourer 1760-1832.* Longmans Green London (17)
2   Hutchinson R, Spriggs EI: A discussion on war bread and its effects on health. Lancet 2: 572-573 (17)
3   Spriggs EI, Weir AB: The digestibility of bread made from two parts of wheat and one part of oats, barley, maize, or rice. Lancet 2: 724-726 (17)

1912
1   Gallant AE: Wheat Bran. Its chemical and physical characteristics in the treatment of chronic constipation. New York Med J 96: 414-417 (12)
2   Newman LF, Robinson GW, Halnan ET et al: Some experiments on the digestibility of white and wholemeal breads. J Hyg Camb 12: 119-143 (12)

1911
1   Edie ES, Simpson GC: Comparative nutritional value of white and standard bread. Br Med J 1: 1151 (11)
2   Edie ES, Simpson GC: The preparation of various foodstuffs (especially wheat and rice). Its effects on the content of organic phosphorus compounds and its relation to disease. Br Med J 1: 1421-1424 (11)
3   Editorial: Standard bread. Br Med J 1: 454-455 (11)

4   Hammond JL, Hammond LB: *The Village Labourer 1760-1832*. Longmans Green London (11)
5   Hill L: A preliminary note on the nutritive value of white and standard bread. Br Med J 1: 1068-1069 (11)
6   Watson C: Comparative nutritive value of white and standard bread (letter). Br Med J 1: 1151 (11)

1900-1905
1   Allinson TR: *Medical Essays* Vol 1-5. LN Fowler London (1900-1905)

1898-1904
1   Bennett R, Elton J: *The History of Corn Milling*. 4 Vols. Simpkins Marshall London (1898-1904)

1892
1   Goodfellow J: *The Dietetic Value of Bread*. Macmillan London (1892).

1888-1889
1   Allinson TR: *The Advantages of Wholemeal Bread*. Reprinted from 'Food'. F Pitman London (1889)
2   Blyth AW: Experiments on the nutritive value of wheat meal. Proc Roy Soc 45: 549-553 (1888-9)

1871
1   Smith E: Dietaries in the workhouses of England and Wales. Br Med J 2: 222 (1871)

1856
1   Dodd, G: *The Food of London*. Longmans Brown and Green and Longmans London (1856)

1849
1   Graham S: *Lectures on the Science of Human Life*. Horsell London (1849).

1847
1   Carr DC: *The Necessity of Brown Bread for Digestion, Nourishment and Sound Health; and the Injurious Effects of White Bread*. Effingham Wilson London (1847)

1837
1   Graham S: *A Treatise on Bread and Bread Making*. Light and Stearns Boston (1837)

1830
1   Cobbett W: *Rural Rides*. W Cobbett London (1830)

1821
1   Accum FC: *Treatise on the Art of Making Good and Wholesome Bread of Wheat, Oats, Rye, Barley and other Farinaceous Grain*. Thomas Boys London (1821)

1610
1   Shakespeare: *Corialanus, Ii*.

Menenius Agrippa: '(The) belly . . . thus answered . . . "I am the store house and the shop of the whole body . . . yet I can make my audit up, that all (parts of the) body do back receive the flour of all and leave me back the bran."'
The bran contains the undigested dietary fibre (H.C.T.)

1542

1   Boorde A: *The Fyrst Boke of the Introduction of Knowledge. A Compendyous Regyment or a Dyetary of Helth.* (1542) (Edited by F J Furnivall. Early English Tract Society London, 1870)

c 430 BC

1   *Hippocrates:* Regimen 2 Chapter 42. Loeb Classical Library. Vol. 4. pages 311-315, New York 1931
2   *Hippocrates:* Regimen 3 Chapter 80. Loeb Classical Library. Vol. 4. pages 407-409, New York 1931.

German Citations
Veröffentlichungen zum Thema 'Ballaststoffe' von Prof. Dr. B. Thomas

1 Die Nähr- und Ballaststoffe der Getreidemehle in ihrer Bedeutung für die Brotnahrung, 256 Seiten, Wissenschaftl. Verlagsgesellschaft Stuttgart (1964)

2 Zur Standardisierung der Rohfaserbestimmung in Getreide und Getreide-produkten gemeinsam mit M. Rothe und L. Tunger. Ernährungsforschung 9: 408-421 (1964)

3 Beiträge zur Nomenklator und Analytik pflanzlicher Zellwandsubstanzen. Getreide Mehl und Brot 26: 158-165 168-169 (1972)

4 Enzymatische Verfahren zur Bestimmung pflanzlicher Gerüstsubstanz und ihrer Zusagekraft. 7 Arbeits- und Diskussionstagung Wien Seite 79-85 der International Cereal Chemistry (1973)

5 Bewertung der Ballaststoffe des Brotes in der kalorienreduzierten Kost. Berichte der 5. Internationalen Tagung: Probleme der modernen Getreide-verarbeitung und Getreidechemie vom 24. 29.9.1973 Bergholz-Rehbrücke (1973)

6 Zur Bewertung der Ballaststoffkomponenten des Brotes. Internationale Zeitschrift für Vitamine und Ernährungsforschung, Beiheft Nr. 14 Qualitätskriterien der Nahrung 53-62 (1974)

7 Möglichkeiten und Grenzen einer Kalorienreduzierung bei Nahrungsmitteln aus Getreide. Getreide Mehl und Brot 28: 213-218 (1974)

8 Enzymatische Rohfaserbestimmung von Getreideprodukten. Getreide Mehl und Brot 29: 115-117 (1975)

9 Ballaststoffe – Lebensnotwendige Bestandteile von Korn und Brot. Erfahrungsheilkunde 24: 1 (1975)

10 Die Balaststoffe des Getreides im Dienste der Ernährungsprophylaxe. Biologische Medizin 4: 234-235 (1975)

11 Schlackrenreiche Kost als Diätform. Deutsche Krankenpflegezeitschrift 29: 425-429 (1976)

12 Die Rohfaseraufnahme in den letzten 100 Jahren. Gemeinsam mit U. Rienermann. Ernährungsumschau 23: 301-303 (1976)

13 Funktionelle Wirkungen und Veränderungen der Ballaststoffe des Weizens während des Verdauungsablaufes. Gemeinsam mit M. Elchazly. Qual. Plantarum 26: 1-3 211-226 (1976)

14 Zur Problematik der Rohfaserbestimmung. Gemeinsam mit M. Elchazly. Getreide Mehl und Brot 30: 252-255 (1976)

15 Verteilung der Ballaststoffe in den Geweben des Weizenkornes. Gemeinsam mit M. Elchazly. Getreide Mehl und Brot 30: 265-269 (1976)

16 Unverdauliche Stoffe im Brot. Die Brotindustrie 19: 340-346 (1976)

17 Einfluss der Ballaststoffe auf die Energieaufnahme. Gemeinsam mit M. Elchazly. Die Mühle 113: 50/51 737-741 (1976)

18 Ober eine biochemische Methode zum Bestimmen der Ballaststoffe und ihrer Komponenten in pflanzlichen Lebensmitteln. Gemeinsam mit M. Elchazly. Zeitschrift für Lebensmitteluntersuchung und -forschung 162: 329-340 (1976)

19 Einflussnahme von Ballaststoffen auf Stoffwechselvorgänge. Gemeinsam mit M. Elchazly und J. Bernasek. Aktuelle Ernährungsmedizin 2: 35-42 (1977)

Author Index

Clarke C (75) 101
Claude R (77) 166
Clayton DG (77) 107
Cleave TL (77) 25, 26;
    (76) 24; (75) 21; (74) 9-12
    (73) 11, 12; (72) 9;
    (69) 2; (66) 1; (62) 4;
    (60) 1; (59) 1; (57) 1;
    (56) 2
Colebourne K W (72) 21
Collinson E (76) 122
Connell AM (77) 27, 28;
    (76) 25; (75) 22
Connor WE (77) 144; (70) 4
Copeland CL (75) 23, 24
Corridan JP (77) 29
Corke M (77) 159
Coste T (76) 26; (75) 25
Cove-Smith JR (75) 26
Crofts TJ (75) 27
Crooks H (65) 6
Crowther JS (73) 13
Cummings JH (77) 10, 30,
    31, 100; (76) 27-30, 35,
    161; (75) 28, 56; (74) 35;
    (73) 14

D'Appolonia BL (77) 113
Davidson LM (77) 87;
    (74) 43
Davies NT (77) 32
Davies PJ (71) 5
Davies PS (77) 6; (75) 123
Davis MB (31) 3
Dawbarn MC (49) 3
Dawson (Lord) (21) 1
Day AA (42) 9
Deer N (49) 4
De Géry A (77) 33
De Groot AP (63) 2
Dekker W (75) 118
De Klerk WA (75) 29
Delbarre F (77) 33
De Moraes Filho JP (75) 30
Denbesten L (70) 4
De Romana GL (76) 86
Desai HG (74) 2
Devereux DF (77) 34
Devi KS (73) 62

Devroede G (77) 35
De Wijn JF (65) 8
De Wit JP (70) 5
Dickson JA (64) 4
Dilawari JB (77) 36
Dimock EM (37) 1; (36) 3
Dinesen K (77) 162;
    (76) 160
Dixon DG (66) 9
Dixon M (77) 116
Dobbs RJ (77) 37
Dodd G (1856) 1
Dodd H (64) 5
Dodds C (72) 10; (54) 2
Dolman W (77) 38
Donefer E (76) 31
Doraiswamy TR (71) 15
Dorfman SH (76) 32
Douglass J (76) 33
Douglass JM (75) 31
Drasar BS (76) 34, 35;
    (75) 50; (73) 13, 15, 31
Dreyer JJ (70) 3
Drossman DA (77) 39
Drummond JC (57) 2;
    (45) 5; (39) 1
Du Bruyn DB (75) 29
Dunlap FL (45) 1
Du Plessis JP (71) 10
Durnin JV (70) 13; (61) 2
Durrington PN (76) 36;
    (75) 32
Duthie HL (76) 133

Eastwood J (76) 38
Eastwood MA (77) 40, 41,
    42, 43, 44, 134; (76) 38,
    39, 40, 53, 96; (75) 33,
    34, 35; (74) 13, 14, 15,
    16, 23, 45, 46; (73) 16, 17,
    18, 19; (70) 6, 7; (69) 4;
    (68) 1, 2, 3; (67) 1
Edie ES (1911) 1, 2
Edwards CS (73) 20
Eggleston FC (74) 17
Egglestone EL (28) 2
Eheart JF (70) 8
Eiseman WR (65) 3
Elchazly M (76) 41, 137

Elias J (76) 14/
Ellis FR (77) 118; (74) 18
Ellis R. (76) 98
Elton J (1898-1904) 1
Enishi A (74) 39
Erfmann R (43) 6
Erikson S (70) 6
Ershoff BH (77) 49;
    (75) 39; (74) 19, 20, 21;
    (62) 5
Escourrau J (77) 167

Fahrenbach MJ (67) 8;
    (66) 2, 10
Falaiye JM (74) 22
Falcon-Lesses M (30) 3
Fantus B (41) 4, 5; (40) 2
Faradji B (77) 66, 67;
    (76) 108; (75) 86
Fassett-Cornelius G (76) 125
Fehrsen GS (77) 80
Fellingham SA (71) 10
Feruglio FS (77) 179
Fettel M (75) 54
Field AC (73) 21
Fielding JF (77) 50
Filippini L (77) 170
Findlay JM (74) 23, 24, 25
Finegold SM (72) 2
Fisher H (67) 2; (66) 3, 5;
    (65) 2
Fisher N (76) 42; (74) 14;
    (73) 22; (72) 10
Flett AA (77) 32
Floch MH (77) 5; (76) 32,
    43, 76
Flynn J (77) 51; (75) 72
Folscroft J (77) 3
Fønns-Bech P (76) 103;
    (75) 82
Forman DT (65) 3
Forrester JM (77) 52
Förster H (77) 53
Fox FW (64) 6; (48) 3
Fox HM (77) 8
Francis B (73) 43
Frankl W (41) 4, 5
Fraser JR (59) 2; (58) 3;
    (57) 3; (56) 5, 6; (51) 2

Frexinos J (77) 167
Frey JW (28) 3
Frohn MJ (76) 44
Fuchs HF (77) 175
Fuchs HM (77) 5; (76) 45,
76
Funnell EH (36) 4
Fuyino Y (77) 89

Gackle D (73) 51
Gajjar D (77) 158
Gallant AE (1912) 1
Galton L (76) 46
Garg KN (77) 15
Garvin JE (65) 3
Gassul MA (77) 36, 68,
69, 71, 72; (76) 47, 48,
71, 84; (75) 63
Gear JS (77) 54
Gearty GF (70) 2
Gehrke CW (75) 52
Gelfand M (76) 49
Gibson N (73) 37
Gilmore OJ (73) 32
Girdwood RH (68) 2
Glasby M (76) 50
Glaser EM (48) 1
Glober GA (77) 55; (74) 26
Gnauck R (77) 170
Goddard J (77) 57
Goddard P (73) 13
Godding EW (76) 51, 52;
(72) 16
Goering HK (73) 23; (70) 9
Goff DV (76) 47, 72
Goldsmith HS (77) 56;
(75) 40
Goldstein F (73) 11
Goodfellow J (1892) 1
Gouffier E (75) 25
Goy JA (76) 53
Graff J (70) 15, 16
Graham GG (76) 86
Graham S (1849) 1;
(1837) 1
Graham-Stewart CW (75) 15
Grande F (65) 4; (61) 3;
(60) 2
Grant WC (66) 2

Greaves JP (66) 4
Greenwood CT (74) 14;
(72) 10
Grimes DS (77) 57; (76) 54
Griminger P (67) 2; (66) 3,
5; (65) 2
Groen JJ (65) 5; (64) 7
Gross SD (77) 56
Gudmand-Høyer E (76)
115, 116
Guinet R (77) 169
Gunby P (77) 58
Gunnin BE (76) 58
Guzman MA (76) 97

Haber GB (77) 59
Haisman P (76) 47
Hall RC (76) 55; (75) 41
Halliday H (24) 2
Halnan ET (1912) 2
Hamilton D (68) 3
Hamilton RM (76) 56
Hamilton T (73) 18;
(72) 12
Hammond JL (1917) 1;
(1911) 4
Hammond LB (1917) 1;
(1911) 4
Hansen LP (75) 51
Hansen OH (76) 57
Hansen HH (77) 172
Hanszen A (36) 2
Hardinge MG (65) 6;
(58) 4
Hardy TL (36) 5
Hart GR (76) 58
Hart JT (74) 27
Hartog M (76) 62
Hartwell GA (24) 3
Harvey RF (77) 93;
(73) 24
Hawkins WW (76) 59
Haworth R (76) 74
Hay WH (35) 2
Hayden DW (75) 62
Heald M (74) 52
Heaton KW (77) 59, 60, 61,
93; (76) 60, 61, 62, 89,
90, 104, 162, 163; (75) 32,

42, 43, 44, 45, 46, 81;
(74) 28, 29, 58; (73) 2,
24, 25, 26, 27, 28, 44;
(72) 13; (71) 6
Heaton ST (71) 6
Harvey RF (76) 90;
(73) 25
Hegsted DM (76) 63
Hellendoorn EW (76) 64;
(75) 47; (73) 29
Hensley GW (65) 1
Herbert P (42) 3
Herrera AF (76) 65
Herxheimer A (76) 66
Hewson AD (57) 4
Heywood PF (75) 48
Higginson J (56) 1; (54) 1
Hill L (1911) 5
Hill MJ (76) 28, 123;
(75) 49. 50; (74) 30
Hill MS (75) 56
Hindhede M (20) 1
Hippocrates (c430 BC) 1, 2
Hipsley EH (74) 31;
(53) 1; (48) 2; (49) 5
Hiromi K (74) 37
Hirschberg N (41) 5
Hobbs JT (76) 64
Hodder RG (41) 6
Hodges RE (64) 1
Hodgson J (77) 62; (74) 32
Hockaday TD (77) 70
Hoelzel F (49) 1
Hollingsworth DF (66) 4
Holloway WD (77) 63
Holm CN (75) 51
Holmes DC (59) 2; (57) 3;
(56) 5, 6
Holmes G (34) 2
Holmgreen GO (72) 14
Holst DO (75) 52
Hoose I (77) 53
Hoppert CA (45) 2; (42) 2
Hopson J (68) 4
Horder (Lord) (54) 2
Horowitz DL (77) 106;
(75) 53
Hosoi K (28) 4
Houston H (77) 31, 73

164

Additional Index

*See also British Medical Journal, Lancet

Addendum

1976

Brooks, P. M., Bremner, W. F., Third, F. H.: Bran, hypertriglyceridaemia and urate clearance. *Med. J. Aust.* **2** 753–756 (76) [1.11*, 2.1*, 5.5*]

Trowell, H. C.: *Dietary fibre and colonic diseases*. 2nd ed. London, Norgine Ltd. (The present state of knowledge; no. 6.) (76) [1.7, 1.8, 6]

1977

Gotestam, K. G.: A double-blind comparison of two bulk laxatives on geriatric patients. *Scand. J. Soc. Med. Suppl.* **14:** 141–145 (77) [1.1*]

McDougall, R. M., Walker, K., Thurston, O. G.: Effect of increased dietary fiber on biliary cholesterol in patients with gallstones. *Surg. Forum* **28:** 416–418 (77) [1.13*, 2.1]

Leveille, G. A.: The role of dietary fiber in nutrition and health †: 84–93 (77) [6]

Nitschke, K. D., Fiero, T. H.: The metabolism of methylcellulose gums †: 57–68 (77) [1.1, 1.11, 5.2*]

Towle, G. A.: Metabolism of natural and certain cellulosic gums †: 44–56 (77) [1.11*, 4.1*]

Van Campen, D. R., Hood, L. F.: Dietary carbohydrates and mineral nutrition †: 94–108 (77) [1.11]

Van Soest, P. J., Robertson, J. B.: Analytical problems of fiber †: 69–83 (77) [4.1*, 1.11]

†Hood, L. F., Wardrip, E. K., Bollenback, G. N., eds: *Carbohydrates and health*. Westport, Connecticut, AVI Publishing Co Inc (77)

DIETARY FIBRE IN HUMAN NUTRITION: A BIBLIOGRAPHY FOR 1978–1982

Alison AVENELL, Anthony R. LEEDS and Hugh C. TROWELL*
Department of Nutrition, Queen Elizabeth College, (University of London),
London, W8 7AH and
*Windhover, Woodgreen, Nr Fordingbridge, Hants. SP6 2AZ, UK.

Dietary fibre has been defined as the residues derived from the traditional foods of man that are not digested by the endogenous secretions of the human alimentary tract. The term 'edible fibre' encompasses dietary fibre and also undigested partially synthetic polysaccharides, such as methyl cellulose; undigested animal polysaccharides, such as aminopolysaccharides present in connective tissues (as eaten by certain ethnic groups); and undigested pharmaceutical preparations from plants not eaten by man as food, eg isphagula bark.

This bibliography includes citations on edible fibre in human nutrition and animal work which may be relevant to human disease. The format follows that of 'Dietary fibre in human nutrition: a bibliography' (H. Trowell editor, John Libbey, 1978), which is reprinted with very slight corrections in this book and which covers the period up to and including 1977. although certain alterations have been made to the subject index. The subject index precedes the citations, with those in foreign languages listed separately. The bibliography is completed by an author index.

Citations have been obtained from the following sources:
(1) Cumulated Index Medicus: 1978–1984.
(2) Nutrition Abstracts and Reviews, Series A (Human and Experimental), prepared by the Commonwealth Bureau of Nutrition, Aberdeen: 1978–1984.
(3) US National Library of Medicine Annual Accumulations (Monographs and Serials): 1978–1983.
(4) Medical Books and Serials in Print (RR Bowker Company, New York and London): 1978–1983.
(5) Cumulative Book Index (HW Wilson Company, New York): 1978–1983.
(6) British National Bibliography: 1978–1983.

In addition, the following journals were searched in order to include references not listed by the above sources:
American Journal of Clinical Nutrition
Annals de Nutrition et Alimentation
British Food Journal
British Medical Journal
Cereal Chemistry
Cereal Foods World
Diabetes

Gastroenterology
Gut
Journal of the American Dietetic Association
Journal of Food Science
Journal of Nutrition
Journal of Plant Foods
Journal of the Science of Food and Agriculture
Modern Geriatrics, becoming Geriatric Medicine after April 1979
Nutrition Bulletin
South African Medical Journal
Scandinavian Journal of Gastroenterology
World Medicine
WHO Technical Report Series

The references are given in the style of Index Medicus, with two initials only for each author, and journal abbreviations are based on British Standard 4148:1970 (for further details see BIOSIS, Chemical Abstracts Service and Engineering Index, Inc., 1974; Bibliographic Guide for Editors and Authors; Biological Abstracts, Philadelphia; Chemical Abstracts, Columbus, Ohio; Engineering Index, Inc., New York). Books on fibre are listed not only by editor or author but also by individual article. A number of citations are taken from the Third Kellogg Nutrition Symposium (see ref 152, 1978). These are also reprinted in the Journal of Plant Foods 1978; 3(1 + 2) and in the same book published by John Libbey in 1979. The more important citations are listed in the subject index with an asterisk, which generally denotes a more extensive review or original research. Relatively few references on phytate or saponins have been included in the bibliography.

Many thanks go to Jane Fitzgerald, Uta Finken, Sheila Legat, Anna Rainbird, the Health Education Council and the many librarians who gave their assistance.

(1) GASTROINTESTINAL
- (1.1) Colonic function, faecal weight, transit time, constipation
- (1.2) Diverticular disease
- (1.3) Irritable bowel syndrome
- (1.4) Large bowel cancer, colonic and faecal bacteria
- (1.5) Appendicitis
- (1.6) Ulcerative colitis, Crohn's disease
- (1.7) The group of large bowel disorders
- (1.8) Hiatus hernia
- (1.9) Stomach, gastric ulcer, small intestine, duodenal ulcer
- (1.10) Dumping syndrome
- (1.11) Digestibility and digestion of fibre; absorption of nutrients, minerals and drugs
- (1.12) Ileostomy
- (1.13) Gallstones, bile salt metabolism
- (1.14) Phytobezoars
- (1.15) Miscellaneous gastrointestinal

(2) CARDIOVASCULAR
- (2.1) Lipid metabolism, cholesterol, triglycerides
- (2.2) Atherosclerosis, ischaemic heart disease
- (2.3) Venous thrombosis, varicose veins, haemorrhoids
- (2.4) Hypertension

(3) METABOLIC
- (3.1) Diabetes mellitus, carbohydrate metabolism
- (3.2) Obesity

(4) FIBRE AND FOOD
- (4.1) Fibre: definition, terminology, composition, analysis
- (4.2) Fibre in the diet and food, except cereals
- (4.3) Fibre in cereal and cereal foods
- (4.4) Modern dietary change

(5) MISCELLANEOUS
- (5.1) Antitoxic action
- (5.2) Ill-effects
- (5.3) Early views on whole foods and dietary fibre before 1940
- (5.4) Experimental methods
- (5.5) Other

(6) DIETARY FIBRE HYPOTHESES, GENERAL PRESENTATION

(7) BOOKS, SYMPOSIA, THESES
- (7.1) Books for the public
- (7.2) Books for the scientist

(1) GASTROINTESTINAL

(2) *CARDIOVASCULAR*
   (2.1) Lipid metabolism, cholesterol, triglycerides
          1*, 4*, 7*, 30, 59*, 60, 64, 65, 75, 94, 95, 108, 110*, 113, 117*, 124*, 126,
          145, 146, 157*, 161, 165, 167, 182*, 185, 190, 194, 197*, 207, 210*, 211, 212,
          213*, 214, 215*, 216*, 218, 220, 226, 230, 231*, 248, 252*, 266, 270, 272,
          276*, 281*, 290*, 292, 294, 295, 297*, 301, 306, 308, 312*, 318, 326*, 330,
          331, 346, 369, 370, 373*, 384, 385*, 388*, 389, 402, 409, 420, 434*, 453,
          454*, 462*

   (2.2) Atherosclerosis, ischaemic heart disease
          28, 125, 140, 150, 210*, 211, 214, 215*, 216*, 265, 266*, 288, 303, 318, 331,
          381, 409, 411, 474

   (2.3) Venous thrombosis, varicose veins, haemorrhoids
          14*, 54*, 221*, 418

   (2.4) Hypertension
          130*, 339

(3) *METABOLIC*
   (3.1) Diabetes mellitus, carbohydrate metabolism
          3*, 4*, 5*, 8, 11, 12, 13*, 17, 18, 30, 32, 41, 60, 61, 78, 83, 139*, 140*, 141,
          145, 149, 153*, 165, 175, 180*, 181*, 182*, 195, 224, 255, 256, 260*, 271,
          272, 302, 306, 307, 308, 316, 376, 379*, 390, 402, 406, 421, 425, 426*, 469

   (3.2) Obesity
          3*, 29, 92*, 96, 112, 141, 142, 149, 153*, 155*, 161, 170*, 177, 195, 326*,
          356, 371*, 390*, 399*, 401*, 405, 466*

(4) *FIBRE AND FOOD*
   (4.1) Fibre: definition, terminology, composition, analysis
          6, 10, 20*, 22, 23*, 44, 57*, 118, 138*, 148*, 157*, 158*, 189, 227*, 245*,
          257, 258*, 284, 298*, 320, 321*, 322, 336*, 338*, 344, 349, 354*, 355*, 357*,
          359*, 360*, 364*, 377, 396*, 397, 398*, 448, 453, 463*, 464, 467, 475*, 477*,
          480

   (4.2) Fibre in the diet and food, except cereals
          5*, 29, 71, 75, 89, 126, 134, 136, 144*, 147, 160, 183, 198, 204, 243, 266, 267,
          273, 295, 300*, 322, 323, 328, 347*, 354*, 355*, 359, 404, 423, 448, 453*,
          467, 478

   (4.3) Fibre in cereal and cereal foods
          5*, 12, 13*, 109, 136, 141, 148, 183, 187*, 243, 257, 258, 259, 266*, 274, 284,
          287, 300*, 320, 336*, 345, 347*, 353, 354*, 355*, 359, 376*, 403*, 410, 412,
          426, 435, 438, 448, 463, 467

   (4.4) Modern dietary change
          159*, 191, 209*, 295, 323, 358*

(5) *MISCELLANEOUS*
   (5.1) Antitoxic action
          39, 60, 62*, 391, 453

   (5.2) Ill-effects
          21*, 61, 234, 277, 387, 407, 413, 416*, 449*

   (5.3) Early views on whole foods and dietary fibre before 1940
          187

   (5.4) Experimental methods
          40*, 42*, 69*, 70, 74, 123, 135, 160*, 219, 237, 269*, 292, 344, 422, 433, 447

   (5.5) Other
          25, 30, 156, 178, 322, 326, 332, 380*

(6) DIETARY FIBRE HYPOTHESES, GENERAL PRESENTATION
9, 31, 53*, 72, 97*+, 98*+, 103*, 144*, 158, 160, 187*, 196, 198, 243, 247,
249, 322. 332, 334*, 362*, 378*, 382*, 383*, 429, 442, 444*, 446, 451*, 452,
457, 459, 468, 481

(7) BOOKS, SYMPOSIA, THESES
   (7.1)   Books for the public
          188, 304, 348

   (7.2)   Books for the scientist
          133*, 152*, 289*, 300*, 365*

+ Identical articles.

THE REFERENCES

(1) Akiba Y, Matsumoto T. Effects of force-feeding and dietary cellulose on liver lipid accumulation and lipid composition of liver and plasma in growing chicks. J Nutr 1978 May; 108 (5): 739-48.

(2) Albert KS, Ayres JW, DiSanto AR, Weidler DJ, Sakmar E, Hallmark MR, Stoll RG, DeSante KA, Wagner JG. Influence of kaolin-pectin suspension on digoxin bioavailability. J Pharm Sci 1978 Nov; 67 (11): 1582-6.

(3) Albrink MJ. Dietary fiber, plasma insulin, and obesity. Am J Clin Nutr 1978 Oct; 31 (10 Suppl): S277-9.

(4) Anderson JW, Ward K. Long-term effects of high-carbohydrate, high-fiber diets on glucose and lipid metabolism: a preliminary report on patients with diabetes. Diabetes Care 1978 Mar-Apr; 1 (2): 77-82.

(5) Anderson JW, Lin W-J, Ward K. Composition of foods commonly used in diets for persons with diabetes. Diabetes Care 1978 Sep-Oct; 1(5): 293-302.

(6) Andersson H, Hallgren B, Hulthen L, Isaksson B, Sandberg AS. Dietary fibre in food and ileostomy contents (abstract). In: Abstracts and Free Communications of XI International Congress of Nutrition. Rio De Janeiro: Executive Committee of XI International Congress of Nutrition, 1978: 595.

(7) Angelico F, Clemente P, Menotti A, Ricci G, Urbinati G. Bran and changes in serum lipids: observations during a project of primary prevention of coronary heart disease. In: Carlson LA, Paoletti R, Sirtori CR, Weber G, eds. International Conference on Atherosclerosis. New York: Raven Press, 1978: 205-7.

(8) Anonymous. What beans may mean to you. Balance 1978; 43: 1.

(9) Anonymous. Dietary fibre. More facts and fallacies. Br Food J 1978 Jul-Aug; 80: 110-2.

(10) Anonymous. New modular system for fibre determination. Grass 1978, 22: 20.

(11) Anonymous. Diabetes and dietary fiber. Nutr Rev 1978 Sep; 36 (9): 273-5.

(12) Apling EC, Khan P, Ellis PR. The formulation, preparation and properties of a guar/wheat bread for therapeutic use: experiences and prospects (abstract). Cereal Foods World 1978 Aug; 23 (8): 460.

(13) Apling EC, Khan P, Ellis P. Guar/wheat bread for therapeutic use. Cereal Foods World 1978 Nov; 23 (11): 640-4.

(14) Arabi Y, Makuria T, Buchmann P, Alexander-Williams J, Keighley MR. Trial of a high fibre diet or local treatment for patients with haemorrhoids (abstract). Gut 1978 Oct; 19 (10): A987.

(15) Araujo PE. Evaluation of the effects of cellulose on fecal and intestinal characteristics of mice. J Food Sci 1978; 43 (3): 1040, 1042.

(16) Archampong EQ, Christian F, Badoe EA. Diverticular disease in an indigenous African community. Ann R Coll Surg Engl 1978 Nov; 60 (6): 464-70.

(17) Arky RA. Current principles of dietary therapy of diabetes mellitus. Med Clin North Am 1978 Jul; 62 (4): 655-62.

(18) Arky RA. Diet and diabetes mellitus: concepts and objectives. Postgrad Med 1978 Jun; 63 (6): 72-8.

(19) Asp N-G, Bauer H, Dahlqvist A, Fredlund P, Oste R. Dietary fibre and experimental colon cancer in the rat. Naringsforskning 1978; 22 (16 Suppl): 64-8.

(20) Asp N-G. Critical evaluation of some suggested methods of assay of dietary fibre. In: Heaton KW, ed. Third Kellogg Nutrition Symposium. Dietary fibre: current developments of importance to health. London: Newman Publishing Ltd, 1978: 21-6.

(21) Bachmann E, Weber E, Post M, Zbinden G. Biochemical effects of gum arabic, gum tragacanth, methylcellulose and carboxymethylcellulose-sodium in rat heart and liver. Pharmacology 1978; 17 (1): 39-49.

(22) Bacon JS. The digestion and metabolism of polysaccharides by man and other animals. In: Heaton KW, ed. Third Kellogg Nutrition Symposium. Dietary fibre: current developments of importance to health. London: Newman Publishing Ltd, 1978: 27-34.

(23) Bailey RW, Chesson A, Monro J. Plant cell wall fractionation and structural analysis. Am J Clin Nutr 1978 Oct; 31 (10 Suppl): S77-81.

176

(24) Baldwin JA. Cholelithiasis and hiatus hernia (letter). Lancet 1978 Nov 4; 2 (8097): 992.

(25) Bansal BR, Rhoads JE Jr, Bansal SC. Effect of diet on colon carcinogenesis and the immune system in rats treated with 1,2-dimethylhydrazine. Cancer Res 1978 Oct; 38 (10): 3293-303.

(26) Barbolt TA, Abraham R. The effect of bran on dimethylhydrazine-induced colon carcinogenesis in the rat. Proc Soc Exp Biol Med 1978 Apr; 157 (4): 656-9.

(27) Bassett ML, Goulston KJ. False positive hemoccult reactions on a high fibre restricted diet. Aust NZ J Med 1978 Oct; 8 (5): 556.

(28) Bassler TJ. Hard water, food fibre, and silicon (letter). Br Med J 1978 Apr 8; 1 (6117): 919.

(29) Beereboom J. Low calorie bulking agents. In: Dwivedi BK, ed. Low calorie and special dietary foods. CRC Press Inc, 1978: 39-50.

(30) Behall KM, Kelsay JL, Prather ES. Effect of fiber from fruits and vegetables on serum levels of triglycerides, free fatty acids, cholesterol, glucose, lactate, insulin, growth hormone, cortisol, and phosphorus of human subjects (abstract). Fed Proc 1978; 37 (3): 543.

(31) Bellows JG, Bellows RT. Dietary fiber in disease (editorial). Compr Ther 1978 May; 4 (5): 3.

(32) Bellows JG. Diabetes mellitus—a fiber deficiency disease (editorial). Compr Ther 1978 Jul; 4 (7): 3-4.

(33) Beyer PL, Flynn MA. Effects of high-and low-fiber diets on human feces. J Am Diet Assoc 1978 Mar; 72 (3): 271-7.

(34) Bjorneklett A, Fausa O, Lovik A, Ritland S, Gjone E. Fibre tablets as effective alternative to wheat bran in constipation (abstract). Acta Med Scand 1978; Suppl 621: 45.

(35) Bokkenheuser VD, Winter J, Kelly WG. Metabolism of biliary steroids by human fecal flora. Am J Clin Nutr 1978 Oct; 31 (10 Suppl): S221-6.

(36) Bond JH, Levitt MD. Effect of dietary fiber on intestinal gas production and small bowel transit time in man. Am J Clin Nutr 1978 Oct; 31 (10 Suppl): S169-74.

(37) Bond JH, Levitt MD. Gaseousness and intestinal gas. Med Clin North Am 1978 Jan; 62 (1): 155-64.

(38) Bornside GH. Stability of human fecal flora. Am J Clin Nutr 1978 Oct; 31 (10 Suppl): S141-44.

(39) Bounous G, Pageau R, Regoli D. The role of diet on 5-fluorouracil toxicity. Int J Clin Pharmacol Biopharm 1978 Nov; 16 (11): 519-22.

(40) Branch WJ, Cummings JH. Comparison of radio-opaque pellets and chromium sesquioxide as inert markers in studies requiring accurate faecal collections. Gut 1978 May; 19 (5): 371-6.

(41) Briggs S, Spiller GA. Dietary fiber, glucose tolerance, and diabetes related; new diet therapy emerges. Food Prod Dev 1978; 12 (3): 81-2, 86-8.

(42) Bright-See E, Rao AV, Li S, Tang T. A system for studying the biological effects of dietary fibers. Nutr Rep Int 1978 Dec; 18 (6): 671-5.

(43) Brodribb AJ, Groves C. Effect of bran particle size on stool weight. Gut 1978 Jan; 19 (1): 60-3.

(44) Brodribb AJ, Gear J. Dietary fibre and colonic function (letter). J R Soc Med 1978 Apr; 71 (4): 304-5.

(45) Brodribb AJ. The treatment of diverticular disease with dietary fibre. In: Heaton KW, ed. Third Kellogg Nutrition Symposium. Dietary fibre: current developments of importance to health. London: Newman Publishing Ltd, 1978: 63-73.

(46) Brown RC, Kelleher J, Losowsky MS. Effect of pectin on small bowel structure and function (abstract). Gut 1978 May; 19 (5): A454-5.

(47) Brown SM, Falk HL. Dietary fibre and chemically induced bowel tumours (letter). Lancet 1978 Dec 9; 2 (8102): 1252.

(48) Bruckstein AH. Laxatives and cathartics. Uses and abuses. NY State J Med 1978 Jun; 78 (7): 1078-82.

(49) Bryant MP. Cellulose digesting bacteria from human feces. Am J Clin Nutr 1978 Oct; 31 (10 Suppl): S113-5.

(50) Budd DC, McCreary ML. Gastric phytobezoar: still another postgastrectomy syndrome. Am Surg 1978 Feb; 44 (2): 104-7.

(51) Burkitt DP. Colonic-rectal cancer: fiber and other dietary factors. Am J Clin Nutr 1978 Oct; 31 (10 Suppl): S58-64.

(52) Burkitt DP. Workshop V—Fiber and cancer. Summary and recommendations. Am J Clin Nutr 1978 Oct; 31 (10 Suppl): S213-5.

(53) Burkitt D. A discarded protection. Dietary Fibre. Ir Med J 1978 May 26; 71 (8): 244-7.

(54) Burkitt DP. Mechanical effects of fibre with reference to appendicitis, hiatus hernia, haemorrhoids and varicose veins. In: Heaton KW, ed. Third Kellogg Nutrition Symposium. Dietary fibre: current developments of importance to health. London: Newman Publishing Ltd, 1978: 35-44.

(55) Calder JF, Wasunna AE. Diverticular disease of the colon in Kenyan Africans. East Afr Med J 1978 Dec; 55 (12): 579-81.

(56) Calloway DH, Kretsch MJ. Protein and energy utilization in men given a rural Guatemalan diet and egg formulas with and without added oat bran. Am J Clin Nutr 1978 Jul; 31 (7): 1118-26.

(57) Campbell LA, Palmer GH. Pectin. In: Spiller GA, ed. Topics in dietary fiber research. New York and London: Plenum Press, 1978: 105-15.

(58) Capron J-P, Payenneville H, Dumont M, Dupas J-L, Lorriaux A. Evidence for an association between cholelithiasis and hiatus hernia. Lancet 1978 Aug 12; 2 (8085): 329-31.

(59) Carroll KK, Hamilton RM, Huff MW, Falconer AD. Dietary fiber and cholesterol metabolism in rabbits and rats. Am J Clin Nutr 1978 Oct; 31 (10 Suppl): S203-7.

(60) Caster WO, Hoff LA, Wade AE. Effect of major nutrient substitutions on body weight gain, blood glucose and cholesterol levels, and the rate of drug metabolism in the liver. Int J Vitam Nutr Res 1978; 48 (1): 54-61.

(61) Catellani J, Collins RJ. Drug labelling (letter). Lancet 1978 Jul 8; 2 (8080): 98.

(62) Chadwick RW, Copeland MF, Chadwick CJ. Enhanced pesticide metabolism, a previously unreported effect of dietary fibre in mammals. Food Cosmet Toxicol 1978 Jun; 16 (3): 217-25.

(63) Chakrabarty PB, Mohan Rao S. 'Kendu' bezoar. J Indian Med Assoc 1978 Mar 1; 70 (5): 111-2.

(64) Chang ML, Johnson MA. Effect of lignin versus cellulose on the absorption of taurocholic acid and lipid metabolism in rats fed cholesterol diet (abstract). Fed Proc 1978; 37 (3): 542.

(65) Chang ML, Johnson MA. Effect of dietary vegetable and type of carbohydrate on lipid metabolism in rats. Nutr Rep Int 1978 Sep; 18 (3): 337-44.

(66) Cheeke PR, Patton NM. Effect of alfalfa and dietary fiber on the growth performance of weanling rabbits. Lab Anim Sci 1978; 28 (2): 167-72.

(67) Chellappa M, Ahmad K. Phytobezoar: a case report. Med J Malaysia 1978 Mar; 32 (3): 245-6.

(68) Chen W-F, Patchefsky AS, Goldsmith HS. Colonic protection from dimethylhydrazine by a high fiber diet. Surg Gynecol Obstet 1978 Oct; 147 (4): 503-6.

(69) Clinton SK, Truex R, Visek WJ. A model system for evaluating the role of dietary fiber in chemical carcinogenesis. Biochem Pharmacol 1978 May 1; 27 (9): 1393-6.

(70) Clinton SK, Visek WJ. A model system for examining the role of dietary fiber in chemical carcinogenesis (abstract). Fed Proc 1978; 37 (3): 263.

(71) Cliver DO. Potential fiber source (letter). Am J Clin Nutr 1978 Jul; 31 (7): 1111-2.

(72) Colmey JC. High-fiber foods in the American diet. Food Technol 1978; 32 (3): 42, 47.

(73) Connell AM. The effects of dietary fiber on gastrointestinal motor function. Am J Clin Nutr 1978 Oct; 31 (10 Suppl): S152-6.

(74) Connell AM. Tests of gastrointestinal motility. Clin Gastroenterol 1978 May; 7 (2): 317-28.

(75) Connor WE, Cerqueira MT, Connor RW, Wallace RB, Malinow MR, Casdorph HR. The plasma lipids, lipoproteins, and diet of the Tarahumara Indians of Mexico. Am J Clin Nutr 1978 Jul; 31 (7): 1131-42.

(76) Corley JR, Easter RA, Roos MA, Fahey GC Jr. Effect of various fiber sources on gain, feed efficiency and nitrogen retention in the weanling pig. Nutr Rep Int 1978 Aug; 18 (2): 135-42.

(77) Correa P, Haenszel W. The epidemiology of large-bowel cancer. Adv Cancer Res 1978; 26: 1-141.

(78) Cressey D, Barbosa J. The effect of complex carbohydrates on plasma glucose in normal and insulin-independent diabetics (abstract). In: Abstracts and Free Communications of XI International Congress of Nutrition. Rio de Janeiro: Executive Committee of XI International Congress of Nutrition, 1978: 232.

(79) Cruse JP, Lewin MR, Ferulano GP, Clark CG. Dietary fibre, Vivonex, cholesterol and experimental colon cancer (abstract). Gut 1978 Oct; 19 (10): A983-4.

(80) Cruse JP, Lewin MR, Clark CG. Dietary fibre and experimental colon cancer (letter). Lancet 1978 Oct 14; 2 (8094): 843-4.

(81) Cruse JP, Lewin MR, Clark CG. Failure of bran to protect against experimental colon cancer in rats. Lancet 1978 Dec 16; 2 (8103): 1278-80.

(82) Cullen RW, Oace SM. Methylmalonic acid and vitamin B12 excretion of rats consuming diets varying in cellulose and pectin. J Nutr 1978 Apr; 108 (4): 640-7.

(83) Cummings JH. Nutritional implications of dietary fiber. Am J Clin Nutr 1978 Oct; 31 (10 Suppl): S21-9.

(84) Cummings JH. Dietary factors in the aetiology of gastrointestinal cancer. J Hum Nutr 1978 Dec; 32 (6): 455-65.

(85) Cummings JH. Dietary fibre and colonic function (editorial). J R Soc Med 1978 Feb; 71 (2): 81-4.

(86) Cummings JH, Southgate DA, Branch W, Houston H, Jenkins DJ, James WP. Colonic response to dietary fibre from carrot, cabbage, apple, bran and guar gum. Lancet 1978 Jan 7; 1 (8054): 5-9.

(87) Cummings JH. Diet and transit through the gut. In: Heaton KW, ed. Third Kellogg Nutrition Symposium. Dietary fibre: current developments of importance to health. London: Newman Publishing Ltd, 1978: 83-95.

(88) Dalhamn T, Nilsson LH, Graf W. The effect of sterculia bulk on the viscosity of stomal output from 12 patients with ileostomy. Scand J Gastroenterol 1978; 13 (4): 485-8.

(89) Davies NT. The effects of dietary fibre on mineral availability. In: Heaton KW, ed. Third Kellogg Nutrition Symposium. Dietary fibre: current developments of importance to health. London: Newman Publishing Ltd, 1978: 113-23.

(90) Davies PS, Rhodes J. Maintenance of remission in ulcerative colitis with sulphasalazine or a high-fibre diet: a clinical trial. Br Med J 1978 Jun 10; 1 (6126): 1524-5.

(91) Davies PS, Rhodes J. Maintenance of remission in ulcerative colitis with sulphasalazine or a high-fibre diet. In: Heaton KW, ed. Third Kellogg Nutrition Symposium. Dietary fibre: current developments of importance to health. London: Newman Publishing Ltd, 1978: 125-7.

(92) Davis JD, Collins BJ. Distention of the small intestine, satiety, and the control of food intake. Am J Clin Nutr 1978 Oct; 31 (10 Suppl): S255-8.

(93) Devroede G. Dietary fiber, bowel habits, and colonic function. Am J Clin Nutr 1978 Oct; 31 (10 Suppl): S157-60.

(94) Dixon M. Bran and HDL-cholesterol (letter). Br Med J 1978 Mar 4; 1 (6112): 578.

(95) Domingo FM, Carreon DT, Ocoma EP, Cilindro PA. Dietary fiber, a hypocholesterolemic agent? Food Nutr Res Inst Sem Rep Ser 1978; 4: 8.

(96) Durrant ML, Royston P. The effect of preloads of varying energy density and methyl cellulose on hunger, appetite and salivation (abstract). Proc Nutr Soc 1978 Dec; 37 (3): 87A.

(97)+ Dwyer JT, Goldin BG, Gorbach S, Patterson J. Drug therapy reviews: dietary fiber and fiber supplements in the therapy of gastrointestinal disorders. Am J Hosp Pharm 1978 Mar; 35 (3): 278-87.

+ Identical articles

(98)+ Dwyer JT, Goldin BG, Gorbach S, Patterson J. Dietary fiber and fiber supplements in the therapy of gastrointestinal disorders. J Maine Med Assoc 1978 Feb; 69 (2): 51-60, 62.

(99) Eastwood MA. Fiber in the gastrointestinal tract. Am J Clin Nutr 1978 Oct; 31 (10 Suppl): S30-2.

(100) Eastwood MA. Fiber and the gastrointestinal tract. In: Nutrition Products Division. Dietary Fiber. Volume 1. Chicago, Illinois: Masonite Corporation, 1978: 12-8.

(101) Eastwood MA, Smith AN. Treatment of diverticular disease with hydrophilic colloids. In: Duthie HL, ed. Proceedings of Sixth International Symposium on Gastrointestinal Motility. Lancaster: MTP Press Ltd, 1978: 95-9.

(102) Eastwood MA, Smith AN, Brydon WG, Pritchard J. Comparison of bran, isphagula, and lactulose on colonic function in diverticular disease. Gut 1978 Dec; 19 (12): 1144-7.

(103) Eastwood MA, Robertson JA. The place of dietary fibre in our diet. J Hum Nutr 1978 Feb; 32 (1): 53-61.

(104) Eastwood MA, Smith AN, Brydon WG, Pritchard J. Colonic function in patients with diverticular disease. Lancet 1978 Jun 3; 1 (8075): 1181-2.

(105) Eastwood M. Epidemiology of diverticular disease. In: Heaton KW, ed. Third Kellogg Nutrition Symposium. Dietary fibre: current developments of importance to health. London: Newman Publishing Ltd, 1978: 75-82.

(106) Ecknauer RE, Sircar B, Lichtenberger LM, Johnson LR. Role of food-bulk in maintaining mucosal morphology in rat small intestine (abstract). Gastroenterology 1978 May; 74 (5 Pt 2): 1030.

(107) Ekwueme O. Bowel habits in Ugandan villagers. Trop Geogr Med 1978 Jun; 30 (2): 247-51.

(108) Elliott J, Kritchevsky D, Mulvihill B, Duncan C, Forsythe R. Effect of vegetable processing wastes and common dietary fiber sources on serum cholesterol in the rat (abstract). Fed Proc 1978; 37 (3): 630.

(109) Ellis R, Morris ER. Low-phytate wheat bran as dietary source of iron and zinc for rats (abstract). Fed Proc 1978; 37 (3): 585.

(110) Erdman JW Jr, O'Reilly TC. Hypercholesterolemia in rats fed cholesterol in agar gel diets. Lipids 1978 Sep; 13 (9): 588-93.

(111) Eshchar J. Constipation and education (editorial). Arch Intern Med 1978 May; 138 (5): 690-1.

(112) Evans E, Miller DS. Slimming aids. J Hum Nutr 1978 Dec; 32 (6): 433-8.

(113) Fahey GC Jr, Miller BL, Hadfield HW. Metabolic factors affected by feeding various types of fiber to guinea pigs (abstract). Fed Proc 1978; 37 (3): 849.

(114) Fahey GC Jr. Evaluation of chemical fractions isolated from wood hemicellulose extracts. Nutr Rep Int 1978 Jan; 17 (1): 1-5.

(115) Fakunle YM, Ajagbonna SO, Ani OE, Awofeso O. Diarrhoea, constipation and intestinal transit in a northern Nigerian population. J Trop Med Hyg 1978 Jul; 81 (7): 137-8.

(116) Falaiye JM. The dietary fibre theory and bile salt pattern in Nigerians. Afr J Med Med Sci 1978 Sep; 7 (3): 157-61.

(117) Farrell DJ, Girle L, Arthur J. Effects of dietary fibre on the apparent digestibility of major food components and on blood lipids in men. Aust J Exp Biol Med Sci 1978 Aug; 56 (4): 469-79.

(118) Fassett-Cornelius G, Spiller GA. Plantix versus dietary fiber: a reply to Trowell (letter). Am J Clin Nutr 1978 Feb; 31 (2): 200-1.

(119) Finegold SM, Sutter VL. Fecal flora in different populations with special reference to diet. Am J Clin Nutr 1978 Oct; 31 (10 Suppl): S116-22.

(120) Fleiszer D, Murray D, MacFarlane J, Brown RA. Protective effect of dietary fibre against chemically induced bowel tumours in rats. Lancet 1978 Sep 9; 2 (8089): 552-3.

(121) Floch MH, Fuchs H-M. Modification of stool content by increased bran intake. Am J Clin Nutr 1978 Oct; 31 (10 Suppl): S185-9.

(122)   Floyd RA. Digoxin interaction with bran and high fiber foods (letter). Am J Hosp
        Pharm 1978 Jun; 35 (6): 660.
(123)   Forman LP, Schneeman BO, Weir WC. Correlation of chromium sequioxide and [14C]
        cellulose as fecal markers in rats. Proc Soc Exp Biol Med 1978 Mar; 157 (3): 418-20.
(124)   Forsythe WA, Chenoweth WL, Bennink MR. Laxation and serum cholesterol in rats
        fed plant fibers. J Food Sci 1978; 43 (5): 1470-2.
(125)   Foster KJ, Holdstock G, Whorwell PJ, Guyer P, Wright R. Prevalence of diverticular
        disease of the colon in patients with ischaemic heart disease. Gut 1978 Nov; 19 (11):
        1054-6.
(126)   Frank GC, Berenson GS, Webber LS. Dietary studies and the relationship of diet to
        cardiovascular disease risk factor variables in 10-year-old children — The Bogalusa
        Heart Study. Am J Clin Nutr 1978 Feb; 31 (2): 328-40.
(127)   Freeman HJ, Spiller GA, Kim YS. A double-blind study on the effect of purified
        cellulose dietary fiber on 1,2-dimethylhydrazine-induced rat colonic neoplasia. Cancer
        Res 1978 Sep; 38 (9): 2912-7.
(128)   Freeman HJ, Kim YS, Spiller GA. Effect of chemically defined dietary fiber on rat
        colonic neoplasia induced by 1,2-dimethylhydrazine (abstract). Gastroenterology 1978
        May; 74 (5 Pt 2): 1036.
(129)   Fritz JC, Pla GW, Clark GA. Effect of wheat bran on utilization of powdered metallic
        iron (abstract). Fed Proc 1978; 37 (3): 488.
(130)   Gardey T, Burstyn PG, Taylor TG. Fat induced hypertension in rabbits. 1. The effects
        of fibre on the blood pressure increase induced by coconut oil (abstract). Proc Nutr
        Soc 1978 Dec; 37 (3): 97A.
(131)   Garrison MV, Reid RL, Fawley P, Breidenstein CP. Comparative digestibility of acid
        detergent fiber by laboratory albino and wild Polynesian rats. J Nutr 1978 Feb; 108
        (2): 191-5.
(132)   Gear JS, Ware AC, Nolan DJ, Fursdon PS, Brodribb AJ, Mann JI. Dietary fibre and
        asymptomatic diverticular disease of the colon (abstract). Proc Nutr Soc 1978 May; 37
        (1): 13A.
(133)   Gear JS. Epidemiological studies of the role of dietary fibre in the aetiology of disease.
        Oxford, England: University of Oxford, 1978. Thesis.
(134)   Gear JS. Dietary fibre and asymptomatic diverticular disease of the colon. In : Heaton
        KW, ed. Third Kellogg Nutrition Symposium. Dietary fibre: current developments of
        importance to health. London: Newman Publishing Ltd, 1978: 57-62.
. (135) George JR, Reeves RD, Harbers LH. Digestion of fiber in rats as observed by scanning
        electron microscopy (abstract). Fed Proc 1978; 37 (3): 756.
(136)   Gibney MJ, Upton PK. The Irish diet. 2. Intakes and sources of fat, individual fatty
        acids, cholesterol, dietary fibre and crude fibre. Ir J Food Sci Technol 1978; 2 (1):
        13-9.
(137)   Goldin B, Dwyer J, Gorbach SL, Gordon W, Swenson L. Influence of diet and age on
        fecal bacterial enzymes. Am J Clin Nutr 1978 Oct; 31 (10 Suppl): S136-40.
(138)   Gordon AJ. The chemical structure of lignin and quantitative and qualitative methods
        of analysis in foodstuffs. In: Spiller GA, ed. Topics in dietary fiber research. New
        York and London: Plenum Press, 1978: 59-103.
(139)   Goulder TJ, Alberti KG, Jenkins DJ. Effect of added fiber on the glucose and
        metabolic response to a mixed meal in normal and diabetic subjects. Diabetes Care
        1978 Nov-Dec; 1 (6): 351-5.
(140)   Goulder TJ, Alberti KG. Dietary fibre and diabetes (editorial). Diabetologia 1978 Oct;
        15 (4): 285-7.
(141)   Grimes DS, Gordon C. Satiety value of wholemeal and white bread. Lancet 1978 Jul 8;
        2 (8080): 106.
(142)   Grovum WL, Phillips GD. Factors affecting the voluntary intake of food by sheep. 1.
        The role of distension, flow-rate of digesta and propulsive motility in the intestines. Br
        J Nutr 1978 Sep; 40 (2): 323-36.
(143)   Guthrie BE, Robinson MF. Zinc balance studies during wheat bran supplementation
        (abstract). Fed Proc 1978; 37 (3): 254.

(144) Hardinge MG. Plant fibers and human health. In: Spiller GA, ed. Topics in dietary fiber research. New York and London: Plenum Press, 1978: 117-26.

(145) Harland BF, O'Dell RG, Stone CL, Prosky L. Metabolic effects of altered fiber, phytate and increased zinc in wheat bran fractions fed to rats (abstract). Fed Proc 1978; 37 (3): 756.

(146) Harland BF, Connor DH, Stringfellow DE, Heggie CM, Reardon MJ, Foster WD, Stafford EE, Stone CL, Wear DJ. Blood and fecal metabolic response in humans consuming self-selected diets with wheat bran supplement (abstract). In: Abstracts and Free Communications of XI International Congress of Nutrition. Rio de Janeiro: Executive Committee of XI International Congress of Nutrition, 1978: 63.

(147) Harland BF, Peterson M. Nutritional status of lacto-ovo vegetarian Trappist monks. J Am Diet Assoc 1978 Mar; 72 (3): 259-64.

(148) Hartley RD. The lignin fraction of plant cell walls. Am J Clin Nutr 1978 Oct; 31 (10 Suppl): S90-3.

(149) Heaton KW, Haber GB, Burroughs L, Murphy D. How fiber may prevent obesity: promotion of satiety and prevention of rebound hypoglycaemia (abstract). Am J Clin Nutr 1978 Oct; 31 (10 Suppl): S280.

(150) Heaton KW, Low-Beer TS. Diet and heart disease (letter). Br Med J 1978 Jan 21; 1 (6106): 170.

(151) Heaton KW, Williamson RC. Dietary fibre and experimental colon cancer (letter). Lancet 1978 Oct 7; 2 (8093): 784-5.

(152) Heaton KW, ed. Third Kellogg Nutrition Symposium. Dietary Fibre: current developments of importance to health. London: Newman Publishing Ltd, 1978.

(153) Heaton KW. Fibre, satiety and insulin — a new approach to overnutrition and obesity. In: Heaton KW, ed. Third Kellogg Nutrition Symposium. Dietary fibre: current developments of importance to health. London: Newman Publishing Ltd, 1978: 141-9.

(154) Heaton KW. Are gallstones preventable? World Med 1978 Jul 12; 13 (20): 21-3.

(155) Heaton KW. Tough line on sugar. World Med 1978 Oct 18; 14 (2): 19-22.

(156) Hedge SN, Rolls BA, Turvey A, Coates ME. The effects on chicks of dietary fibre from different sources: a growth factor in wheat bran. Br J Nutr 1978 Jul; 40 (1): 63-8.

(157) Hellendoorn EW. Fermentation as the principal cause of the physiological activity of indigestible food residue. In: Spiller GA, ed. Topics in dietary fiber research. New York and London: Plenum Press, 1978: 127-68.

(158) Hellendoorn EW. Some critical observations in relation to 'dietary fibre', the methods for its determination and the current hypotheses for the explanation of its physiological action. Voeding 1978; 39 (8): 230-5.

(159) Heller SN, Hackler LR. Changes in the crude fiber content of the American diet. Am J Clin Nutr 1978 Sep; 31 (9): 1510-4.

(160) Hendrikx ME. Practical dietary research design and applications for Southwestern American Indians. In: Spiller GA, ed. Topics in dietary fiber research. New York and London: Plenum Press, 1978: 169-80.

(161) Henry RW, Stout RW, Love AH. Lack of effect of bran enriched bread on plasma lipids, calcium, glucose and body weight. Ir J Med Sci 1978 Jul; 147 (7): 249-51.

(162) Hill M. Nutrition and cancer. The role of nutrition in the causation of cancer. Nutr Bull 1978; 4 (4): 234-46.

(163) Hill MJ. Some leads to the etiology of cancer of the large bowel. Surg Annu 1978; 10: 135-49.

(164) Hintz HF, Schryver HF, Stevens CE. Digestion and absorption in the hindgut of non-ruminant herbivores. J Anim Sci 1978 Jun; 46 (6): 1789-99.

(165) Hockaday TD, Hockaday JM, Mann JI, Turner RC. Prospective comparison of modified-fat-high-carbohydrate with standard low-carbohydrate dietary advice in the treatment of diabetes: one year follow-up study. Br J Nutr 1978 Mar; 39 (2): 357-62.

(166) Holloway WD, Tasman-Jones C, Lee SP. Digestion of certain fractions of dietary fiber in humans. Am J Clin Nutr 1978 Jun; 31 (6): 927-30.

(167) Howard AN. The hypocholesterolaemic effect of psyllium seed (abstract). In: Abstracts and Free Communications of XI International Congress of Nutrition. Rio De Janeiro: Executive Committee of XI International Congress of Nutrition, 1978: 233.

(168) Howell DA, Crow HC, Almy TP, Ramsey WH. A controlled double-blind study of sigmoid motility using psyllium mucilloid in diverticular disease (DD) (abstract). Gastroenterology 1978 May; 74 (5 Pt 2): 1046.

(169) Huang CT, Gopalakrishna GS, Nichols BL. Fiber, intestinal sterols, and colon cancer. Am J Clin Nutr 1978 Mar; 31 (3): 516-26.

(170) Hunt JN, Cash R, Newland P. Energy density of food, gastric emptying, and obesity. Am J Clin Nutr 1978 Oct; 31 (10 Suppl): S259-60.

(171) Hussain Rathore A. Recurrent acute intestinal obstruction due to multiple enteroliths. JPMA 1978 Nov; 28 (11): 169-70.

(172) Huybregts A, van de Werf S, van Berge Henegouwen GP, Hectors M. Effect of bran ingestion on biliary lipids and bile acid kinetics in man (abstract). Gastroenterology 1978 May; 74 (5 Pt 2): 1047.

(173) Hyland J, Darby C, Hammond P, Taylor I. Comparison of colonic motor function in diverticular disease and the irritable colon syndrome (abstract). Gut 1978 Oct; 19 (10): A995.

(174) Imoto S, Namioka S. VFA production in the pig large intestine. J Anim Sci 1978 Aug; 47 (2): 467-78.

(175) Jackson WP, Campbell GD, Joffe BI, Goldberg MD. Hyperglycaemia among vegetarians (letter). S Afr Med J 1978 Jun 3; 53 (22): 880-1.

(176) James IM. When the diagnosis is true constipation. Mod Geriatr 1978 Mar; 8 (3): 11-5.

(177) James IM. Diet still the best therapy in obesity. Mod Geriatr 1978 May; 8 (5): 40-4.

(178) James WP. United Kingdom nutrition and the Dunn. Am J Clin Nutr 1978 Aug; 31 (8): 1419-20.

(179) James WP, Branch WJ, Southgate DA. Calcium binding by dietary fibre. Lancet 1978 Mar 25; 1 (8065): 638-9.

(180) Jenkins DJ, Wolever TM, Leeds AR, Gassull MA, Haisman P, Dilawari J, Goff DV, Metz GL, Alberti KG. Dietary fibres, fibre analogues, and glucose tolerance: importance of viscosity. Br Med J 1978 May 27; 1 (6124): 1392-4.

(181) Jenkins DJ, Wolever TM, Nineham R, Taylor R, Metz GL, Bacon S, Hockaday TD. Guar crispbread in the diabetic diet. Br Med J 1978 Dec 23-30; 2 (6154): 1744-6.

(182) Jenkins DJ. Action of dietary fiber in lowering fasting serum cholesterol and reducing postprandial glycaemia: gastrointestinal mechanisms. In: Carlson LA, Paoletti R, Sirtori CR, Weber G, eds. International Conference on Atherosclerosis. New York: Raven Press, 1978: 173-82.

(183) Johnson CK, Kolasa K. Factors which influence the dietary fiber intake of older women enrolled in a meal program in southeastern Michigan (abstract). Fed Proc 1978; 37 (3): 756.

(184) Johnson JR. Pathogenesis of acute appendicitis (letter). Br Med J 1978 Feb 4; 1 (6108): 305.

(185) Johnson MA, Chang ML. The hypocholesteremic effect of pectin as influenced by type of dietary fat in rats fed a cholesterol-containing diet (abstract). Fed Proc 1978; 37 (3): 542.

(186) Jones FA. Diet and intestinal disease. In: Yudkin J, ed. Diet of man: needs and wants. London: Applied Science Publishers Ltd, 1978: 109-26.

(187) Jones FA. Presidential address. Lettsom, food and fibre. Trans Med Soc Lond 1977-78; 94: 1-14.

(188) Jones J. The fabulous fibre cookbook. London: Pitman Publishing, 1978.

(189) Jones LH. Mineral components of plant cell walls. Am J Clin Nutr 1978 Oct; 31 (10 Suppl): S94-8.

(190) Judd PA, Truswell AS. The effect of rolled oats on plasma lipids (abstract). In: Abstracts and Free Communications of XI International Congress of Nutrition. Rio de Janeiro: Executive Committee of XI International Congress of Nutrition, 1978: 256.

(191) Kagawa Y. Impact of Westernization on the nutrition of Japanese: changes in physique, cancer, longevity and centenarians. Prev Med 1978 Jun; 7 (2): 205-17.

(192) Kakande I, Kavuma J, Kayondo J. Appendicitis in Mulago hospital, Kampala. East Afr Med J 1978 Apr; 55 (4): 172-6.

(193) Kasper H, Zilly W. Influence of dietary fiber on retinol and digoxin absorption (abstract). In: Abstracts and Free Communications of XI International Congress of Nutrition. Rio De Janeior: Executive Committee of XI International Congress of Nutrition, 1978: 62.

(194) Kay RM, Judd PA, Truswell AS. The effect of pectin on serum cholesterol (letter). Am J Clin Nutr 1978 Apr; 31 (4): 562-3.

(195) Kay RM. Food form, postprandial glycemia, and satiety (letter). Am J Clin Nutr 1978 May; 31 (5): 738-9.

(196) Kay RM, Strasberg SM. Origin, chemistry, physiological effects and clinical importance of dietary fibre. Clin Invest Med 1978; 1 (1): 9-24.

(197) Kelley JJ, Tsai AC. Effect of pectin, gum arabic and agar on cholesterol absorption, synthesis, and turnover in rats. J Nutr 1978 Apr; 108 (4): 630-9.

(198) Kelsay JL. A review of research on effects of fiber intake in man. Am J Clin Nutr 1978 Jan; 31 (1): 142-59.

(199) Kelsay JL, Behall KM, Prather ES. Effect of fiber from fruits and vegetables on metabolic responses of human subjects. 1. Bowel transit time, number of defecations, fecal weight, urinary excretions of energy and nitrogen and apparent digestibilities of energy, nitrogen and fat. Am J Clin Nutr 1978 Jul; 31 (7): 1149-53.

(200) Kelsay JL, Behall KM, Prather ES. Effect of fiber from fruits and vegetables on calcium, magnesium, iron, silicon and vitamin A balances of human subjects (abstract). Fed Proc 1978; 37 (3): 755.

(201) Keltz FR, Kies C, Fox HM. Urinary ascorbic acid excretion in the human as affected by dietary fiber and zinc. Am J Clin Nutr 1978 Jul; 31 (7): 1167-71.

(202) Kern F Jr, Birkner HJ, Ostrower VS. Binding of bile acids by dietary fiber. Am J Clin Nutr 1978 Oct; 31 (10 Suppl): S175-9.

(203) Keynes M. Dietary fibre and colonic function (letter). J R Soc Med 1978 May; 71 (5): 386-7.

(204) Khan MA, Eggum BO. The nutritive value of some Pakistani diets. J Sci Food Agric 1978 Dec; 29 (12): 1023-9.

(205) Kidder DE, Manners MJ. Digestion in the pig. Bristol: Scientechnica, 1978.

(206) Kies C, Fox HM. Fiber and protein nutritional status. Cereal Foods World 1978 May; 23 (5): 249-52.

(207) Kies C, Fox HM, Vaughan L. Wheat bran supplementary effects on nutritional status (abstract). Cereal Foods World 1978 Aug; 23 (8): 490.

(208) Kies C, Drews L, Fox HM. Copper, zinc and magnesium nutritional status of adolescent boys as affected by dietary fiber (abstract). In: Abstracts and Free Communications of XI International Congress of Nutrition. Rio De Janeiro: Executive Committee of XI International Congress of Nutrition, 1978: 133.

(209) Kliks M. Paleodietetics: a review of the role of dietary fiber in preagricultural human diets. In: Spiller GA, ed. Topics in dietary fiber research. New York and London: Plenum Press, 1978: 181-202.

(210) Kritchevsky D. Fiber, lipids, and atherosclerosis. Am J Clin Nutr 1978 Oct; 31 (10 Suppl): S65-74.

(211) Kritchevsky D. Workshop IV — Fiber, lipids and cardiovascular disease. Am J Clin Nutr 1978 Oct; 31 (10 Suppl): S190.

(212) Kritchevsky D. Food products and hyperlipidemia. Arch Surg 1978 Jan; 113 (1): 52-4.

(213) Kritchevsky D. Dietary fiber and its effect on lipid metabolism. In: Nutrition Products Division. Dietary fiber. Volume 1. Chicago, Illinois: Masonite Corporation, 1978: 19-22.

(214) Kritchevsky D. Are dietary components risk factors in atherosclerosis? Geriatrics 1978 May; 33 (5): 35-9.

(215) Kritchevsky D. Effect of dietary fiber on lipid metabolism and atherosclerosis. In: Carlson LA, Paoletti R, Sirtori CR, Weber G, eds. International Congress on Atherosclerosis. New York: Raven Press, 1978: 169-72.

(216) Kritchevsky D, Story JA. Fiber, hypercholesterolemia, and atherosclerosis. Lipids 1978 May; 13 (5): 366-9.

(217) Kritchevsky D. Influence of dietary fiber on bile acid metabolism. Lipids 1978 Dec; 13 (12): 982-5.

(218) Kuppurajan K, Rajagopalan SS, Koteswara Rao T, Sitaraman R. Effect of guggulu (Commiphora mukul — Engl.) on serum lipids in obese, hypercholesterolemic and hyperlipemic cases. J Assoc Physicians India 1978 May; 26 (5): 367-73.

(219) Ladisch MR, Tsai GT, Ladisch CM. Protein determination in the presence of cellulose. Biotechnol Bioeng 1978; 20 (3): 461-2.

(220 Lang JA. Dietary fiber — the influence of the physical form of diets (abstract). In: Abstracts and Free Communications of XI International Congress of Nutrition. Rio De Janeiro: Executive Committee of XI International Congress of Nutrition, 1978: 61.

(221) Latto C. Practical experiences in fibre. In: Heaton KW, ed. Third Kellogg Nutrition Symposium. Dietary fibre: current developments of importance to health. London: Newman Publishing Ltd, 1978: 151-5.

(222) Leeds AR, Jenkins DJ, Metz G, Ralphs DN. Treatment of the dumping syndrome with thickened 'slow release' meals (abstract). In: Abstracts and Free Communications of XI International Congress of Nutrition. Rio De Janeiro: Executive Committee of XI International Congress of Nutrition, 1978: 96.

(223) Leeds AR, Ralphs DN, Boulos P, Ebied F, Metz G, Dilawari JB, Elliott A, Jenkins DJ. Pectin and gastric emptying in the dumping syndrome (abstract). Proc Nutr Soc 1978 May; 37 (1): 23A.

(224) Leeds AR, Bolster N, Truswell AS. Guar gum and glucose absorption: absence of evidence for malabsorption (abstract). Proc Nutr Soc 1978 Dec; 37 (3): 89A.

(225) Leng E. Absorption of inorganic ions and volatile fatty acids in the rabbit caecum. Br J Nutr 1978 Nov; 40 (3): 509-19.

(226) Letchford P, Zabroja R, Arthur J, Farrell DJ. Manipulation of plasma cholesterol in man and its suppression by wheat fibre (abstract). Proc Nutr Soc Aust 1978; 3: 97.

(227) Lewis BA. Physical and biological properties of structural and other nondigestible carbohydrates. Am J Clin Nutr 1978 Oct; 31 (10 Suppl): S82-5.

(228) Lewis EA, Kale OO. Bowel habit in a Yoruba rural community: preliminary report. Afr J Med Med Sci 1978 Sep; 7 (3): 157-61.

(229) Lewis EA, Ashley-Dejo OF. Bowel habit in an urban population sample. Niger Med J 1978 Jul; 8 (4): 343-8.

(230) Lin WJ, Anderson JW. Effects of guar gum and wheat bran on lipid metabolism of rats (abstract). Fed Proc 1978; 37 (3): 542.

(231) Looney MA, Lei KY. Dietary fiber, zinc and copper: effects on serum and liver cholesterol levels in the rat. Nutr Rep Int 1978 Mar; 17 (3): 329-37.

(232) Losowsky MS. Effects of dietary fibre on intestinal absorption. In: Heaton KW, ed. Third Kellogg Nutrition Symposium. Dietary fibre: current developments of importance to health. London: Newman Publishing Ltd, 1978: 124-39.

(233) Low AG, Partridge IG, Sambrook IE. Studies on digestion and absorption in the intestines of growing pigs. 2. Measurements of the flow of dry matter, ash and water. Br J Nutr 1978 May; 39 (3): 515-26.

(234) Lutz WK, Brandle E, Zbinden G. Effect of gum arabic on aminopyrine demethylation in rats. Experientia 1978 Dec 15; 34 (12): 1609-10.

(235) Lyon JL, Sorenson AW. Colon cancer in a low-risk population. Am J Clin Nutr 1978 Oct; 31 (10 Suppl): S227-30.

(236) Lyon JL. Diet fiber and colonic cancer (letter). N Engl J Med 1978 Jan 12; 298 (2): 110-1.

(237) Malagelada J-R, Carlson GL, Carter S. Development and preliminary evaluation of a radiolabelled fiber marker (abstract). Gastroenterology 1978 May; 74 (5 Pt 2): 1059.

(238) Malhotra SL. New approaches to the pathogenesis of peptic ulcer based on the protective action of saliva with special reference to roughage, vegetable fibre and fermented milk products. Med Hypotheses 1978 Jan-Feb; 4 (1): 1-14.

(239) Malhotra SL. A comparison of unrefined wheat and rice diets in the management of duodenal ulcer. Postgrad Med J 1978 Jan; 54 (627): 6-9.

(240) Mangold D, Woolam GL, Garcia-Rinaldi R. Intestinal|obstruction due to phytobezoars. Observations in two patients with hypothyroidism and previous gastric surgery. Arch Surg 1978 Aug; 113 (8): 1001-3.

(241) Marigo C, Correa P, Haenszel W. Cancer and 'cancer-related' colorectal lesions in Sao Paulo, Brazil. Int J Cancer 1978 Dec; 22 (6): 645-54.

(242) Martelli H, Devroede G, Arhan P, Duguay C, Dornic C, Faverdin C. Some parameters of large bowel motility in normal man. Gastroenterology 1978 Oct; 75 (4): 612-8.

(243) Martin CR. Dietary fibre. Facts and fallacy. Br Food J 1978 Jan-Feb; 80: 18-21.

(244) Mathur MS, Ram H, Chadda VS. Effect of bran on intestinal transit time in normal Indians and in intestinal amoebiasis. Am J Proctol Gastroenterol Colon Rectal Surg 1978 Nov-Dec; 29 (6): 30-2, 34.

(245) Matthee V, Appledorf H. Effect of cooking on vegetable fiber. J Food Sci 1978; 43 (4): 1344-5.

(246) Mattsson H, Forsum E. Chemical and biological determination of metabolizable energy in mixed diets (abstract). In: Abstracts and Free Communications of XI International Congress of Nutrition. Rio De Janeiro: Executive Committee of XI International Congress of Nutrition, 1978: 77.

(247) Matzkies F, Berg G. Dietary fiber syndrome as the cause of disease in civilised societies. Acta Hepatogastroenterol (Stuttg) 1978 Oct; 25 (5): 402-7.

(248) Maurice DV, Jensen LS. Effect of dietary cereal on liver and plasma lipids in laying Japanese quail. Br Poult Sci 1978; 19(2): 199-205.

(249) Mendeloff AI. Workship III — Fiber and the gastrointestinal tract. Summary and recommendations. Am J Clin Nutr 1978 Oct; 31 (10 Suppl): S145-7.

(250 Mendeloff AI. Dietary fiber and gastrointestinal diseases. Some facts and fancies. Med Clin North Am 1978 Jan; 62 (1): 165-71.

(251) Mendeloff AI. Diet fiber and colonic cancer (letter). N Engl J Med 1978 Jan 12; 298 (2): 111.

(252) Miettinen TA. Effect of dietary fibers and ion-exchange resins on cholesterol metabolism in man. In: Carlson LA, Paoletti R, Sirtori CR, Weber G, eds. International Conference on Atherosclerosis. New York: Raven Press, 1978: 193-8.

(253) Miettinen TA, Tarpila S. Fecal β-sitosterol in patients with diverticular disease of the colon and vegetarians. Scand J Gastroenterol 1978 May; 13 (5): 573-6.

(254) Miller AB. Epidemiology and colorectal cancer. Can J Surg 1978 May; 21 (3): 209-10.

(255) Miranda PM, Horwitz DL. High-fiber diets in the treatment of diabetes mellitus. Ann Intern Med 1978 Apr; 88 (4): 482-6.

(256) Mirouze J, Monnier L, Bringer J, Pham TC, Orsetti A. Plasma glucagon levels in chemical diabetes with reactive hypoglycaemia before and after correction by pectin (abstract). In: Abstracts and Free Communications of XI International Congress of Nutrition. Rio De Janeiro: Executive Committee of XI International Congress of Nutrition, 1978: 253.

(257) Miyazawa T, Tazawa H, Fujino Y. Molecular species of triglyceride in rice bran. Cereal Chem 1978; 55 (2): 138-45.

(258) Mod RR, Conkerton EJ, Ory RL, Normand FL. Hemicellulose composition of dietary fiber of milled rice and rice bran. J Agric Food Chem 1978; 26 (5): 1031-5.

(259) Mongeau R, Brassard R. Content of insoluble dietary fibre, hemicellulose, cellulose and lignin in various breads (abstract). Cereal Foods World 1978 Aug; 23 (8): 460.

(260) Monnier L, Pham TC, Aguirre L, Orsetti A, Mirouze J. Influence of indigestible fibers on glucose tolerance. Diabetes Care 1978 Mar-Apr; 1 (2): 83-8.

(261) Monnier L, Aguirre L, Colette C, Mirouze J. Effects of indigestible fibers on the intestinal iron absorption in patients with idiopathic hemochromatosis (abstract). In: Abstracts and Free Communications of XI International Congress of Nutrition. Rio De Janeiro: Executive Committee of XI International Congress of Nutrition, 1978: 141.

(262) Moore WE, Cato EP, Holdeman LV. Some current concepts in intestinal bacteriology. Am J Clin Nutr 1978 Oct; 31 (10 Suppl): S33-42.

(263) Moore WE. Workshop II — Fiber and bacteria in the gut. Summary and recommendations. Am J Clin Nutr 1978 Oct; 31 (10 Suppl): S111-2.

(264) Morin ML, Renquist DM, Knapka J, Judge FJ. The effect of dietary crude fiber levels on Rhesus monkeys during quarantine. Lab Anim Sci 1978; 28 (4): 405-11.

(265) Morris JN, Marr JW, Clayton DG. Diet and heart disease (letter). Br Med J 1978 May 6; 1 (6121): 1213.

(266) Morris JN, Marr JW, Clayton DG. Dietary fibre from cereals and the incidence of coronary heart disease. In: Heaton KW, ed. Third Kellogg Nutrition Symposium. Dietary fibre: current developments of importance to health. London: Newman Publishing Ltd, 1978: 45-56.

(267) Morse E. Cellulose: the versatile dietary fiber. Cereal Foods World 1978 Nov; 23 (11): 645-59.

(268) Moskovitz M, White C, Floch MH. Acid and neutral sterol excretion in carcinoma of the colon and control subjects (abstract). Am J Clin Nutr 1978 Apr; 31 (4): 714.

(269) Mullen JD. Dietary fiber sources for human studies. Am J Clin Nutr 1978 Oct; 31 (10 Suppl): S103-6.

(270) Munoz JM, Sandstead HH, Jacob RA, Logan GM Jr, Klevay LM. Effects of dietary fiber on plasma lipids of normal men (abstract). Am J Clin Nutr 1978 Apr; 31 (4): 696.

(271) Munoz JM, Sandstead HH, Jacob RA, Logan GM Jr, Klevay LM. Improvement of oral glucose tolerance test and peripheral insulin activity by dietary fiber (abstract). Am J Clin Nutr 1978 Apr; 31 (4): 715.

(272) Munoz JM, Sandstead HH, Jacob RA, Logan GM Jr, Klevay LM. Effects of some cereal brans on glucose tolerance and plasma lipids of normal men (abstract). Fed Proc 1978; 37 (3): 755.

(273) Murphy EW, Marsh AC, Willis BW. Nutrient content of spices and herbs. J Am Diet Assoc 1978 Feb; 72 (2): 174-6.

(274) McCallum G, Ballinger BR, Presly AS. A trial of bran and bran biscuits for constipation in mentally handicapped and psychogeriatric patients. J Hum Nutr 1978 Oct; 32 (5): 369-72.

(275) MacDonald IA, Webb GR, Mahouny DE. Fecal hydroxysteroid dehydrogenase activities in vegetarian Seventh-Day Adventists, control subjects, and bowel cancer patients. Am J Clin Nutr 1978 Oct; 31 (10 Suppl): S232-8.

(276) McDougall RM, Yakymyshyn M, Walker K, Thurston OG. Effect of wheat bran on serum lipoproteins and biliary lipids. Can J Surg 1978 Sep; 21 (5): 433-5.

(277) McGill HC Jr, Sprinz H. Carrageenan and necrotizing enterocolitis of the newborn (letter). Gastroenterology 1978 Jan; 74 (1): 161-2.

(278) McLeish JA, Johnson AG. Dietary fibre depletion produces abnormal motility responses in the duodenum and the colon. Aust NZ J Med 1978 Oct; 8 (5): 555-6.

(279) McLeish JA, Johnson AG. Low residue diet affects motility of the duodenum as well as the colon. In: Duthie HL, ed. Proceedings of the Sixth International Symposium on Gastrointestinal Motility. Lancaster: MTP Press Ltd, 1978: 185-94.

(280) MacLennan R, Jensen OM, Mosbech J, Vuori H. Diet, transit time, stool weight, and colon cancer in two Scandinavian populations. Am J Clin Nutr 1978 Oct; 31 (10 Suppl): S239-42.

(281) McNaughton JL. Effect of dietary fiber on egg yolk, liver, and plasma cholesterol concentrations of the laying hen. J Nutr 1978 Nov; 108 (11): 1842-8.

(282) McNeil NI, Cummings JH, James WP. Short chain fatty acid absorption by the human large intestine. Gut 1978 Sep; 19 (9): 819-22.

(283) Nahapetian A, Bagheri SM. Effect of fiber and phytate on physiological availability of iron in normal rats (abstract). In: Abstracts and Free Communications of XI International Congress of Nutrition. Rio De Janeiro: Executive Committee of XI International Congress of Nutrition, 1978: 129.

(284) Naivikul O, D'Appolonia BL. Comparison of legume and wheat flour carbohydrates. 1. Sugar analysis. Cereal Chem 1978; 55 (6): 913-8.

(285) Navrrette DA, Elias LG, Bressani R. Effect of forms of consumption on the digestibility of black beans (Phaseolus vulgaris) (abstract). In: Abstracts and Free Communications of XI International Congress of Nutrition. Rio De Janeiro: Executive Committee of XI International Congress of Nutrition, 1978: 76.

(286) Newton CR. Effect of codeine phosphate, Lomotil, and Isogel on ileostomy function. Gut 1978 May; 19 (5): 377-83.

(287) Nicol BM, Phillips PG. The utilization of proteins and amino acids in diets based on cassava (Manihot utilissima), rice or sorghum (Sorghum sativa) by young Nigerian men of low income. Br J Nutr 1978 Mar; 39 (2): 271-87.

(288) Norum KR. Some present concepts concerning diet and prevention of coronary heart disease. Nutr Rev 1978 Jun; 36 (6): 194-8.

(289) Nutrition Products Division. Dietary fiber. Volume 1. Chicago, Illinois: Masonite Corporation, 1978.

(290) Oakenfull DG, Fenwick DE. Adsorption of bile salts from aqueous solution by plant fibre and cholestyramine. Br J Nutr 1978 Sep; 40 (2): 299-309.

(291) Oakenfull D, Fenwick DE. The role of saponins in the adsorption of bile acids by dietary fibre (abstract). Proc Nutr Soc Aust 1978; 3: 67.

(292) O'Dell BL, Knehans AW. Dietary fiber evaluation by use of a guinea pig assay (abstract). In: Abstracts and Free Communications of XI International Congress of Nutrition. Rio De Janeiro: Executive Committee of XI International Congress of Nutrition, 1978: 62.

(293) Ogunbiyi TA. Whole-gut transit rates and wet stool weight in an urban Nigerian population. World J Surg 1978 May; 2 (3): 387-93.

(294) O'Moore RR, Flanagan M, McGill AR, Wright EA, Little C, Weir DG. Diet and heart disease (letter). Br Med J 1978 May 6; 1 (6121): 1213.

(295) Ostwald R, Gebre-Medhin M. Westernization of diet and serum lipids in Ethiopians. Am J Clin Nutr 1978 Jun; 31 (6): 1028-40.

(296) Painter NS. Dietary fibre and colonic function (letter). J R Soc Med 1978 Apr; 71 (4): 305-6.

(297) Palumbo PJ, Briones ER, Nelson RA. High fiber diet in hyperlipemia. Comparison with cholestyramine treatment in type IIa hyperlipoproteinemia. JAMA 1978 Jul 21; 240 (3): 223-7.

(298) Parrot ME, Thrall BE. Functional properties of various fibers: physical properties. J Food Sci 1978; 43 (3): 759-63, 766.

(299) Partridge IG. Studies on digestion and absorption in the intestines of growing pigs. 4. Effects of dietary cellulose and sodium levels on mineral absorption. Br J Nutr 1978 May; 39 (3): 539-45.

(300) Paul AA, Southgate DA. McCance and Widdowson's the composition of foods. London: HMSO, 1978.

(301) Peifer JJ, Karp LA. Comparative ability of dietary fibers to promote losses of fecal bile acids, sterols and fatty acids by the rat (abstract). Fed Proc 1978; 37 (3): 755.

(302) Peng B, Tsai AC. Effect of locust bean gum on glucose tolerance in rats (abstract). Fed Proc 1978; 37 (3): 542.

(303) Phillips RL, Lemon FR, Beeson WL, Kuzma JW. Coronary heart disease mortality among Seventh-Day Adventists with differing dietary habits: a preliminary report. Am J Clin Nutr 1978 Oct; 31 (10 Suppl): S191-8.

(304) Plageman K. Natural fibre cooking. London: Thorsons, 1978. (Self-help series.)

(305) Pollman JW, Morris JJ, Rose PN. Is fiber the answer to constipation problems in the elderly? A review of the literature. Int J Nurs Stud 1978; 15 (3): 107-14.

(306) Prosky L, Harland BF, O'Dell RG, Stone CL. Year-long study of rats fed wheat bran and Alphacel (abstract). Fed Proc 1978; 37 (3): 755.

(307) Putney JD, Trout DL, Johnson DA, Michaelis OE IV. Effect of xanthan gel on hepatic lipogenesis in starved refed rats (abstract). Fed Proc 1978; 37 (3): 543.

(308) Putney JD, Trout DL, Johnson DA, Moy NL, Michaelis OE IV. Effect of xanthan gel on hepatic lipogenesis in starved-refed rats. Nutr Rep Int 1978 Dec; 18 (6): 659-69.

(309) Rahmanifar A, Chenoweth WL. Mineral utilization in rats fed purified fiber and wheat bran (abstract). Fed Proc 1978; 37 (3): 756.

(310) Ralphs DN, Lawaetz O, Brown NJ, Leeds AR. Effect of dietary fibre on gastric emptying in dumpers (abstract). Gut 1978 Oct; 19 (10): A986-7.

(311) Ranhotra GS, Lee C, Gelroth JA. Bioavailability of iron in high-fiber bread (abstract). Cereal Foods World 1978 Aug; 23 (8): 460.

(312) Ranhotra GS, Loewe RJ, Puyat LV. Effect of wheat bran and its subfractions on lipid metabolism in cholesterol-fed rats. J Food Sci 1978; 43 (6): 1829-31.

(313) Rashed-Mohassel MA. Report of a case of a giant phytobezoar in a patient with a duodenal bulb ulcer. Acta Trop (Basel) 1978 Dec; 35 (4): 373-7.

(314) Reddy BS, Hedges AR, Laakso K, Wynder EL. Metabolic epidemiology of large bowel cancer. Fecal bulk and constituents of high-risk North American and low-risk Finnish population. Cancer 1978 Dec; 42 (6): 2832-8.

(315) Reddy BS, Hedges AR, Laakso K, Wynder EL. Fecal constituents of a high-risk North American and a low-risk Finnish population for the development of large bowel cancer. Cancer Lett 1978 Apr; 4 (4): 217-22.

(316) Reiser S. The role of cereal fiber in human nutrition and health: glucose tolerance and diabetes. In: Proceedings of 10th National Conference on Wheat Utilization Research. Berkeley, California: Science and Education Administration, 1978: 39-50.

(317) Rerat A. Digestion and absorption of carbohydrates and nitrogenous matters in the hindgut of the omnivorous nonruminant animal. J Anim Sci 1978 Jun; 46 (6): 1807-37.

(318) Rhodes J, Jones GR, Newcombe RG, Davies D. Effect of dietary bran on serum lipids in patients with previous myocardial infarction, with gallstones, and in normal subjects. Curr Med Res Opin 1977-8; 5 (4): 310-4.

(319) Ritchie JA, Truelove SC. Therapeutic trial of Ativan, Buscopan and Fybogel in the irritable bowel syndrome (abstract). Gut 1978 Oct; 19 (10): A975.

(320) Roberts RL. Composition and taste evaluation of rice milled to different degrees. J Food Sci 1978; 44 (1): 127-9.

(321) Robertson JB. The detergent system of fiber analysis. In: Spiller GA, ed. Topics in dietary fiber research. New York and London: Plenum Press, 1978: 1-42.

(322) Robinson RK, Khan P. The potential dietetic importance of stabilisers, with special reference to guar gum. Plant Foods for Man 1978; 2 (3 + 4): 113-9.

(323) Robson JR. Fruit in the human diet. Fruit in the diet of prehistoric man and of the hunter-gatherer. J Hum Nutr 1978 Feb; 32 (1): 19-26.

(324) Roe DA, Wrick K, McLain D, Van Soest P. Effects of dietary fiber sources on riboflavin absorption (abstract). Fed Proc 1978: 37 (3): 756.

(325) Rolls BA, Turvey A, Coates ME. The influence of the gut microflora and of dietary fibre on epithelial cell migration in the chick intestine. Br J Nutr 1978 Jan; 39 (1): 91-8.

(326) Rotenberg S, Jakobsen PE. The effect of dietary pectin on lipid composition of blood, skeletal muscle and internal organs of rats. J Nutr 1978 Sep; 108 (9): 1384-92.

(327) Roxas BV, Loyola AS, Reyes EL. The effect of different degrees of rice milling on nitrogen digestibility and retention. Philipp J Nutr 1978; 31 (2): 110-3.

(328) Saito Y, Suzuki M, Ohsawa A, Dokiya Y. The study on thiamine, ascorbic acid, mineral element and fiber contents in edible wild plants (abstract). In: Abstracts and Free Communications of XI International Congress of Nutrition. Rio De Janeiro: Executive Committee of XI International Congress of Nutrition, 1978: 364.

(329) Salyers AA, Palmer JK, Wilkins TD. Degradation of polysaccharides by intestinal bacterial enzymes. Am J Clin Nutr 1978 Oct; 31 (10 Suppl): S128-30.

(330) Samuel P, Watermeyer G, Meilman E, Fehrsen S. The relationship between serum cholesterol and fecal 7α-dehydroxylase activity in three ethnic groups in South Africa. Atherosclerosis 1978 Oct; 31 (2): 177-84.

(331) Sanders TA, Ellis FR, Dickerson JW. Studies of vegans: the fatty acid composition of plasma choline phosphoglycerides, erythrocytes, adipose tissue, and breast milk, and some indications of susceptibility to ischemic heart disease in vegans and omnivore controls. Am J Clin Nutr 1978 May; 31 (5): 805-13.

(332) Sanders TA. The health and nutritional status of vegans. Plant Foods for Man 1978; 2 (3 + 4): 181-93.

(333) Sandstead HH, Munoz JM, Jacob RA, Klevay LM, Reck SJ, Logan GM, Dintzis FR, Inglett GE, Shuey WC. Influence of dietary fiber on trace element balance. Am J Clin Nutr 1978 Oct; 31 (10 Suppl): S180-4.

(334)   Saperstein S, Spiller GA. Dietary fiber. Am J Dis Child 1978 Jul; 132 (7): 657-60.

(335)   Saunders RM. A relationship between crude fiber and digestibility of wheat milling fractions in rats. Am J Clin Nutr 1978 Dec; 31 (12): 2136-9.

(336)   Saunders RM. Wheat bran: composition and digestibility. In: Spiller GA, ed. Topics in dietary fiber research. New York and London: Plenum Press, 1978: 43-58.

(337)   Savage DC. Factors involved in colonization of the gut epithelial surface. Am J Clin Nutr 1978 Oct; 31 (10 Suppl): S131-5.

(338)   Schaller D. Fiber content and structure in foods. Am J Clin Nutr 1978 Oct; 31 (10 Suppl): S99-102.

(339)   Schemmel R, Crissey S, Ziegler T. Blood pressure in rats fed semi-purified diets (abstract). In: Abstracts and Free Communications of XI International Congress of Nutrition. Rio De Janeiro: Executive Committee of XI International Congress of Nutrition, 1978: 257.

(340)   Schneeman BO, Gallaher D. Loss of lipase activity with fiber treatment (abstract). Fed Proc 1978; 37 (3): 849.

(341)   Schneeman BO. Effect of plant fiber on lipase, trypsin and chymotrypsin activity. J Food Sci 1978; 43 (2): 634-5.

(342)   Schneider RE, Pineda O, Camargo CL, Calloway DH. Changes observed in the digestive capacity, expired hydrogen concentration and fecal flora observed in rural Guatemalans under different dietary conditions (abstract). In: Abstracts and Free Communications of XI International Congress of Nutrition. Rio De Janeiro: Executive Committee of XI International Congress of Nutrition, 1978: 223.

(343)   Segal I, Ou Tim L, Solomon A, Giraud A. Diverticular disease in urban blacks (letter). S Afr Med J 1978 Jun 10; 53 (23): 922.

(344)   Seibert GR, Benjaminson MA, Hoffman H. A conjugate of cellulose with fluorescein isothiocyanate: a specific stain for cellulose. Stain Technol 1978 Mar; 53 (2): 103-6.

(345)   Shafer MA, Zabik ME. Dietary fiber sources for baked products: comparison of wheat brans and other cereal brans in layer cakes. J Food Sci 1978; 43 (2): 371-9.

(346)   Shier NW, Conley T, Davis C, Fealk F, Hubbard M, Hyszczak O, Hyszczak R, Justice B. Human serum cholesterol and triglyceride responses to the consumption of a diet high in cellulose (abstract). Fed Proc 1978; 37 (3): 542.

(347)   Shipley EA. Dietary fibre content of foods. In: Spiller GA, ed. Topics in dietary fiber research. New York and London: Plenum Press, 1978: 203-12.

(348)   Siegal S. Dr Siegal's natural fiber cookbook. New York: Dell Publishing Company, 1978.

(349)   Sills V, Wallace GM. Methodology in dietary fibre analysis (abstract). Proc Nutr Soc NZ 1978; 3 (2): 130.

(350)   Slavin JL, Marlett JA. The effect of purified cellulose on human bowel function (abstract). Fed Proc 1978; 37 (3): 756.

(351)   Smith AN. Effect of bulk additives on constipation and in diverticular disease. In: Heaton KW, ed. Third Kellogg Nutrition Symposium. Dietary fibre: current developments of importance to health. London: Newman Publishing Ltd, 1978: 97-104.

(352)   Solomons N, Pineda O, Viteri F, Jacob R, Sandstead H. Bioavailability of inorganic zinc: influence of a typical Guatemalan meal and of the iron fortifying agent, NaFeEDTA (abstract). In: Abstracts and Free Communications of XI International Congress of Nutrition. Rio De Janeiro: Executive Committee of XI International Congress of Nutrition, 1978: 71.

(353)   Smith DA, Hawrysh ZJ. Quality characteristics of wheat-bran chiffon cakes. J Am Diet Assoc 1978 Jun; 72 (6): 599-603.

(354)   Southgate DA. Dietary fiber: analysis and food sources. Am J Clin Nutr 1978 Oct; 31 (10 Suppl): S107-10.

(355)   Southgate DA, Van Soest PJ. Fiber analysis tables. Am J Clin Nutr 1978 Oct; 31 (10 Suppl): S281-4.

(356)   Southgate DA. Has dietary fibre a role in the prevention and treatment of obesity? Bibl Nutr Dieta 1978; (26): 70-6.

(357)   Southgate DA, Hudson GJ, Englyst H. The analysis of dietary fibre — the choices for the analyst. J Sci Food Agric 1978 Nov; 29 (11): 979-88.

(358)   Southgate DA, Bingham S, Robertson J. Dietary fibre in the British diet. Nature 1978 Jul 6; 274 (5666): 51-2.
(359)   Southgate DA. The definition, analysis and properties of dietary fibre. In: Heaton KW, ed. Third Kellogg Nutrition Symposium. Dietary fibre: current developments of importance to health. London: Newman Publishing Ltd, 1978: 9-19.
(360)   Spiller GA, Gates JE. Defining dietary plant fibers in human nutrition. Adv Exp Med Biol 1978; 105: 165-94.
(361)   Spiller GA. Interaction of dietary fiber with other dietary components: a possible factor in certain cancer etiologies. Am J Clin Nutr 1978 Oct; 31 (10 Suppl): S231-2.
(362)   Spiller GA, Shipley EA, Blake JA. Recent progress in dietary fiber (plantix) in human nutrition. CRC Crit Rev Food Sci Nutr 1978 Sep; 10 (1): 31-90.
(363)   Spiller GA, Chernoff MC, Hill RA, Gates JE, Nassar JJ, Shipley EA. Effect on transit time, fecal weight and volatile fatty acids of purified cellulose, pectin and low residue diets in humans (abstract). Fed Proc 1978; 37 (3): 755.
(364)   Spiller GA, Gates JE. Defining dietary plant fibers in human nutrition. In: Friedman M, ed. Nutritional improvement of food and feed proteins. New York: Plenum Publishing Corporation, 1978: 165-94.
(365)   Spiller GA, ed. (Amen RJ, assistant). Topics in dietary fiber research. New York and London: Plenum Press, 1978.
(366)   Stasse-Wolthuis M, Katan MB, Hautvast JG. Fecal weight, transit time, and recommendations for dietary fiber intake (letter). Am J Clin Nutr 1978 Jun; 31 (6): 909-10.
(367)   Stevens CE. Physiological implications of microbial digestion in the large intestine of mammals: relation to dietary factors. Am J Clin Nutr 1978 Oct; 31 (10 Suppl): S161-8.
(368)   Stevenson MH, Unsworth EF. Studies on the absorption of calcium, phosphorus, magnesium, copper and zinc by sheep fed on roughage-cereal diets. Br J Nutr 1978 Nov; 40 (3): 491-6.
(369)   Story JA, Kritchevsky D. Bile acid metabolism and fiber. Am J Clin Nutr 1978 Oct; 31 (10 Suppl): S199-202.
(370)   Sugano M, Fujikawa T, Hiratsuji Y, Hasegawa Y. Hypocholesterolemic effects of chitosan in cholesterol-fed rats. Nutr Rep Int 1978 Nov; 18 (5): 531-7.
(371)   Sullivan AC, Triscari J, Comai K. Caloric compensatory responses to diets containing either nonabsorbable carbohydrate or lipid by obese and lean Zucker rats. Am J Clin Nutr 1978 Oct; 31 (10 Suppl): S261-6.
(372)   Tadesse K, Eastwood MA. Metabolism of dietary fibre components in man assessed by breath hydrogen and methane. Br J Nutr 1978 Sep; 40 (2): 393-6.
(373)   Tarpila S, Miettinen TA, Metsaranta L. Effects of bran on serum cholesterol, faecal mass, fat, bile acids and neutral sterols, and biliary lipids in patients with diverticular disease of the colon. Gut 1978 Feb; 19 (2): 137-45.
(374)   Tasman-Jones C, Jones AL, Owen RL. Jejunal morphological consequences of dietary fiber in rats (abstract). Gastroenterology 1978 May; 74 (5 Pt 2): 1102.
(375)   Taylor I, Duthie HL. The effect of bran on colonic myoelectrical function in diverticular disease. In: Duthie HL, ed. Proceedings of Sixth International Symposium on Gastrointestinal Motility. Lancaster: MTP Press Ltd, 1978: 225-31.
(376)   Tredger J, Ransley J. Guar gum — its acceptability to diabetic patients when incorporated into baked food products. J Hum Nutr 1978 Dec; 32 (6): 427-32.
(377)   Trowell H, Godding E, Spiller G, Briggs G. Fiber bibliographies and terminology (letter). Am J Clin Nutr 1978 Sep; 31 (9): 1489-90.
(378)   Trowell H. The development of the concept of dietary fiber in human nutrition. Am J Clin Nutr 1978 Oct; 31 (10 Suppl): S3-11.
(379)   Trowell H. Diabetes mellitus and dietary fiber of starchy foods. Am J Clin Nutr 1978 Oct; 31 (10 Suppl): S53-7.
(380)   Trowell H, National library of medicine; scientific communications office; national institute of arthritis, metabolism, and digestive diseases. Selected bibliography on dietary fiber. Am J Clin Nutr 1978 Oct; 31 (10 Suppl): S285-91.
(381)   Trowell H. Diet and heart disease (letter). Br Med J 1978 Jan 21; 1 (6106): 170-1.

(382) Trowell HC. Western diseases, Western diets and fibre. East Afr Med J 1978 Jun; 55 (6): 283-9.

(383) Trowell HC. Recent developments in dietary-fibre hypotheses. In: Heaton KW, ed. Third Kellogg Nutrition Symposium. Dietary fibre: current developments of importance to health. London: Newman Publishing Ltd, 1978: 1-8.

(384) Truswell AS. Diet and plasma lipids — a reappraisal. Am J Clin Nutr 1978 Jun; 31 (6): 977-89.

(385) Truswell AS. Effect of different types of dietary fibre on plasma lipids. In: Heaton KW, ed. Third Kellogg Nutrition Symposium. Dietary fibre: current developments of importance to health. London: Newman Publishing Ltd, 1978: 105-12.

(386) Tsai CY, Lei KY. Dietary fiber, zinc and copper: effects on tissue mineral levels in rats (abstract). Fed Proc 1978; 37 (3): 542.

(387) Udall JN, Suskind RM. Carrageenan and necrotizing enterocolitis of the newborn (letter). Gastroenterology 1978 Jan; 74 (1): 161.

(388) Vahouny GV, Roy T, Gallo LL, Story JA, Kritchevsky D, Cassidy M, Grund BM, Treadwell CR. Dietary fiber and lymphatic absorption of cholesterol in the rat. Am J Clin Nutr 1978 Oct; 31 (10 Suppl): S208-10.

(389) Vahouny GV, Roy T, Cassidy M, Gallo LL, Kritchevsky D, Story J, Treadwell CR. Dietary fibers and lymphatic absorption of cholesterol in the rat (abstract). Fed Proc 1978; 37 (3): 755.

(390) Vaisrub S. Dietary fiber for the diabetic (editorial). JAMA 1978 Jul 28; 240 (4): 379.

(391) Vanderborght OL, Van Puymbroeck S, Babakova I. Effect of combined alginate treatments on the distribution and excretion of an old radiostrontium contamination. Health Phys 1978 Aug; 35 (2): 255-8.

(392) Van Itallie T. Dietary fiber and obesity. Am J Clin Nutr 1978 Oct; 31 (10 Suppl): S43-52.

(393) Van Itallie TB. Workshop VI — Fiber and obesity. Summary and recommendations. Am J Clin Nutr 1978 Oct; 31 (10 Suppl): S252-4.

(394) Van Itallie TB, Gale SK, Kissileff HR. The control of food intake in the regulation of depot fat: an overview. In: Katzen HM, Mahler RJ, eds. Diabetes, obesity and vascular disease: metabolic and molecular relationships. New York: John Willey, 1978: 427. (Advances in modern nutrition; Vol 2.)

(395) Van Itallie TB. Diets for weight reduction: mechanisms of action and physiological effects. Int J Obes 1978; 2 (2): 113-22.

(396) Van Soest PJ. Dietary fibers: their definition and nutritional properties. Am J Clin Nutr 1978 Oct; 31 (10 Suppl): S12-20.

(397) Van Soest PJ. Workshop I — Component analysis of fiber in food. Summary and recommendations. Am J Clin Nutr 1978 Oct; 31 (10 Suppl): S75-6.

(398) Van Soest PJ, Robertson JB. Chemical and physical properties of dietary fibre. In: Nutrition Products Division. Dietary fiber. Volume 1. Chicago, Illinois: Masonite Corporation, 1978: 1-11.

(399) Vercellotti JR, Salyers AA, Wilkins TD. Complex carbohydrate breakdown in the human colon. Am J Clin Nutr 1978 Oct; 31 (10 Suppl): S86-9.

(400) Visek WJ. Diet and cell growth modulation by ammonia. Am J Clin Nutr 1978 Oct; 31 (10 Suppl): S216-20.

(401) Visek WJ, Clinton SK, Truex CR. Nutrition and experimental carcinogenesis. Cornell Vet 1978 Jan; 68 (1): 3-39.

(402) Viswanathan M, Snehalatha C, Ramachandran A, Viswanathan M, Sobhana R. Effect of a calorie restricted high carbohydrate, high protein low fat diet on serum lipids in diabetes — a follow up study. J Assoc Physicians India 1978 Mar; 26 (3): 162-8.

(403) Vratanina DL, Zabik ME. Dietary fiber sources for baked products: bran in sugar-snap cookies. J Food Sci 1978; 43 (5): 1590-4.

(404) Wadsworth GR. Fruit in the human diet. The use, dietary significance and production of fruit. J Hum Nutr 1978 Feb; 32 (1): 27-40.

(405) Wagner DD, Thomas OP. Influence of diets containing rye or pectin on the intestinal flora of chicks. Poult Sci 1978 Jul; 57 (4): 971-5.

(406) Wahlqvist ML, Morris M, Bond A, Littlejohn GO, Jackson RV, Wilmshurst EG, Richardson EN. Glucose tolerance in healthy subjects: effect of saccharide chain length and dietary fibre (abstract). Proc Nutr Soc Aust 1978; 3: 99.

(407) Wakabayashi K, Inagaki T, Fujimoto Y, Fukuda Y. Induction by degraded carrageenan of colorectal tumors in rats. Cancer Lett 1978 Mar; 4 (3): 171-6.

(408) Walker AR. The relationship between bowel cancer and fiber content in the diet. Am J Clin Nutr 1978 Oct; 31 (10 Suppl): S248-51.

(409) Walker AR, Walker BF. High high-density-lipoprotein cholesterol in African children and adults in a population free of coronary heart disease. Br Med J 1978 Nov 11; 2 (6148): 1336-7.

(410) Walker AR, du Plessis JP. White and brown breads (editorial). S Afr Med J 1978 Mar 11; 53 (10): 346.

(411) Walker AR. Diet and coronary heart disease. S Afr Med J 1978 Apr 15; 53 (15): 587-90.

(412) Walker AR. Can brown bread significantly prejudice mineral metabolism (editorial). S Afr Med J 1978 Oct 14; 54 (16): 632-3.

(413) Watanabe K, Reddy BS, Wong CQ, Weisburger JH. Effect of dietary undegraded carrageenan on colon carcinogenesis in F344 rats treated with azoxymethane or methylnitrosourea. Cancer Res 1978 Dec; 38 (12): 4427-30.

(414) Watanabe K, Reddy BS, Kritchevsky D. Effect of various dietary fibers and food additives on azoxymethane (AOM) or methylnitrosourea (MNU)-induced colon carcinogenesis in rats (abstract). Fed Proc 1978; 37 (3): 262.

(415) Watkins JB. Fiber and the development of gastrointestinal function. Am J Clin Nutr 1978 Oct; 31 (10 Suppl): S148-51.

(416) Watt J, Marcus AJ. Comparison of the effects of carrageenins and Danish agar on the colon of guinea-pigs (abstract). Proc Nutr Soc 1978 Sep; 37 (2): 39A.

(417) Watts J McK, Jablonski P, Toouli J. The effect of added bran to the diet on the saturation of bile in people without gallstones. Am J Surg 1978 Mar; 135 (3): 321-4.

(418) Webster DJ, Gough DC, Craven JL. The use of bulk evacuant in patients with haemorrhoids. Br J Surg 1978 Apr; 65 (4): 291-2.

(419) Weisburger JH. Environmental cancer: on the causes of the main human cancers. Tex Rep Biol Med 1978; (37): 1-20.

(420) Werner GT, Sareen DK. Serum cholesterol levels in the population of Punjab in north west India. Am J Clin Nutr 1978 Aug; 31 (8): 1479-83.

(421) West KM. Epidemiology of diabetes and its vascular lesions. New York: Elsevier, 1978: 262-4.

(422) West LG, Greger JL. A rapid method for the detection of dietary zinc-complexing agents. Nutr Rep Int 1978 Jul; 18 (1): 117-24.

(423) Evaluation of certain food additives. Geneva: WHO, 1978: 26-7. (WHO Technical Report Series 617.)

(424) Wicks AC, Yeates J, Heaton KW. Bran and bile: time-course of changes in normal young men given a standard dose. Scand J Gastroenterol 1978 May; 13 (3): 289-92.

(425) Wolever TM, Taylor R, Goff DV. Guar: viscosity and efficacy (letter). Lancet 1978 Dec 23-30; 2 (8104-5): 1381.

(426) Wolever TM, Jenkins DJ, Leeds AR, Gassull MA, Diliwari JB, Goff DV, Metz GL, Alberti KG. Dietary fibre and glucose tolerance: importance of viscosity (abstract). Proc Nutr Soc 1978 Sep; 37 (2): 47A.

(427) Wyman JB, Heaton KW, Manning AP, Wicks AC. Variability of colonic function in healthy subjects. Gut 1978 Feb; 19 (2): 146-50.

(428) Yatzidis H. Preliminary studies with locust bean gum: a new sorbent with great potential. Kidney Int 1978 Jun; 8 Suppl: S150-2.

(429) Yudkin J. Carbohydrate confusion. J R Soc Med 1978 Aug; 71 (8): 551-6.

(430) Zimring JG. High-fiber diet versus laxatives in geriatric patient. NY State J Med 1978 Dec; 78 (14): 2223-4.

(431) Zoiopoulos PE, Topps JH, English PR. Digestion by growing pigs of fibrous diets measured over-all and at the terminal ileum (abstract). Proc Nutr Soc 1978 Dec; 37 (3): 78A.

CZECH

(432) Toman R. Colonic diverticulosis (English abstract). Vnitr Lek 1978 Nov; 24 (11): 1043-51.

DANISH

(433) Becker U, Elsborg L, Mosbech J. A new method for measuring intestinal transit time (English abstract). Ugeskr Laeger 1978 Oct 9; 140 (41): 2504-7.

DUTCH

(434) Deurenberg P. Effect of a low-fat, high-carbohydrate diet and of a high-fibre diet on serum lipids in female student dietitians. Voeding 1978; 39 (8): 222-6.

(435) Sinkeldam EJ. Physiological effects of dietary fibre in bread in diets for rats. Voeding 1978; 39 (6): 185.

FRENCH

(436) Abele R, Cochet B, Balant L, Gorgia A, Tinguely D, Estreicher J. Effect of guar on the gastrointestinal absorption of D-xylose: compartmental analysis on a computer (English abstract). Pharm Acta Helv 1978; 53 (9-10): 253-60.

(437) Audigier J-C, Lambert R. Bran in the treatment of constipation. Gastroenterol Clin Biol 1978 Jan; 2 (1): 77-85.

(438) Bernier JJ. The usefulness of bran bread: biological effects of bran (English abstract). Bull Acad Natl Med (Paris) 1978; 162 (3): 238-45.

(439) Cassard P, Chevrel B. The place of vegetable fiber in the treatment of constipation. Med Chir Dig 1978; 7 (3): 279-82.

(440) Coste T, Rautureau J, Paraf A. Treatment of constipation and colonic diverticulosis by bran. Med Chir Dig 1978; 7 (7): 631-4.

(441) Coste T, Karsenti P, Rautureau J, Berta J-L, Cubeau J. Consumption of dietary fiber in 72 cholelithiasis patients (letter). Nouv Presse Med 1978 Dec 23; 7 (46): 4238.

(442) Coste T, Paraf A. Role of dietary fibres in nutrition (English abstract). Rev Med (Paris) 1978; 19 (8): 407-14.

(443) Frexinos J, Louis A. Effect of three dietary fiber-containing products on stool weight. Gastroenterol Clin Biol 1978 Dec; 2 (12): 1055-6.

(444) Frexinos J. Why, when and how dietary fiber will be used in gastrointestinal disorders (English abstract). Nouv Presse Med 1978 Apr 8; 7 (14): 1195-8.

(445) Lambert R. Fiber in the diet and carcinoma. Bull Cancer (Paris) 1978; 65 (1): 71-2.

(446) Lambert R. Cellulose in the diet of man. Bull Soc Sci Vet Med Comp Lyon 1978; 80 (1): 51-4.

(447) Martin MS. Experimental models: nutrition and intestinal cancers (English abstract). Bull Cancer (Paris) 1978; 65 (1): 49-52.

(448) Minaire Y. The origin and nature of cellulose and fibre in plant foods. Bull Soc Sci Vet Med Comp Lyon 1978; 80 (1): 15-19.

(449) Rostan O, Jost A, Loup P. Hazards of mucilaginous laxatives after oesophago-gastric surgery. Rev Med Suisse Romande 1978 Jun; 98 (6): 317-9.

(450) Roy L, Dorion SB, Lord J, Rousseau B. Use of pectin in the treatment of hypo-glycemic dumping syndrome (English abstract). Union Med Can 1978 Aug; 107 (8): 722-3.

GERMAN

(451) Ammann R. Fiber deficiency as a cause of gastrointestinal diseases (English abstract). Praxis 1978 Aug 15; 67 (33): 1210-4.

(452) Anonymous. 'Western Diseases'. MMW 1978 Nov 17; 120 (46): 42, 44.

(453) Bock W, Krause M. Functional and nutritional physiological properties of pectins. Ernahrungsforschung — Wissenschaft und Praxis 1978; 23 (4): 100-5.

(454) Elmadfa I, Domke I. Influence of date seed flour and cellulose on growth, food utilization and parameters of fat metabolism of growing and adult rats (English abstract). Z Ernaehrungswiss 1978 Dec; 17 (4): 197-205.

(455) Franken FH. The irritable colon. Dtsch Med Wochenschr 1978 Apr 14; 103 (15): 665-8.

(456) Gabler H. Plantago ovata as a laxative. Ther Ggw 1978 Sep; 117 (9): 1382-6.

(457) Haenel H, Renger F, Rothe M, Vetter K. Roughage in human nutrition (English abstract). Dtsch Gesundheitswes 1978; 33 (11): 506-10.

(458) Harmuth-Hoene A-E, Jakubick V, Schelenz R. Effect of guar gum in diet on nitrogen balance, protein metabolism and food transit time in rats (English abstract). Nutr Metab 1978; 22 (1): 32-43.

(459) Huth K. Bulk materials. Dtsch Med Wochenschr 1978 Nov 3; 103 (44): 1721-3.

(460) Huth K, Michalsky U, Cremer H-D, Schmahl FW. Body weight and dietary bulk. The prevention and therapy of obesity. Med Welt 1978 Jan 27; 29 (4): 121-3.

(461) Manning AP, Harvey RF, Heaton KW. The irritable bowel. A high fibre diet. Dtsch Med Wochenschr 1978 Jan 6; 103 (1): 5-6.

(462) Matzkies F, Berg G. Cholesterol-lowering activity of a formula diet containing soy proteins, apple pectin and bran. Z Ernaehrungswiss 1978 Dec; 17 (4): 262-9.

(463) Menger A. A review of the current status of physiological and analytical evaluation of dietary cereal fibre. Getreide Mehl Brot 1978; 32 (1): 13-6.

(464) Mossberg R, Alstin F. Fibres in foods and feedingstuffs. Muhle + Mischfuttertechnik 1978; 115 (13): 177-8.

(465) Munzner R, Harmuth-Hoene A-E. Effect of guar gum diet on feces microbiology in rats (English abstract). Nutr Metab 1978; 22 (6): 368-73.

(466) Phillip J. Treatment of diverticular disease of the colon. Dtsch Med Wochenschr 1978 Jun 16; 103 (24): 995-6.

(467) Thomas B, Elchazly M. Crude fibre, ballast and their components in different foods. In: Aktuelle fragen der ernahrungstherapie in nephrologie und gastroenterologie. Stuttgart, German Federal Republic: Georg Thieme Verlag, 1978: 120-8.

HEBREW

(468) Guggenheim K. Dietary fiber and human health. Harefuah 1978 May 1; 94 (9): 288-93.

(469) Kanter Y, Eitan N, Barzilai D. High dietary fiber and diabetics (editorial). Harefuah 1978 Feb; 94 (3-4): 148-9.

ITALIAN

(470) Di Gesu G, Leo P, Guardino V. Two cases of phytobezoar of gastric & gastrointestinal localization (English abstract). Minerva Dietol Gastroenterol 1978 Jan-Mar; 24 (1): 57-69.

(471) Ricci PD, Angeli R. Plantago ovata and defecation disorders in the aged. Effects of the administration of powdered Plantago ovata seeds on defecation disorders in the aged. (English abstract). Clin Ter 1978 Sep 15; 86 (5): 434-9.

NORWEGIAN

(472) Bjorneklett A, Fausa O, Lovik A. Comparative study of the laxative effect of wheat bran and dietary fiber tablets (Dumovital) (English abstract). Tidsskr Nor Laegeforen 1978 May 30; 98 (15): 776-8.

POLISH

(473) Butruk E, Bartnik W. Long-term treatment of functional disorders of the intestines with bran (English abstract). Pol Arch Med Wewn 1978 Dec; 60 (6): 497-502.

(474) Cybulska B, Szostak WB. The food antiatherosclerotic factors. Przegl Lek 1978; 35 (7): 649-53.

(475) Garszel J, Piekarska J. Methods of cellulose determination in food products (English abstract). Rocz Panstw Zakl Hig 1978; 29 (4): 365-70.

(476) Krygier T. Prevention of cholelithiasis — new concepts. Pol Tyg Lek 1978; 33 (43): 1699-701.

(477) Piekarska J. The content and composition of fibre in foodstuffs. Przegl Lek 1978; 35 (4-5): 561-4.

(478) Szponar L, Ostapczuk J. The consumption of fat, cellulose, and cholesterol in daily food rations of women in rural areas (English abstract). Przegl Lek 1978; 35 (4-5): 514-5.

SPANISH
(479) Flores-Espinosa J, Flores De Masvidal G, Zanolini L. Diverticular disease of the colon. Saccharine disease of Cleave and Saint's triad. Gac Med Mex 1978 Nov; 114 (11): 515-23.

SWEDISH
(480) Asp NG, Dahlqvist A, Johansson CG. Evaluation of different methods proposed for the analysis of dietary fibre. Naringsforskning 1978; 22 (2): 186-7.
(481) Theander O. Structure and properties of dietary fibre. Naringsforskning 1978; 22 (3): 204-11.

197

Mathur MS: 244
Matsumoto T: 1
Matthee V: 245
Mattsson H: 246
Matzkies F: 462
Maurice DV: 248
Meilman E: 330
Mendeloff AI: 249, 250, 251
Menger A: 463
Menotti A: 7
Metsaranta L: 373
Metz GL: 180, 181, 222,
    223, 426
Michaelis OE IV: 307, 308
Michalsky U: 460
Miettinen TA: 252, 253 373
Miller AB: 254
Miller BL: 113
Miller DS: 112
Minaire Y: 448
Miranda PM: 255
Mirouze J: 256, 260, 261
Miyazawa T: 257
Mod RR: 258
Mohan Rao S: 63
Mongeau R: 259
Monnier L: 256, 260, 261
Monro J: 23
Moore WE: 262, 263
Morin ML: 264
Morris ER: 109
Morris JJ: 305
Morris JN: 265, 266
Morris M: 406
Morse E: 267
Mosbech J: 280, 433
Moskovitz M: 268
Mossberg R: 464
Moy NL: 308
Mullen JD: 269
Mulvihille E: 108
Munoz JM: 270, 271, 272,
    333
Munzner R: 465
Murphy D: 149
Murphy EW: 273
Murray D: 120
McCallum G: 274
McCreary ML: 50
MacDonald IA: 275
McDougall RM: 276
MacFarlane J: 120
McGill AR: 294
McGill HC Jr: 277
McLain D: 324
McLeish JA: 278, 279
MacLennan R: 280

McNaughton JL: 281
McNeil NI: 282

Nahapetain A: 283
Naivikul O: 284
Namioka S: 174
Nassar JJ: 363
Navrrette DA: 285
Nelson RA: 297
Newcombe RG: 318
Newland P: 170
Newton CR: 286
Nichols BL: 169
Nicol BM: 287
Nilsson LH: 88
Nineham R: 181
Nolan DJ: 132
Normand FL: 258
Norum KR: 288

Oace JM: 82
Oakenfull DG: 290, 291
Ocoma EP: 95
O'Dell BL: 292
O'Dell RG: 145, 306
Ogunbiyi TA: 293
Ohsawa A: 328
O'Moore RR: 294
O'Reilly TC: 110
Orsetti A: 256, 260
Ory RL: 258
Ostapczuk J: 478
Oste R: 19
Ostrower VS: 202
Ostwald R: 295
Ou Tim L: 343
Owen RL: 374

Pageau R: 39
Painter NS: 296
Palmer GH: 57
Palmer JK: 329
Palumbo PJ: 297
Paraf A: 440, 442
Parrot ME: 298
Partridge IG: 233, 299
Patchefsky AS: 68
Patterson J: 97, 98
Patton NM: 66
Paul AA: 300
Payenneville H: 58
Peifer JJ: 301
Peng B: 302
Peterson M: 147
Pham TC: 256, 260
Phillip J: 466

Phillips GD: 142
Phillips PG: 287
Phillips RL: 303
Peikarska J: 475, 477
Pineda O: 342, 352
Pla GW: 129
Plageman K: 304
Pollman JW: 305
Post M: 21
Prather ES: 30, 199, 200
Presly AS: 274
Pritchard J: 102, 104
Prosky L: 145, 306
Putney JD: 307, 308
Puyat LV: 312

Rahmanifar A: 309
Rajagopalan SS: 218
Ralphs DN: 222, 223, 310
Ram H: 244
Ramachandran A: 402
Ramsey WH: 168
Ranhotra GS: 311, 312
Ransley J: 376
Rao AV: 42
Rashed-Mohassel MA: 313
Rautureau J: 440, 441
Reardon MJ: 146
Reck SJ: 333
Reddy BS: 314, 315, 413,
    414
Reeves RD: 135
Regoli D: 39
Reid RL: 131
Reiser S: 316
Renger F: 457
Renquist DM: 264
Rerat A: 317
Reyes EL: 327
Rhoads JE Jr: 25
Rhodes J: 90, 91, 318
Ricci G: 7
Ricci PD: 471
Richardson EN: 406
Ritchie JA: 319
Ritland S: 34
Roberts RL: 320
Robertson J: 358
Robertson JA: 103
Robertson JB: 321, 398
Robinson MF: 143
Robinson RK: 322
Robson JR: 323
Roe DA: 324
Rolls BA: 156, 325
Roos MA: 76
Rose PN: 305

(1) GASTROINTESTINAL

THE REFERENCES

(1) Achord JL. Irritable bowel syndrome and dietary fiber. J Am Diet Assoc 1979 Oct; 75 (4): 452-3.

(2) Adelstein P, Baldwin JA, Fedrich J. Cancers of the large bowel. Associated disorders in individuals. Cancer 1979 Jun; 43 (6): 2553-7.

(3) Akpapunam MA, Markakis P. Oligosaccharides of 13 American cultivars of cowpeas (Vigna sinensis). J Food Sci 1979; 44 (5): 1317-8.

(4) Albrink MJ, Newman T, Davidson PC. Effect of high- and low-fiber diets on plasma lipids and insulin. Am J Clin Nutr 1979 Jul; 32 (7): 1486-91.

(5) Aman P. Carbohydrates in raw and germinated seeds from mung bean and chick pea. J Sci Food Agric 1979 Sep; 30 (9): 869-75.

(6) American Diabetes Association. Special Report. Principles of nutrition and dietary recommendations for individuals with diabetes mellitus: 1979. Diabetes 1979 Nov; 28 (11): 1027-30.

(7) Anderson JW. High carbohydrate, high fiber diets for patients with diabetes. Adv Exp Med Biol 1979; 119: 263-73.

(8) Anderson J, Alberti KG, Tobin J, Barbosa J, Camerini-Davalos R, Lebovitz H, Clements R, Reaven GM, Gerritsen G. Diet therapy. Discussion. Adv Exp Med Biol 1979; 119: 281-6.

(9) Anderson JW, Chen W-J. Plant fiber. Carbohydrate and lipid metabolism. Am J Clin Nutr 1979 Feb; 32 (2): 346-63.

(10) Anderson JW. Triglyceride lowering effects of high fiber diets (abstract). Am J Clin Nutr 1979 Apr; 32 (4): 933.

(11) Anderson JW, Ward K. High-carbohydrate, high-fiber diets for insulin-treated men with diabetes mellitus. Am J Clin Nutr 1979 Mar; 32 (11): 2312-21.

(12) Anderson JW, Sieling B, Ferguson S. Long-term effects of high-fiber diets on mineral and fat soluble vitamin status in persons with diabetes (abstract). Diabetes 1979; 28 (Program): 384.

(13) Anderson JW, Midgley WR, Wedman B. Fiber and diabetes. Diabetes Care 1979 Jul-Aug; 2 (4): 369-77.

(14) Andersson H, Bosaeus I, Falkheden T, Melkersson M. Transit time in constipated geriatric patients during treatment with a bulk laxative and bran: a comparison. Scand J Gastroenterol 1979; 14 (7): 821-6.

(15) Andersson N, Griffiths H, Murphy J, Roll R, Serenyi A, Swann I, Cockroft A, Myers J, St Leger A. Is appendicitis familial? Br Med J 1979 Sep 22; 2 (6192): 697-8.

(16) Anonymous. Can a constipated adult with coeliac disease who has been advised to have a gluten-free diet use bran? Br Med J 1979 Jul 7; 2 (6181): 24.

(17) Anonymous. Fresh horizon's fiber source challenged. Cereal Foods World 1979 Apr; 24 (4): 156.

(18) Anonymous. Oat bran bread. Cereal Foods World 1979 Jun; 24 (6): 245.

(19) Anonymous. Effects of fiber intake on nutrition studied. Cereal Foods World 1979 Aug; 24 (8): 355.

(20) Anonymous. Bran reduces cholesterol saturation of bile. JAMA 1979 Mar 16; 241 (11): 1088.

(21) Anonymous. Is there such a thing as roughage? J Hum Nutr 1979 Feb; 33 (1): 1-2.

(22) Anonymous. Keep taking your bran (editorial). Lancet 1979 Jun 2; 1 (8127): 1175.

(23) Anonymous. Guar gum, dietary fiber and diabetes. Med Lett Drugs Ther 1979 Jun 15; 21 (12): 51-2.

(24) Anonymous. Dietary fiber and vitamin B_{12} balance. Nutr Rev 1979 Apr; 37 (4): 116-8.

(25) Appledorf H, Kelly LS. Proximate and mineral content of fast foods. J Am Diet Assoc 1979 Jan; 74 (1): 35-40.

(26) Araujo PE, Norden AR. Response of mouse intestinal microflora to dietary cellulose, starch and sucrose. J Food Sci 1979; 44 (1): 308-9.

(27) Araujo PE. Effect of glucose and fructose on incubation glycogenic capacity in tissue from mice previously consuming various carbohydrates. J Food Sci 1979; 44 (3): 742-4.

206

(28) Archampong EQ. Diverticular disease in urban Kenyans (letter). Br Med J 1979 Sep 15; 2 (6191): 672-3.

(29) Archbold A, Parks TG. Fybogel; its effect on colonic motility and intestinal transit in diverticular disease (abstract).|Ir J Med Sci 1979 Jan; 148 (1): 27.

(30) Augustin J, Toma RB, True RH, Shaw RL, Teitzel C, Johnson SR, Orr P. Composition of raw and cooked potato peel and flesh: proximate and vitamin composition. J Food Sci 1979; 44 (3): 805-6.

(31) Baig MM, Burgin C, Cerda JJ. Use of galactose oxidase tritiated potassium borohydride method for labelling pectic polysaccharides (abstract). Am J Clin Nutr 1979 Jun; 32 (6): xviii.

(32) Baig MM, Cerda JJ. Use of galactose oxidase tritiated-potassium borohydride method for labeling pectic polysaccharides. Anal Biochem 1979 Oct 1; 98 (2): 429-32.

(33) Baker D, Norris KH, Li BW. Food fiber analysis: advances in methodology. In: Inglett GE, Falkehag SI, eds. Dietary fibers: chemistry and nutrition. New York: Academic Press, 1979: 67-78.

(34) Banta CA, Clemens ET, Krinsky MM, Sheffy BE. Sites of organic acid production and patterns of digesta movement in the gastrointestinal tract of dogs. J Nutr 1979 Sep; 109 (9): 1592-1600.

(35) Bauer HG, Asp N-G, Oste R, Dahlqvist A, Fredlund PE. Effect of dietary fiber on the induction of colorectal tumors and fecal β-glucuronidase activity in the rat. Cancer Res 1979 Sep; 39 (9): 3752-6.

(36) Becker U, Elsborg L. A new method for the determination of gastrointestinal transit times. Scand J Gastroenterol 1979; 14 (3): 355-9.

(37) Beereboom JJ. Low calorie bulking agents. CRC Crit Rev Food Sci Nutr 1979 May; 11 (4): 401-13.

(38) Behall KM, Kelsay JL, Prather ES. Effects of four diets with different fiber content from fruits and vegetables on fasting serum levels of glucose, lipids and hormones of human subjects (abstract). Am J Clin Nutr 1979 Apr; 32 (4): 947.

(39) Benjamin IS. Cholelithiasis and hiatus hernia (letter). Lancet 1979 Jun 30; 1 (8131): 1411-2.

(40) Bierman EL. Carbohydrates, sucrose, and human disease. Am J Clin Nutr 1979 Dec; 32 (12 Suppl): S2712-22.

(41) Bingham S, Cummings JH, McNeil NI. Intakes and sources of dietary fiber in the British population. Am J Clin Nutr 1979 Jun; 32 (6): 1313-9.

(42) Bingham S, Williams DR, Cole TJ, James WP. Dietary fibre and regional large-bowel cancer mortality in Britain. Br J Cancer 1979 Sep; 40 (3): 456-63.

(43) Bingham S. Low-residue diets: a reappraisal of their meaning and content. J Hum Nutr 1979 Feb; 33 (1): 5-16.

(44) Blanshard JM, Mitchell JR, eds. Polysaccharides in food. London: Butterworth and Co Ltd, 1979.

(45) Borgman RF, Lightsey SF. Lipid metabolism and cholelithiasis in rabbits fed plant materials. Am J Vet Res 1979 Jan; 40 (1): 150-3.

(46) Bose T. High dietary fibre in routine Bengalee diet - a check to diabetes mellitus? Indian J Nutr Diet 1979; 16 (8): 312-5.

(47) Brauer PM, Marlett JA. Apparent digestibility of dietary fiber in elderly subjects (abstract). Fed Proc 1979; 38 (3 Pt I): 768.

(48) Brillouet JM, Mercier C. Fractionation procedure and composition of hemicelluloses of wheat bran (abstract). Cereal Foods World 1979 Sep; 24 (9): 464.

(49) Brodribb AJ, Condon RE, Cowles V, DeCosse JJ. Effect of dietary fiber on intraluminal pressure and myoelectrical activity of left colon in monkeys. Gastroenterology 1979 Jul; 77 (1): 70-4.

(50) Brown RC, Kelleher J, Walker BE, Losowsky MS. The effect of wheat bran and pectin on paracetamol absorption in the rat. Br J Nutr 1979 May; 41 (3): 455-64.

(51) Brown RC, Kelleher J, Losowsky MS. The effect of pectin on the structure and function of the rat small intestine. Br J Nutr 1979 Nov; 42 (3): 357-65.

(52) Brown W. Interactions of small molecules with hydrated polymer networks. In: Inglett GE, Falkehag SI, eds. Dietary fibers: chemistry and nutrition. New York: Academic Press, 1979: 1-13.

(53) Brydon WG, Borup-Christensen S, Van der Linden W, Eastwood MA. The effect of dietary psyllium hydrocolloid on bile. Z Ernaehrungswiss 1979 Jul; 18 (2): 77-80.

(54) Bryson E, Dore C, Garrow JS. Wholemeal bread and satiety (letter). Lancet 1979 Aug 4; 2 (8136): 260-1.

(55) Burczak JD, Kellogg TF. Binding of cholate, deoxycholate, and chenodeoxycholate in vitro by various types and sizes of fibrous materials. Nutr Rep Int 1979 Feb; 19 (2): 261-6.

(56) Burkitt DP, Trowell HC. Nutritional intake, adiposity, and diabetes (letter). Br Med J 1979 Apr 21; 1 (6170): 1083-4.

(57) Burkitt D. Don't forget fibre in your diet. To help avoid many of our commonest diseases. London: Martin Dunitz Ltd, 1979.

(58) Burkitt DP. Epidemiological features of gastrointestinal cancer. Front Gastrointest Res 1979; 4: 86-95.

(59) Burkitt DP, Meisner P. How to manage constipation with high-fiber diet. Geriatrics 1979 Feb; 34 (2): 33-5, 38-40.

(60) Burkitt D. Managing constipation by a fibre-rich diet. Mod Geriatr 1979 Jan; 9 (1): 69-70.

(61) Burkitt DP. Some neglected leads to cancer causation. Natl Cancer Inst Monogr 1979 Sep; (52): 5-12. Article reprinted from JNCI 1971 Nov; 47 (5): 913-9, with new addendum.

(62) Burkitt DP. Large-bowel cancer: an epidemiologic jigsaw puzzle. Natl Cancer Inst Monogr 1979 Sep; (52): 137-41. Article reprinted from JNCI 1975 Jan; 54 (1): 3-6, with new addendum.

(63) Burkitt DP. The protective value of plant fibre against many modern western diseases. Qual Plant Plant Foods Hum Nutr 1979; 29 (1-2): 39-48.

(64) Burrows CF, Merrit AM. The effect of changing dietary fiber on canine colonic motility (abstract). Gastroenterology 1979 May; 76 (5 Pt 2): 1109.

(65) Busk GC Jr, Labuza TP. A dye diffusion technique to evaluate gel properties. J Food Sci 1979; 44 (5): 1369-72.

(66) Calder JF. Diverticular disease of the colon in Africans. Br Med J 1979 Jun 2; 1 (6176): 1465-6.

(67) Calder JF. Diverticular disease in Kenyan Africans (letter). Br Med J 1979 Aug 25; 2 (6188): 498.

(68) Castleden WM. Diet in the aetiology of carcinoma of the large bowel. London: University of London, 1979. Thesis.

(69) Cerqueira MT, Fry MM, Connor WE. The food and nutrient intakes of the Tarahumara Indians of Mexico. Am J Clin Nutr 1979 Apr; 32 (4): 905-15.

(70) Chang GW, Fukumoto HE, Gyory CP, Block AP, Kretsch MJ, Calloway DH. Effects of diet on the gut microflora: fecal enzymes and bacterial metabolites (abstract). Fed Proc 1979; 38 (3 Pt I): 767.

(71) Chang J-J, Hash JH. The use of an amino acid analyzer for the rapid identification and quantitative determination of chitosan oligosaccharides. Anal Biochem 1979 Jun; 95 (2): 563-7.

(72) Chang ML, Johnson MA, Baker D. Effects of whole wheat flour and mill-fractions on lipid metabolism in rats. Proc Soc Exp Biol Med 1979 Jan; 160 (1): 88-93.

(73) Chatterjee AK, Buchanan GE, Behrens MK, Starr MP. Synthesis and excretion of polygalacturonic acid trans-eliminase in Erwinia, Yersinia, and Klebsiella species. Can J Microbiol 1979 Jan; 25 (1): 94-102.

(74) Chen W-J, Anderson JW. Influence of guar gum, oat bran and pectin on lipid metabolism in rats (abstract). Fed Proc 1979; 38 (3 Pt I): 548.

(75) Chen W-J, Anderson JW. Effects of guar gum and wheat bran on lipid metabolism of rats. J Nutr 1979 Jun; 109 (6): 1028-34.

(76)   Chen W-J, Anderson JW. Effects of plant fiber in decreasing plasma total cholesterol and increasing high-density lipoprotein cholesterol. Proc Soc Exp Biol Med 1979 Nov; 162 (2): 310-3.

(77)   Cleave TL. Aetiology of appendicitis (letter). Br Med J 1979 Mar 24; 1 (6166): 820.

(78)   Cleave TL. Nutritional intake, adiposity, and diabetes (letter). Br Med J 1979 May 5; 1 (6172): 1214.

(79)   Clinton SK, Edes TE, Truex CR, Visek WJ. Wheat bran and the induction of intestinal aryl hydrocarbon hydroxylase (abstract). Fed Proc 1979; 38 (3 Pt I): 713.

(80)   Coccodrilli G Jr, Shah N, Sommer S, Ali R. Bioavailability of zinc from ready-to-eat breakfast cereals, wheat bran, and defatted peanut flour (abstract). Fed Proc 1979; 38 (3 Pt I): 558.

(81)   Cohen M, Martin FI. Guar crispbread in the diabetic diet (letter). Br Med J 1979 Mar 3; 1 (6163): 616-7.

(82)   Collins TF, Black TN, Prew JH. Effects of calcium and sodium carrageenans and ι-carrageenan on hamster foetal development. Food Cosmet Toxicol 1979 Oct; 17 (5): 443-9.

(83)   The committee of diet and heart disease of the national heart foundation of Australia. Diet and coronary heart disease: a review. Med J Aust 1979 Sep 22; 2 (6): 294-307.

(84)   Compston J. Rickets in Asian immigrants (letter). Br Med J 1979 Sep 8; 2 (6190): 612.

(85)   Crofts TJ. Bran and experimental colon cancer (letter). Lancet 1979 Jan 13; 1 (8107): 108.

(86)   Cruse P, Lewin M, Clark C. Dietary fibre and experimental colon cancer (letter). Lancet 1979 Feb 17; 1 (8112): 376.

(87)   Cruse P, Lewin M, Clark CG. Cholesterol and colon cancer (letter). Lancet 1979 Jul 7; 2 (8132): 43-4.

(88)   Cummings JH, Hill MJ, Jivraj T, Houston H, Branch WJ, Jenkins DJ. The effect of meat protein and dietary fiber on colonic function and metabolism. I. Changes in bowel habit, bile acid excretion, and calcium absorption. Am J Clin Nutr 1979 Oct; 32 (10): 2086-93.

(89)   Cummings JH, Hill MJ, Bone ES, Branch WJ, Jenkins DJ. The effect of meat protein and dietary fiber on colonic function and metabolism. II. Bacterial metabolites in feces and urine. Am J Clin Nutr 1979 Oct; 32 (10): 2094-101.

(90)   Cummings JH, Southgate DA, Branch WJ, Wiggins HS, Houston H, Jenkins DJ, Jivraj T, Hill MJ. The digestion of pectin in the human gut and its effect on calcium absorption and large bowel function. Br J Nutr 1979 May; 41 (3): 477-85.

(91)   Cummings JH, Stephen AM, Wayman B, Chapman G. Influence of age, sex and dose on colonic response to dietary fiber from bread (abstract). Gastroenterology 1979 May; 76 (5 Pt 2): 1116.

(92)   Dales LG, Friedman GD, Ury HK, Grossman S, Williams S. A case-control study of relationships of diet and other traits to colorectal cancer in American blacks. Am J Epidemiol 1979 Feb; 109 (2): 132-44.

(93)   Dea IC. Interactions of ordered polysaccharide structures — synergism and freeze-thaw phenomena. In: Blanshard JM, Mitchell JR, eds. Polysaccharides in food. London: Butterworth and Co Ltd, 1979: 229-47.

(94)   Dekker RF. The hemicellulase group of enzymes. In: Blanshard JM, Mitchell JR, eds. Polysaccharides in food. London: Butterworth and Co Ltd, 1979: 93-108.

(95)   Devi MA, Venkataraman LV, Rajasekaran T. Hypocholesterolemic effect of diets containing algae on albino rats. Nutr Rep Int 1979 Jul; 20 (1): 83-90.

(96)   Dewar J, Garcia-Webb P, Shenfield GM. Guar and diabetes (letter). Lancet 1979 Mar 17; 1 (8116): 612-3.

(97)   Dintzis FR, Legg LM, Deatherage WL, Baker FL, Inglett GE, Jacob RA, Reck SJ, Munoz JM, Klevay LM, Sandstead HH, Shuey WC. Human gastrointestinal action on wheat, corn, and soy hull bran — preliminary findings. Cereal Chem 1979; 56 (3): 123-7.

(98) Dintzis FR, McBrien JB, Baker FL, Inglett GE, Jacob RA, Munoz JM, Klevay LM, Sandstead HH, Shuey WC. Some effects of baking and human gastrointestinal action upon a hard red wheat bran. In: Inglett GE, Falkehag SI, eds. Dietary fibers: chemistry and nutrition. New York: Academic Press, 1979: 157-71.

(99) Dippe SE, Cook JE. The birth of fiber and the death of fat. Ariz Med 1979 Feb; 36 (2): 113-5.

(100) Doi K, Matsuura M, Kawara A, Baba S. Treatment of diabetes with glucomannan (konjac mannan) (letter). Lancet May 5; 1 (8123): 987-8.

(101) Dolan PA, Thompson BW. Management of persimmon bezoars (diosopyrobezoars). South Med J 1979 Dec; 72 (12): 1527-8, 1531.

(102) Drews LM, Kies C, Fox HM. Effect of dietary fiber on copper, zinc, and magnesium utilization by adolescent boys. Am J Clin Nutr 1979 Sep; 32 (6): 1893-7.

(103) Dreyer JJ, de Klerk WA, van der Walt WH. In vivo determination of indigestible dry matter in foodstuffs (letter). Am J Clin Nutr 1979 Oct; 32 (10): 1980-2.

(104) Duggan JM. Ischaemic heart disease — an hypothesis to integrate the role of insulin, fibre and sucrose. Med Hypotheses 1979 Feb; 5 (2): 209-19.

(105) Durrant M, Royston P. Short-term effects of energy density on salivation, hunger and appetite in obese subjects. Int J Obes 1979; 3 (4): 335-47.

(106) Eastwood MA, Kay RM. An hypothesis for the action of dietary fiber along the gastrointestinal tract. Am J Clin Nutr 1979 Feb; 32 (2): 364-7.

(107) Ebihara K, Kiriyama S, Manabe M. Cholesterol-lowering activity of various natural pectins and synthetic pectin-derivatives with different physico-chemical properties. Nutr Rep Int 1979 Oct; 20 (4): 519-26.

(108) Eide TJ, Stalsberg H. Diverticular disease of the large intestine in Northern Norway. Gut 1979 Jul; 20 (7): 609-15.

(109) Elfak AM, Pass G, Phillips GO. The effect of shear rate on the viscosity of solutions of guar gum and locust bean gum. J Sci Food Agric 1979 Apr; 30 (4): 439-44.

(110) Elfak AM, Pass G, Phillips GO. The effect of shear rate on the viscosity of solutions of sodium carboxymethylcellulose and κ-carrageenan. J Sci Food Agric 1979 Jul; 30 (7): 724-30.

(111) El Tinay AH, Abdel Gadir AM, El Hidai M. Sorghum fermented Kisra bread. 1 — Nutritive value of Kisra. J Sci Food Agric 1979 Sep; 30 (9): 859-63.

(112) Englyst H, Wiggins H. Measurement of the carbohydrate component of dietary fibre (non-starch polysaccharides) (abstract). Gut 1979 Oct; 20 (10): A935.

(113) Fahey GC Jr. The nutritional significance of chemically defined dietary fibers. In: Inglett GE, Falkehag SI, eds. Dietary fibers: chemistry and nutrition. New York: Academic Press, 1979: 117-46.

(114) Fahey GC Jr, Miller BL, Hadfield HW. Metabolic parameters affected by feeding various types of fiber to guinea pigs. J Nutr 1979 Jan; 109 (1): 77-83.

(115) Fedail SS, Harvey RF, Burns-Cox CJ. Abdominal and thoracic pressures during defaecation. Br Med J 1979 Jan 13; 1 (6156): 91.

(116) Fetzer SG, Kies C, Fox HM. Gastric disappearance of dietary fiber by adolescent boys. Cereal Chem 1979; 56 (1): 34-7.

(117) Fielding JF, Melvin K. Dietary fibre and the irritable bowel syndrome. J Hum Nutr 1979 Aug; 33 (4): 243-7.

(118) Fingl E, Freston JW. Antidiarrheal agents and laxatives: changing concepts. Clin Gastroenterol 1979 Jan; 8 (1): 161-85.

(119) Ford CW. Simultaneous quantitative determination of sucrose, raffinose and stachyose by invertase hydrolysis and gas-liquid chromotography. J Sci Food Agric 1979 Sep; 30 (9): 853-8.

(120) Forman LP, Scuri LM, Schneeman BO. Influence of dietary pectin and fat on adaptation of pancreatic digestive enzymes in the rat (abstract). Fed Proc 1979; 38 (3 pt I): 549.

(121) Foster GE, Bolwell JS, Wright J, Hardcastle JD. Controlled trial of bulk forming evacuants in the treatment of patients with haemorrhoids (abstract). Gut 1979 May; 20 (5): A452-3.

210

(122) Frank HA, Green LC. Successful use of a bulk laxative to control the diarrhea of tube feeding. Scand J Plast Reconstr Surg 1979; 13 (1): 193-4.

(123) Freeman HJ. Dietary fibre and colonic neoplasia. Can Med Assoc J 1979 Aug 4; 121 (3): 291-6.

(124) Furda I. Interaction of pectinaceous dietary fiber with some metals and lipids. In: Inglett GE, Falkehag SI, eds. Dietary fibers: chemistry and nutrition. New York: Academic Press, 1979: 31-48.

(125) Gallaher D, Schneeman BO. Effect of a high fiber diet on enzyme activity in the pancreas and small intestine (abstract). Fed Proc 1979; 38 (3 Pt I): 549.

(126) Gear JS, Ware A, Fursdon P, Mann JI, Nolan DJ, Brodribb AJ, Vessey MP. Symptomless diverticular disease and intake of dietary fibre. Lancet 1979 Mar 10; 1 (8115): 511-4.

(127) Geervani P, Theophilus F. Flatus inducing effect of processed legumes in pre-school children. Indian J Med Res 1979 Nov; 70: 750-5.

(128) George JR, Harbers LH, Reeves RD. Digestion of wheat bran in rats as observed by scanning electron microscopy (abstract). Fed Proc 1979; 38 (3 Pt I): 767.

(129) Ginter E, Kubec FJ, Vozar J, Bobek P. Natural hypocholesterolemic agent: pectin plus ascorbic acid. Int J Vitam Nutr Res 1979; 49 (4): 406-12.

(130) Glass RL. Use of a high bulk diet after a small bowel bypass operation for obesity. Case reports. Mo Med 1979 Jan; 76 (1): 34-5.

(131) Glauert HP, Sander CH, Sanger VL, Bennink MR. Influence of dietary agar and tallow on colon carcinogenesis (abstract). Fed Proc 1979; 38 (3 Pt I): 714.

(132) Glicksman M. Gelling hydrocolloids in food product applications. In: Blanshard JM, Mitchell JR, eds. Polysaccharides in food. London: Butterworth and Co Ltd, 1979: 185-204.

(133) Godding EW. Fibre in the traditional Eskimo diet (letter). Br Med J 1979 May 26; 1 (6175): 1428.

(134) Gomez MI, Kothary M. Studies on the production of red-kidney-bean Tempeh. J Plant Foods 1979; 3 (3): 191-8.

(135) Gormley TR, Kevany J, O'Donnell B, McFarlane R. Effect of peas on serum cholesterol levels in humans. Ir J Food Sci Technol 1979; 3 (2): 101-9.

(136) Goulder TJ. Guar and diabetes (letter). Lancet 1979 Mar 17; 1 (8116): 612.

(137) Goulding NJ, Husbands DR, Burstyn PG, Taylor TG. The effect of feeding cellulose to rats and rabbits on the fragility of the erythrocyte membrane (abstract). Proc Nutr Soc 1979 Sep; 38 (2): 31A.

(138) Graham GG, Morales E, Placko RP, MacLean WC Jr. Nutritive value of brown and black beans for infants and small children. Am J Clin Nutr 1979 Nov; 32 (11): 2362-6.

(139) Graham S, Haenszel W, Bock FG, Lyon JL. Need to pursue new leads in the epidemiology of colorectal cancer. JNCI 1979 Oct; 63 (4): 879-81.

(140) Gray C. Fibre diets: separating factual grain from fictional chaff. Can Med Assoc J 1979 Apr 7; 120 (7): 865-9.

(141) Gruden N, Buben M, Ciganovic M. The effect of cellulose and zinc on ^{65}Zn absorption in infant rats. Nutr Rep Int 1979 Dec; 20 (6): 757-63.

(142) Guild RT, Cerda JJ, Burgin CW. A model for the evaluation of bile salt-pectin interaction (abstract). Am J Clin Nutr 1979 Apr; 32 (4): 951.

(143) Haider SQ, Wheeler M. Nutritive intake of black and Hispanic mothers in a Brooklyn ghetto. J Am Diet Assoc 1979 Dec; 75 (6): 670-2.

(144) Hall SE, Bolton TM, Hetenyi G Jr. Can bran increase insulin sensitivity (abstract). Diabetes 1979; 28 (Program): 385.

(145) Hanley HG. Prescription for a better British diet (letter). Br Med J 1979 Apr 7; 1 (6168): 953.

(146) Harada T. Curdlan: a gel-forming β-1,3-glucan. In: Blanshard JM, Mitchell JR, eds. Polysaccharides in food. London: Butterworth and Co Ltd, 1979: 283-300.

(147) Harland BF, Prosky L. Development of dietary fiber values for foods. Cereal Foods World 1979 Sep; 24 (9): 387-94.

(148)   Harland BF, Stringfellow DE, Connor DH, Foster WD, Heggie CM. Lowered plasma zinc in humans ingesting wheat bran products (abstract). Fed Proc 1979; 38 (3 Pt I): 548.

(149)   Harmuth-Hoene A-E, Schwerdtfeger E. Effect of indigestible polysaccharides on protein digestibility and nitrogen retention in growing rats. Nutr Metab 1979; 23 (5): 399-407.

(150)   Harverson G. Diverticular disease in Kenyan Africans (letter). Br Med J 1979 Aug 25; 2 (6188): 498-9.

(151)   Heaton KW. Fiber: new terminology or new concepts (letter). Am J Clin Nutr 1979 Dec; 32 (12): 2373-4.

(152)   Heaton KW, Thornton JR, Emmett PM. Treatment of Crohn's disease with an unrefined-carbohydrate, fibre-rich diet. Br Med J 1979 Sep 29; 2 (6193): 764-6.

(153)   Heaton KW. Diet and gallstones. In: Fisher MM, Goresky CA, Shaffer EA, Strasberg SM, eds. Gallstones. New York: Plenum Press, 1979: 371-89. (Hepatology - research and clinical issues; vol 4.)

(154)   Heaton KW. Dietary fibre in clinical practice. Welwyn Garden City, Hertfordshire, England: Smith Kline and French Laboratories Limited. (GI for the GP 1979 Nov; vol 1; no 7.)

(155)   Heaton KW. Fibre, satiety, and energy balance (letter). Lancet 1979 Sep 15; 2 (8142): 593-4.

(156)   Hellendoorn EW. Beneficial physiological activity of leguminous seeds. Qual Plant Plant Foods Hum Nutr 1979; 29 (1-2): 227-44.

(157)   Helms P. Vegetable carbohydrates in human food. Preventive, prophylactic and epidemiological aspects. Qual Plant Plant Foods Hum Nutr 1979; 29 (1-2): 95-108.

(158)   Hetherington RJ. Half-remembered (letter). World Med 1979 Mar 10; 14 (11): 95.

(159)   Hill MA, Leeds AR. High-fibre foods: a feasibility study using guar gum. J Hum Nutr 1979 Aug; 33 (4): 253-8.

(160)   Hill M, MacLennan R, Newcombe R. Diet and large-bowel cancer in three socioeconomic groups in Hong Kong (letter). Lancet 1979 Feb 24; 1 (8113): 436.

(161)   Hockaday TD, Jenkins DJ, Wolever TM, Nineham R, Taylor R, Bacon S. Guar crispbread in the diabetic diet (letter). Br Med J 1979 May 19; 1 (6174): 1353.

(162)   Holt S, Heading RC, Carter DC, Prescott LF, Tothill P. Effect of gel fibre on gastric emptying and absorption of glucose and paracetamol. Lancet 1979 Mar 24; 1 (8117): 636-9.

(163)   Honig DH, Rackis JJ. Determination of the total pepsin-pancreatin indigestible content (dietary fiber) of soybean products, wheat bran, and corn bran. J Agric Food Chem 1979 Nov-Dec; 27 (6): 1262-6.

(164)   Honore LH. Cholelithiasis and hiatus hernia (letter). Lancet 1979 Apr 28; 1 (8122): 927-8.

(165)   Honore LH. Cholelithiasis and hiatus hernia (letter). Lancet 1979 Jun 30; 1 (8131): 1412.

(166)   Horwitz DL, Schoeller DA, Niu HC, Schneider JF, Klein PD. Effects of high-cellulose bread on glucose absorption and utilization (abstract). Am J Clin Nutr 1979 Apr; 32 (4): 953.

(167)   Hove EL, King S. Effects of pectin and cellulose on growth, feed efficiency, and protein utilization, and their contribution to energy requirement and cecal VFA in rats. J Nutr 1979 Jul; 109 (7): 1274-8.

(168)   Hughes RE, Jones E. A Welsh diet for Britain (letter). Br Med J 1979 Apr 28; 1 (6171): 1145.

(169)   Hunt PS, Sali A. The prevention of colorectal cancer. Med J Aust 1979 Jun 30; 1 (13): 613-6.

(170)   Hutt MS. Epidemiology of chronic intestinal disease in middle Africa. Isr J Med Sci 1979 Apr; 15 (4): 314-7.

(171)   Hyland JM, Taylor I. Diverticular disease — has its natural history altered (abstract). Gut 1979 May; 20 (5): A441-2.

(172) Inglett GE, Falkehag SI, eds. Dietary fibers: chemistry and nutrition. New York: Academic Press, 1979.

(173) Institute of food technologists' expert panel on food safety and nutrition and the committee on public information. Dietary fiber. Food Technol 1979 Jan; 33 (1): 35-9.

(174) Ishii S, Kiho K, Sugiyama S, Sugimoto H. Low-methoxyl pectin prepared by pectinesterase from Aspergillus japonicus. J Food Sci 1979; 44 (2): 611-4.

(175) Jacobs GP, Simes R. The gamma irradiation of tragacanth: effect on microbial contamination and rheology. J Pharm Pharmacol 1979 May; 31 (5): 333-4.

(176) James JR. Trends in duodenal ulcer (letter). Br Med J 1979 Mar 24; 1 (6166): 820.

(177) James R. Dangerous diets (letter). World Med 1979 Mar 24; 14 (12): 18.

(178) Jaya TV, Naik HS, Venkataraman LV. Effect of germinated legumes on the rate of in vitro gas production by Clostridium perfringens. Nutr Rep Int 1979 Sep; 20 (3): 393-401.

(179) Jayakumari N, Kurup PA. Dietary fiber and cholesterol metabolism in rats fed a high cholesterol diet. Atherosclerosis 1979 May; 33 (1): 41-7.

(180) Jeltema MS, Zabik ME. Fiber components — quantitation and relationship to cake quality. J Food Sci 1979; 44 (6): 1732-5.

(181) Jenkins DJ, Wolever TM, Nineham R, Bacon S, Smith R, Hockaday TD. Dietary fiber and diabetic therapy: a progressive effect with time. Adv Exp Med Biol 1979; 119: 275-9.

(182) Jenkins DJ, Leeds AR, Slavin B, Mann J, Jepson EM. Dietary fiber and blood lipids: reduction of serum cholesterol in type II hyperlipidemia by guar gum. Am J Clin Nutr 1979 Jan; 32 (1): 16-8.

(183) Jenkins DJ, Reynolds D, Leeds AR, Waller AL, Cummings JH. Hypocholesterolemic action of dietary fiber unrelated to fecal bulking effect. Am J Clin Nutr 1979 Dec; 32 (12): 2430-5.

(184) Jenkins DJ, Hockaday TD, Wolever TM, Nineham R, Goff DV, Haisman P, Charnock R, Taylor RH, Bacon S. Dietary fibre and ketone bodies: reduced urinary 3-hydroxybutyrate excretion in diabetics on guar. Br Med J 1979 Dec 15; 2 (6204): 1555.

(185) Jenkins DJ. Dietary fiber: potential therapeutic and prophylactic roles. Compr Ther 1979 Dec; 5 (12): 36-44.

(186) Jenkins DJ, Nineham R, Craddock C, Craig-McFeely P, Donaldson K, Leigh T, Snook J. Fibre and diabetes (letter). Lancet 1979 Feb 24; 1 (8113): 434-5.

(187) Jenkins DJ, Taylor RH, Nineham R, Goff DV, Bloom SR, Sarson D, Alberti KG. Combined use of guar and acarbose in reduction of postprandial glycaemia. Lancet 1979 Nov 3; 2 (8149): 924-7.

(188) Jenkins DJ. Dietary fibre, diabetes, and hyperlipidaemia. Progress and prospects. Lancet 1979 Dec 15; 2 (8155): 1287-90.

(189) Jenkins DJ, Reynolds D, Slavin B, Leeds AR, Waller AL, Jepson EM. Reduction of blood lipids by guar crispbread (abstract). Proc Nutr Soc 1979 Sep; 38 (2): 86A.

(190) Jensen OM, MacLennan R. Dietary factors and colorectal cancer in Scandinavia. Isr J Med Sci 1979 Apr; 15 (4): 329-34.

(191) Jones RW, Krull LH, Blessin CW, Inglett GE. Neutral sugars of hemicellulose fractions of pith from stalks of selected plants. Cereal Chem 1979; 56 (5): 441-2.

(192) Jwuang W-L, Zabik ME. Enzyme neutral detergent fiber analysis of selected commercial and home-prepared foods. J Food Sci 1979; 44 (3): 924-5.

(193) Kang JY, Doe WF. Unprocessed bran causing intestinal obstruction. Br Med J 1979 May 12; 1 (6173): 1249-50.

(194) Karbassi A, Luh BS. Some characteristics of an endo-pectate lyase produced by a thermophilic bacillus isolated from olives. J Food Sci 1979; 44 (4): 1156-61.

(195) Karp M, Faiman G, Flexer Z. Blood glucose and clinical response to fiber-supplemented meals in young insulin-dependent diabetics. In: Laron Z, Tikva P, Karp M, eds. Nutrition and the diabetic child. Basel: S Karger, 1979: 77-82. (Pediatric and adolescent endocrinology; vol 7.)

(196) Kasper H, Rabast U, Fassl H, Fehle F. The effect of dietary fiber on the postprandial serum vitamin A concentration in man. Am J Clin Nutr 1979 Sep; 32 (9): 1847-9.

(197) Kasper H, Sommer H. Dietary fiber and nutrient intake in Crohn's disease. Am J Clin Nutr 1979 Sep; 32 (9): 1898-901.

(198) Kasper H, Zilly W, Fassl H, Fehle F. The effect of dietary fiber on postprandial serum digoxin concentration in man. Am J Clin Nutr 1979 Dec; 32 (12): 2436-8.

(199) Kay RM, Strasberg SM, Petrunka CN, Wayman M. Differential adsorption of bile acids by lignins. In: Inglett GE, Falkehag SI, eds. Dietary fibers: chemistry and nutrition. New York: Academic Press, 1979: 57-65.

(200) Kay RM, Wayman M, Strasberg SM. Effect of autohydrolysed lignin and lactulose on gallbladder bile (GB) composition in the hamster (abstract). Gastroenterology 1979 May; 76 (5 Pt 2): 1167.

(201) Keagy PM, Shane B, Oace SM. Dietary fiber effects on folacin bioavailability (abstract). Cereal Foods World 1979 Sep; 24 (9): 461.

(202) Keighley MR, Buchmann P, Minervini S, Arabi Y, Alexander-Williams J. Prospective trials of minor surgical procedures and high-fibre diet for haemorrhoids. Br Med J 1979 Oct 20; 2 (6196): 967-9.

(203) Keim K, Kies C. Effects of dietary fiber on nutritional status of weanling mice. Cereal Chem 1979; 56 (2): 73-8.

(204) Kelsay JL, Behall KM, Prather ES. Effect of fiber from fruits and vegetables on metabolic responses of human subjects. II. Calcium, magnesium, iron, and silicon balances. Am J Clin Nutr 1979 Sep; 32 (9): 1876-80.

(205) Kelsay JL, Jacob RA, Prather ES. Effect of fiber from fruits and vegetables on metabolic responses of human subjects. III. Zinc, copper, and phosphorus balances. Am J Clin Nutr 1979 Nov; 32 (11): 2307-11.

(206) Kelsay JL. Effect of level of fiber in the diet on bowel function and trace mineral balances of human subjects (abstract). Cereal Foods World 1979 Sep; 24 (9): 445-6.

(207) Kelsay JL, Clark WM, Herbst BJ, Prather ES. Response of human subjects to three levels of fiber intake from fruits and vegetables (abstract). Fed Proc 1979; 38 (3 Pt I): 767.

(208) Khan P, Macraie R, Robinson RK. The novel use of a chromatography refractive index detector for monitoring model dialysis experiments. Lab Pract 1979; 28: 260.

(209) Kies C, Fox HM. Blood serum lipids of adolescent humans as affected by dietary fiber (abstract). Am J Clin Nutr 1979 Jun; 32 (6): xviii.

(210) Kies C, Fox HM, Beshgetoor D. Effect of various levels of dietary hemicellulose on zinc nutritional status of men. Cereal Chem 1979; 56 (3): 133-6.

(211) Knehans AW, Kincaid RL, Regan WO, O'Dell BL. An unrecognised dietary factor for guinea pigs associated with the fibrous fractions of plant products. J Nutr 1979 Mar; 109 (3): 418-25.

(212) Kobayashi T, Otsuka S, Yugari, Y. Effect of chitosan and serum and liver cholesterol levels in cholesterol-fed rats. Nutr Rep Int 1979 Mar; 19 (3): 327-34.

(213) Kochen M. Dietary fiber (letter). West J Med 1979 Apr; 130 (4): 375-6.

(214) Koopman JP, Kennis HM, Lankhorst A, Prins RA. Influence of the composition of the diet on some parameters connected with gastro-intestinal colonization resistance in mice. Z Versuchstierkd 1979; 21 (1): 21-6.

(215) Kosakai M, Yosizawa Z. A partial modification of the carbazole method of Bitter and Muir for quantitation of hexuronic acids. Anal Biochem 1979 Mar; 93 (2): 295-8.

(216) Kratzer FH, Shariff G, Vohra P. Effect of gums and pectin on growth of Tribolium castaneum larvae, chickens and Japanese quail (abstract). Fed Proc 1979; 38 (3 Pt I): 549.

(217) Kretsch MJ, Crawford L, Calloway DH. Some aspects of bile acid and urobilinogen excretion and fecal elimination in men given a rural Guatemalan diet and egg formulas with and without added oat bran. Am J Clin Nutr 1979 Jul; 32 (7): 1492-6.

(218) Kritchevsky D. Dietary fiber and research. Compr Ther 1979 Dec; 5 (12): 31-5.

(219) Kritchevsky D. Dietary interactions. In: Levy RI, Rifkind BM, Dennis BH, Ernst N, eds. Nutrition, lipids and coronary heart disease. A global view. New York: Raven Press, 1979: 229-46. (Nutrition in health and disease; vol 1.)

214

(220)   Kritchevsky D. Metabolic effects of dietary fiber. West J Med 1979 Feb; 130 (2): 123-7.

(221)   Labuza TP, Busk GC. An analysis of the water binding in gels. J Food Sci 1979; 44 (5): 1379-85.

(222)   Lang JA, Bray DL, Reyes PS, Henika RG, Lambert MR, Briggs GM. An experimental technique to optimize levels of a growth factor from alfalfa and dietary fiber in a guinea pig diet (abstract). Fed Proc 1979; 38 (3 Pt I): 549.

(223)   Latto C. Postoperative deep vein thrombosis in Nigerians on high-fibre diets (letter). Br Med J 1979 Jan 20; 1 (6157): 199.

(224)   Ledward DA. Protein-polysaccharide interactions. In: Blanshard JM, Mitchell JR, eds. Polysaccharides in food. London: Butterworth and Co Ltd, 1979: 205-17.

(225)   Lee WY, Bennink MR, Chenoweth WL. Steroid metabolism, transit time, and cecal bacteria in rats fed corn or wheat bran. Cereal Chem 1979; 56 (4): 279-83.

(226)   Leeds AR. Gastric emptying, fibre, and absorption (letter). Lancet 1979 Apr 21; 1 (8121): 872-3.

(227)   Leeds AR, Bolster NR, Andrews R, Truswell AR. Meal viscosity, gastric emptying and glucose absorption in the rat (abstract). Proc Nutr Soc 1979 Sep; 38 (2): 44A.

(228)   Leeds AR. The dietary management of diabetes in adults. Proc Nutr Soc 1979 Dec; 38 (3): 365-71.

(229)   Leff EI. Meckel's diverticulitis secondary to orange pulp bezoar. South Med J 1979 Jul; 72 (7): 888-9.

(230)   Leitzmann C, Meier-Ploeger A, Huth K. The influence of lignin on the lipid metabolism of the rat. In: Inglett GE, Falkehag SI, eds. Dietary fibers: chemistry and nutrition. New York: Academic Press, 1979: 273-81.

(231)   Leung HK, Steinberg MP. Water binding of food constituents as determined by NMR, freezing, sorption and dehydration. J Food Sci 1979; 44 (4): 1212-6, 1220.

(232)   Levin B, Horwitz D. Dietary fiber. Med Clin North Am 1979 Sep; 63 (5): 1043-55.

(233)   Levine AS, Silvis SE. Steatorrhea due to high dietary fiber (abstract). Gastroenterology 1979 May; 76 (5 Pt 2): 1183.

(234)   Levine AS. The relationship of diet to intestinal gas. J Med Soc NJ 1979 Dec; 76 (13): 921-2.

(235)   Levine GD, Schwartz SE. Effects of dietary fiber on rat intestinal glucose absorption (abstract). Gastroenterology 1979 May; 76 (5 Pt 2): 1184.

(236)   Lewis B. Cholesterol and colon cancer (letter). Lancet 1979 May 26; 1 (8126): 1136-7.

(237)   Lewis EA, Kale OO. Laxative usage in a Yoruba rural community. Niger Med J 1979 Apr; 9 (4): 449-52.

(238)   Littlewood ER, Ornstein MH. Intestinal transit time estimation by a single abdominal x-ray (abstract). Gut 1979 Oct; 20 (10): A927.

(239)   Liu K, Stamler J, Moss D, Garside D, Persky V, Soltero I. Dietary cholesterol, fat, and fibre, and colon-cancer mortality. An analysis of international data. Lancet 1979 Oct 13; 2 (8146): 782-5.

(240)   Liu YK, Luh BS. Effect of harvest maturity on free amino acids, pectins, ascorbic acid, total nitrogen and minerals in tomato pastes. J Food Sci 1979; 44 (2): 425-8.

(241)   Lo GS, Settle SL, Steinke FH, Hopkins DT. Effect on transit time and fecal output of soy polysaccharides in pigs (abstract). Fed Proc 1979; 38 (3 Pt I): 548.

(242)   Long A. Prescription for a better British diet (letter). Br Med J 1979 Apr 21; 1 (6170): 1090.

(243)   Love MH, Beach PJ, Bloomer CK, Hemphill J. Changes in cake volume produced by high fiber ingredient substitutions (abstract). Cereal Foods World 1979 Sep; 24 (9): 464.

(244)   Low AG. A new automatic method for measuring dry matter and nitrogen flow through re-entrant cannulas in the duodenum of growing pigs (abstract). Proc Nutr Soc 1979 Dec; 38 (3): 129A.

(245)   Lowenfels AB. Bran and experimental colon cancer (letter). Lancet 1979 Jan 13; 1 (8107): 108.

(246) Malinow MR, McLaughlin P, Stafford C, Livingston AL, Kohler GO, Cheeke PR. Comparative effects of alfalfa saponins and alfalfa fiber on cholesterol absorption in rats. Am J Clin Nutr 1979 Sep; 32 (9): 1810-2.

(247) Mann JI, Eaton J. High- and low-carbohydrate diets (letter). Br Med J 1979 Oct 13; 2 (6195): 935.

(248) Mann JI. High-carbohydrate diets and insulin-dependent diabetics (letter). Br Med J 1979 Nov 3; 2 (6198): 1142.

(249) Mann JI. A prudent diet for the nation. J Hum Nutr 1979 Feb; 33 (1): 57-63.

(250) Mannerberg D. Rehabilitation of cardiovascular diseases in a USA centre. Chest Heart Stroke J 1979, 3 (5): 62-5.

(251) Mantel N. Guar crispbread in the diabetic diet (letter). Br Med J 1979 Dec 15; 2 (6204): 1589.

(252) Marya SK, Lal A, Kumar S. Intestinal obstruction due to wheat grains: a case report. Indian J Med Sci 1979 Sep; 33 (9): 238.

(253) Marzio L, Lanfranchi GA, Trento L, Labo G. Anal manometry in constipated patients (letter). Gastroenterology 1979 May; 76 (5 Pt 1): 1080.

(254) Maurice DV, Jensen LS. Hepatic lipid metabolism in domestic fowl as influenced by dietary cereal. J Nutr 1979 May; 109 (5): 872-82.

(255) Meyer PD, DenBesten L, Mason EE. The effects of a high fiber diet on bile acid pool size, bile acid kinetics, and biliary lipid secretory rates in the morbidly obese. Surgery 1979 Mar; 85 (3): 311-6.

(256) Mickelsen O, Makdani DD, Cotton RH, Titcomb ST, Colmey JC, Gatty R. Effects of a high fiber bread diet on weight loss in college-age males. Am J Clin Nutr 1979 Aug; 32 (8): 1703-9.

(257) Miller BS. Note on the evaluation of hard white winter wheat bran. Cereal Chem 1979; 56 (2): 118-9.

(258) Miller LT, Yu M. Effect of wheat bran on fecal caloric and nutrient excretion in men (abstract). Am J Clin Nutr 1979 Jun; 32 (6): xviii.

(259) Miller LT, Lindberg AS, Whanger P, Leklem JE. Effect of wheat bran on the bioavailability of vitamin B_6 and the excretion of selenium in man (abstract). Fed Proc 1979; 38 (3 Pt I): 767.

(260) Miller TL, Wolin MJ. Fermentations by saccharolytic intestinal bacteria. Am J Clin Nutr 1979 Jan; 32 (1): 164-72.

(261) Mitchell JR. Rheology of polysaccharide solutions and gels. In: Blanshard JM, Mitchell JR, eds. Polysaccharides in food. London: Butterworth and Co Ltd, 1979: 51-72.

(262) Mod RR, Conkerton EJ, Ory RL, Normand FL. Composition of water-soluble hemicelluloses in rice bran from four growing areas. Cereal Chem 1979; 56 (4): 356-8.

(263) Modan B. Patterns of gastrointestinal neoplasms in Israel. Isr J Med Sci 1979 Apr; 15 (4): 301-4.

(264) Mongeau R, Brassard R. Determination of neutral detergent fiber, hemicellulose, cellulose, and lignin in breads. Cereal Chem 1979; 56 (5): 437-41.

(265) Moore SW, Robbs JV. Acute appendicitis in the Zulu — an emerging disease (letter). S Afr Med J 1979 Apr 28; 55 (18): 700.

(266) Morgan LM, Goulder TJ, Tsiolakis D, Marks V, Alberti KG. The effect of unabsorbable carbohydrate on gut hormones. Modification of post-prandial GIP secretion by guar. Diabetologia 1979 Aug; 17 (2): 85-9.

(267) Morris ER, Ellis R. Phytate and phosphorus balance in human subjects: dephytinized vs nondephytinized whole wheat bran (abstract). Cereal Foods World 1979 Sep; 24 (9): 461.

(268) Morris ER. Polysaccharide structure and conformation in solutions and gels. In: Blanshard JM, Mitchell JR, eds. Polysaccharides in food. London: Butterworth and Co Ltd, 1979: 15-31.

(269) Moskovitz M, White C, Barnett RN, Stevens S, Russell E, Vargo D, Floch MH. Diet, fecal bile acids, and neutral sterols in carcinoma of the colon. Dig Dis Sci 1979 Oct; 24 (10): 746-51.

(270) Mossberg LR. Fiber determinations in foods and feed — an instrumental approach. Cereal Foods World 1979 March; 24 (3): 90-2.

(271) Mss Information Corporation. Dietary Fiber. Edison, New Jersey: Mss Information Corporation, 1979. (Landmark Series.)

(272) Muirden JC, Naraqi S. Pelvic phleboliths: a study of 528 Melanesian and white patients in Papua New Guinea. Med J Aust 1979 Mar 24; 1 (6): 245-6.

(273) Mullard KS. Abdominal and thoracic pressures during defecation (letter). Br Med J 1979 Feb 3; 1 (6159): 344.

(274) Munoz JM, Sandstead HH, Jacob RA, Logan GM Jr, Reck SJ, Klevay LM, Dintzis FR, Inglett GE, Shuey WC. Effects of some cereal brans and textured vegetable protein on plasma lipids. Am J Clin Nutr 1979 Mar; 32 (3): 580-92.

(275) Munoz JM, Sandstead HH, Jacob RA. Effects of dietary fiber on glucose tolerance of normal men. Diabetes 1979 May; 28 (5): 496-502.

(276) Murat J-C, Paris H, Castilla C. Digestion of carbohydrates in fish: fermentation and volatile fatty acids (abstract). Ann Nutr Aliment 1979; 33 (2): 299-300.

(277) McCarroll AM, Connell AM. Effect of fiber on glucagon and gastrointestinal hormone responses in diabetics (abstract). Diabetes 1979; 28 (Program): 400.

(278) MacDonald I. Polysaccharides and health. In: Blanshard JM, Mitchell JR, eds. Polysaccharides in food. London: Butterworth and Co Ltd, 1979: 331-6.

(279) McHale M, Kies C, Fox HM. Calcium and magnesium nutritional status of adolescent humans fed cellulose or hemicellulose supplements. J Food Sci 1979; 44 (5): 1412-7.

(280) McLaren GA, Bankes PW, Patel TI, Smith TR, Fahey GC Jr, Williams JE, Nomani NZ. Extracted bran as a source of biologically active acid-resistant hemicellulose. Nutr Rep Int 1979 Oct; 20 (4): 469-74.

(281) MacLeod MA, Blacklock NJ. The influence of glucose and crude fibre (wheat bran) on the rate of intestinal ^{47}Ca absorption. The influence of glucose and wheat bran on calcium absorption. J R Nav Med Serv 1979 Win; 65 (3): 143-6.

(282) McLoughlin JC, Love AH, Adgey AA, Gough AD, Varma MP. Intact removal of phytobezoar using fibreoptic endoscope in patient with gastric atony. Br Med J 1979 Jun 2; 1 (6176): 1466.

(283) McMichael AJ, Potter JD, Hetzel BS. Time trends in colo-rectal cancer mortality in relation to food and alcohol consumption: United States, United Kingdom, Australia and New Zealand. Int J Epidemiol 1979 Dec; 8 (4): 295-303.

(284) McQueen RE, Nicholson JW. Modification of the neutral-detergent fiber procedure for cereals and vegetables by using α-amylase. J Assoc Off Anal Chem 1979; 62 (3): 676-80.

(285) Nagyvary JJ, Falk JD, Hill ML, Schmidt ML, Wilkins AK, Bradbury EL. The hypolipidemic activity of chitosan and other polysaccharides in rats. Nutr Rep Int 1979 Nov; 20 (5): 677-88.

(286) Naivikul O, D'Appolonia BL. Carbohydrates of legume flours compared with wheat flour. 3. Nonstarchy polysaccharides. Cereal Chem 1979; 56 (2): 45-9.

(287) Newcombe RG. Bran and experimental colon cancer (letter). Lancet 1979 Jan 13; 1 (8107): 108.

(288) Nigro ND, Bull AW, Klopfer BA, Pak PS, Campbell RL. Effect of dietary fiber on azoxymethane-induced intestinal carcinogenesis in rats. JNCI 1979 Apr; 62 (4): 1097-102.

(289) Nomani MZ, Albrink MJ, Davis GK, Lai H-Y. Changes in the serum cholesterol level of the rat with variable digestible dry matter, as affected by dietary fiber (abstract). Fed Proc 1979; 38 (3 Pt I): 550.

(290) Nomani MZ, Fashandi EF, Davis GK, Bradac CJ. Influence of dietary fiber on the growth and protein metabolism of the rat. J Food Sci 1979; 44 (3): 745-7, 751.

(291) Nomani MZ, Bradac CJ, Lai HL, Watne AL. Effect of dietary fiber fractions on the fecal output and steroids in the rat. Nutr Rep Int 1979 Aug; 20 (2): 269-78.

(292) Nomani MZ, Albrink MJ, Davis GK, Lai HY, Watne AL. Changes in serum cholesterol with the variable digestibility of fiber diets at low energy intake. Nutr Rep Int 1979 Sep; 20 (3): 363-9.

(293) Normand FL, Ory RL, Mod RR. In vitro binding of bile acids by rice hemicelluloses. In: Inglett GE, Falkehag SI, eds. Dietary fibers: chemistry and nutrition. New York: Academic Press, 1979: 203-13.

(294) Northcote DH. Polysaccharides of the plant cell during its growth. In: Blanshard JM, Mitchell JR, eds. Polysaccharides in food. London: Butterworth and Co Ltd, 1979: 3-13.

(295) Norton RA, Philipps E, Feffer J, Matloff D, Braver J, Prentiss D. How to measure intragastric bezoar volumes (abstract). Gastroenterology 1979 May; 76 (5 Pt 2): 1210.

(296) Oakenfull DG, Fenwick DE, Hood RL, Topping DL, Illman RL, Storer GB. Effects of saponins on bile acids and plasma lipids in the rat. Br J Nutr 1979 Sep; 42 (2): 209-16.

(297) O'Brien BC, Reiser R. Comparative effects of purified and human-type diets on cholesterol metabolism in the rat. J Nutr 1979 Jan; 109 (1): 98-104.

(298) Okojie XG. Aetiology of appendicitis (letter). Br Med J 1979 Oct 6; 2 (6194): 865.

(299) O'Mullane NM. High-carbohydrate diets and insulin-dependent diabetics (letter). Br Med J 1979 Sep 29; 2 (6193): 796.

(300) Onderdonk AB, Bartlett JG. Bacteriological studies of experimental ulcerative colitis. Am J Clin Nutr 1979 Jan; 32 (1): 258-65.

(301) Oohashi Y, Kitamura S, Wakabayashi K, Kuwabara N, Fukuda Y. Irreversibility of degraded carrageenan-induced colorectal squamous metaplasia in rats. Gan 1979 Jun; 70 (3): 391-2.

(302) Ornstein MH, Littlewood ER, Cox AG, McLean Baird I, North W. Diverticular disease —is high fibre really necessary (abstract). Gut 1979 Oct; 20 (10): A942.

(303) Ostuzzi R, Micciolo R, Armellini F, Crivellenti G, Bosello O. Effects of bran feeding on body weight and glucose tolerance in man. In: Vague J, Vague P, eds. Proceedings of the fifth International Meeting of Endocrinology. Amsterdam: Excerpta Medica, 1979: 369-72. (International congress series 454.)

(304) Overeem A. Some aspects of food legislation with particular reference to stabilizers, thickeners and gelling agents. In: Blanshard JM, Mitchell JR, eds. Polysaccharides in food. London: Butterworth and Co Ltd, 1979: 301-15.

(305) Painter NS. The treatment of uncomplicated diverticular disease of the colon with a high fibre diet. The reasons for using bran. Acta Chir Belg 1979 Nov-Dec; 78 (6): 359-68.

(306) Painter NS. Haemorrhoids and a high-fibre diet (letter). Br Med J 1979 Nov 17; 2 (6200): 1293.

(307) Palmer HJ, Bennink MR. Oat bran decreases cholesterol synthesis and biological half-life in chicks (abstract). Am J Clin Nutr 1979 Jun; 32 (6): xix.

(308) Papakyrikos H, Kies C, Fox HM. Zinc and magnesium utilization as affected by graded levels of hemicellulose, cellulose and wheat bran (abstract). Fed Proc 1979; 38 (3 Pt I): 549.

(309) Parry EH. Urban change and health in Africa. Ethiop Med J 1979 Oct; 17 (4): 127-42.

(310) Passmore R, Hollingsworth DF, Robertson J. Prescription for a better British diet. Br Med J 1979 Feb 24; 1 (6162): 527-31.

(311) Paul AA, Southgate DA. McCance and Widdowson's 'The composition of foods': dietary fibre in egg, meat and fish dishes. J Hum Nutr 1979 Oct; 33 (5): 335-6.

(312) Pedersen JK. The selection of hydrocolloids to meet functional requirements. In: Blanshard JM, Mitchell JR, eds. Polysaccharides in food. London: Butterworth and Co Ltd, 1979: 219-27.

(313) Pettitt DJ. Xanthan gum. In: Blanshard JM, Mitchell JR, eds. Polysaccharides in food. London: Butterworth and Co Ltd, 1979: 263-82.

(314) Pilnik W, Rombouts FM. Pectic enzymes. In: Blanshard JM, Mitchell JR, eds. Polysaccharides in food. Butterworth and Co Ltd, 1979: 109-26.

(315) Plant A, Kies C, Fox HM. The effect of copper and fiber supplementation on copper utilization in humans (abstract). Fed Proc 1979; 38 (3 Pt I): 549.

(316) Pollmann DS, Danielson DM, Peo ER Jr. Value of high fiber diets for gravid swine. J Anim Sci 1979; 48 (6): 1385-93.

(317) Prynne CJ, Southgate DA. The effects of a supplement of dietary fibre on faecal excretion by human subjects. Br J Nutr 1979 May; 41 (3): 495-503.

(318)   Putney JD, Trout DL, Johnson DA, Malik MA, Szepesi B. Effect of xanthan, pectin, carrageenan, acacia, agar and locust bean gum on hepatic lipogenesis in starved-refed rats (abstract). Fed Proc 1979; 38 (3 Pt I): 769.

(319)   Radcliffe JD, Webster AJ. The effect of varying the quality of dietary protein and energy on food intake and growth in the Zucker rat. Br J Nutr 1979 Jan; 41 (1): 111-24.

(320)   Ranhotra GS, Lee C, Gelroth JA. Bioavailability of iron in high-cellulose bread. Cereal Chem 1979; 56 (3): 156-8.

(321)   Ranhotra GS. Bioavailability of iron in high-fiber bread. Cereal Foods World 1979 Jun; 24 (6): 252-3.

(322)   Ranhotra GS, Lee C, Gelroth JA. Bioavailability of iron in some commerical variety breads. Nutr Rep Int 1979 Jun; 19 (6): 851-7.

(323)   Rao AV, Bright-See E. Effect of graded amounts of dietary pectin on growth parameters of rats. Nutr Rep Int 1979 Mar; 19 (3): 411-7.

(324)   Rasper VF. Chemical and physical characteristics of dietary cereal fiber. In: Inglett GE, Falkehag SI, eds. Dietary fibers: chemistry and nutrition. New York: Academic Press, 1979: 93-115.

(325)   Rasper VF. Chemical and physical properties of dietary cereal fiber. Food Technol 1979 Jan; 33 (1): 40-4.

(326)   Reaven GM, Coulston AM, Marcus RA. Nutritional management of diabetes. Med Clin North Am 1979 Sep; 63 (5): 927-43.

(327)   Reddy PR, Tsen CC. Effect of cereal fibers on nutritive quality (PER) and digestibility of proteins by rat feeding studies (abstract). Cereal Foods World 1979 Sep; 24 (9): 467.

(328)   Reilly C. Zinc, iron and copper binding by dietary fibre. Biochem Soc Trans 1979 Feb; 7 (1): 202-4.

(329)   Reinhold JG, Garcia JS. Fiber of the maize tortilla. Am J Clin Nutr 1979 Jun; 32 (6): 1326-9.

(330)   Reiser S. Effect of dietary fiber on parameters of glucose tolerance in humans. In: Inglett GE, Falkehag SI, eds. Dietary fibers: chemistry and nutrition. New York: Academic Press, 1979: 173-91.

(331)   Rennie J. Unprocessed bran causing intestinal obstruction (letter). Br Med J 1979 Jun 9; 1 (6176): 1491.

(332)   Resurreccion AP, Juliano BO, Tanaka Y. Nutrient content and distribution in milling fractions of rice grain. J Sci Food Agric 1979 May; 30 (5): 475-81.

(333)   Ritchie JA, Truelove SC. Treatment of irritable bowel syndrome with lorazepam, hyoscine butylbromide, and isphagula husk. Br Med J 1979 Feb 10; 1 (6160): 376-8.

(334)   Ritt RS, Jordan HA, Levitz LS. Changes in nutrient intake during a behavioural weight control program. J Am Diet Assoc 1979 Mar; 74 (3): 325-30.

(335)   Robbs JV, Moshal MG. Duodenal ulceration in Indians and Blacks in Durban. S Afr Med J 1979 Jan 13; 55 (2): 39-42.

(336)   Roberts RL. Composition and taste evaluation of rice milled to different degrees. J Food Sci 1979; 44 (1): 127-9.

(337)   Robertson J, Brydon WG, Tadesse K, Wenham P, Walls A, Eastwood MA. The effect of raw carrot on serum lipids and colon function. Am J Clin Nutr 1979 Sep; 32 (9): 1889-92.

(338)   Robertson JA, Eastwood MA, Yeoman MM. An investigation into the dietary fibre content of named varieties of carrot at different developmental ages. J Sci Food Agric 1979 Apr; 30 (4): 388-94.

(339)   Robertson JA, Eastwood MA, Yeoman MM. An investigation of lignin extraction from dietary fibre using acetyl bromide. J Sci Food Agric 1979 Nov; 30 (11): 1039-42.

(340)   Robertson WG, Peacock M, Hodgkinson A. Dietary changes and the incidence of urinary calculi in the UK between 1958 and 1976. J Chronic Dis 1979; 32 (6): 469-76.

(341)   Rolon PA. Gastrointestinal pathology in South America. Isr J Med Sci 1979 Apr; 15 (4): 318-21.

(342) Ross JK, Leklem JE. Effect of bran and pectin on human fecal steroid excretion and activity of B-glucuronidase and 7α-dehydroxylase (abstract). Fed Proc 1979; 38 (3 Pt I): 864.

(343) Rotenberg S, Jakobsen PE. Lipid metabolism in rats fed a diet with high citrus pectin content. Z Tierphysiol Dec; 42 (6): 299-311.

(344) Rubio MA, Pethica BA, Zuman P, Falkehag SI. The interactions of carcinogens and co-carcinogens with lignin and other components of dietary fiber. In: Inglett GE, Falkehag SI, eds. Dietary fibers: chemistry and nutrition. New York: Academic Press, 1979: 251-71.

(345) Ryan GP, Dudrick J, Copeland EM, Johnson LR. Effects of various diets on colonic growth in rats. Gastroenterology 1979 Oct; 77 (4 Pt 1): 658-63.

(346) Saarivirta M, Kreula M. The contents of water-insoluble dietary fibre in Finnish berries and mushrooms. A preliminary study. Z Lebensm Unters Forsch 1979 Aug; 169 (2): 88-9.

(347) Sable-Amplis R, Sicart R, Abadie D. Metabolic changes associated with adding apples to the diet in golden hamsters. Nutr Rep Int 1979 May; 19 (5): 723-32.

(348) Sable-Amplis R, Sicart R, Abadie D. Effects of an apple-supplemented diet on lipid metabolism in golden hamsters (abstract). Ann Nutr Aliment 1979; 33 (4): 552-3.

(349) Saka S, Thomas RJ, Gratzl JS. Lignin distribution by energy dispersive X-ray analysis. In: Inglett GE, Falkehag SI, eds. New York: Academic Press, 1979: 15-29.

(350) Saldana G, Meyer RD, Stephens TS, Lime BJ, del var Petersen H. Nutrient composition of canned beets and tomatoes grown in a subtropical area. J Food Sci 1979; 44 (4): 1001-3, 1007.

(351) Salmon MB. A professional dietitian's natural fiber diet. Englewood Cliffs, New Jersey: Prentice-Hall Inc, 1979.

(352) Salyers AA. Energy sources of major intestinal fermentative anaerobes. Am J Clin Nutr 1979 Jan; 32 (1): 158-63.

(353) Salyers A, Palmer JK, Balascio J. Digestion of plant cell wall polysaccharides by bacteria from the human colon. In: Inglett GE, Falkehag SI, eds. Dietary fibers: chemistry and nutrition. New York: Academic Press, 1979: 193-201.

(354) Sambrook IE. Studies on digestion and absorption in the intestines of growing pigs. 8. Measurements of the flow of total lipid, acid-detergent fibre and volatile fatty acids. Br J Nutr 1979 Sep; 42 (2): 279-87.

(355) Sanders TA. Vegetarian diets. Nutr Bull 1979 Sep; 5 (3): 137-44.

(356) Sanderson JE, Paulis JW, Porcuna FN, Wall JS. Sweet corn: varietal and developmental differences in amino acid content and composition of grain. J Food Sci 1979; 44 (3): 836-8.

(357) Sandford PA. A survey of possible new polysaccharides. In: Blanshard JM, Mitchell JR, eds. Polysaccharides in food. London: Butterworth and Co Ltd, 1979: 251-62.

(358) Sandstead H, Klevay L, Jacob R, Munoz J, Johnson L, Dintzis F, Inglett G. Mineral requirements: influence of fiber and protein (abstract). Am J Clin Nutr 1979 Apr; 32 (4): 933.

(359) Sandstead HH, Klevay LM, Jacob RA, Munoz JM, Logan GM Jr, Reck SJ, Dintzis FR, Inglett GE, Shuey WC. Effects of dietary fiber and protein level on mineral element metabolism. In: Inglett GE, Falkehag SI, eds. Dietary fibers: chemistry and nutrition. New York: Academic Press, 1979: 147-56.

(360) Sauer WC, Eggum BO, Jacobsen I. The influence of level and source of fiber on protein utilisation in rats. Arch Tierernaehr 1979 Sep; 29 (9): 533-40.

(361) Saunders RM, Hautala E. Relationships among crude fiber, neutral detergent fiber, in vitro dietary fiber, and in vivo (rats) dietary fiber in wheat foods. Am J Clin Nutr 1979 Jun; 32 (6): 1188-91.

(362) Saunders RM, Hautala E. Dietary fiber evaluation of wheat products by in vitro and in vivo methods. In: Inglett GE, Falkehag SI, eds. Dietary fibers: chemistry and nutrition. New York: Academic Press, 1979: 79-92.

(363) Schaefer O. Aetiology of appendicitis (letter). Br Med J 1979 May 5; 1 (6172): 1215.

(364) Schaeffer MC, Bennink MR. Nutrient and energy utilization as influenced by dietary fiber (abstract). Fed Proc 1979; 38 (3 Pt I): 767.

(365) Schneeman BO, Gallaher D. Effect of dietary cellulose on bile acid levels in the rat small intestine (abstract). Fed Proc 1979; 38 (3 Pt I): 548.

(366) Schneeman BO. Acute pancreatic and biliary response to protein, cellulose, and pectin. Nutr Rep Int 1979 Jul; 20 (1): 45-8.

(367) Schoeters GE, Van Puymbroeck S, Colard J, Vanderborght OL. Sparing of bone marrow stem cells by long-term administration of Na-alginate to [226]Ra contaminated mice. Int J Radiol 1979 Oct; 36 (4): 379-86.

(368) Schweizer TF, Wursch P. Analysis of dietary fibre. J Sci Food Agric 1979 Jun; 30 (6): 613-9.

(369) Schwerdtfeger E. Problems concerning the assay of dietary fibre. Qual Plant Plant Foods Hum Nutr 1979; 29 (1-2): 19-29.

(370) Scoular RS, Lee SP. Gastric phytobezoar (letter). Aust NZ J Med 1979 Apr; 9 (2): 207.

(371) Selvendran RR, March JF, Ring SG. Determination of aldoses and uronic acid content of vegetable fiber. Anal Biochem 1979 Jul 15; 96 (2): 282-92.

(372) Selvendran RR, Ring SG, Dupont MS. Assessment of procedures used for analysing dietary fibre and some recent developments. Chemistry and Industry 1979; 7: 225-30.

(373) Selvendran RR. The binding of bile salts by vegetable fibre. Qual Plant Plant Foods Hum Nutr 1979; 29 (1-2): 109-33.

(374) Sen'kevich SI, Belavtseva EM, Plashchina IG, Braudo EE, Kamenskaya EV, Tolstoguzov VB. Electron-microscope study of pectin solution. Biophysics 1979 Nov-Dec; 24 (4): 655-9.

(375) Shah BG, Giroux A, Belonje B. Bioavailability of zinc in infant cereals. Nutr Metab 1979; 23 (4): 286-93.

(376) Shogren MD, Pomeranz Y, Finney KF. Counteracting the effects of fiber in breadmaking (abstract). Cereal Foods World 1979 Sep; 24 (9): 448.

(377) Shurpalekar KS, Sundaravalli OE, Rao MN. In vitro and in vivo digestibility of legume carbohydrates. Nutr Rep Int 1979 Jan; 19 (1): 111-7.

(378) Silman AJ. Cereal fibre, total energy intake, and obesity (letter). Lancet 1979 Oct 27; 2 (8148): 905.

(379) Simpson RW, Mann JI, Eaton J, Moore RA, Carter R, Hockaday TD. Improved glucose control in maturity-onset diabetes treated with high-carbohydrate-modified fat diet. Br Med J 1979 Jun 30; 1 (6180): 1753-6.

(380) Simpson RW, Mann JI, Eaton J, Carter RD, Hockaday TD. High-carbohydrate diets and insulin-dependent diabetics. Br Med J 1979 Sep 1; 2 (6189): 523-5.

(381) Sinclair H. Prescription for a better British diet (letter). Br Med J 1979 Apr 7; 1 (6168): 952-3.

(382) Sirtori CR, Gatti E, Mantero O, Conti F, Agradi E, Tremoli E, Sirtori M, Fraterrigo L, Tavazzi L, Kritchevsky D. Clinical experience with the soybean protein diet in the treatment of hypercholesterolemia. Am J Clin Nutr 1979 Aug; 32 (8): 1645-58.

(383) Smith CJ, Bryant MP. Introduction to metabolic activities of intestinal bacteria. Am J Clin Nutr 1979 Jan; 32 (1): 149-57.

(384) Smith DA, Gee MI. A dietary survey to determine the relationship between diet and cholelithiasis. Am J Clin Nutr 1979 Jul; 32 (7): 1519-26.

(385) Solomons N, Viteri F, Pineda O, Jacob R. The effect of the Guatemalan diet on zinc bioavailability (abstract). Am J Clin Nutr 1979 Apr; 32 (4): 932.

(386) Solomons NW, Jacob RA, Pineda O, Viteri FE. Studies on the bioavailability of zinc in man. Effects of the Guatemalan rural diet and of the iron-fortifying agent, NaFe-EDTA. J Nutr 1979 Sep; 109 (9): 1519-28.

(387) Soni GL, Sohal BS, Singh R. Comparative effect of pulses on tissue and plasma cholesterol levels of albino rats. Indian J Biochem Biophys 1979 Dec; 16 (6): 444-6.

(388) Southgate DA, Bingham SA. The contribution of different groups of foodstuffs to the intake of dietary fibre. Qual Plant Plant Foods Hum Nutr 1979; 29 (1-2): 49-58.

(389) Spiller GA, Kay RM. Recommendations and conclusions of the dietary fiber workshop of the XI International Congress of Nutrition, Rio De Janeiro, 1978. Am J Clin Nutr 1979 Oct; 32 (10): 2102-3.

(390) Spiller GA, Briggs G. Reply to letter by Heaton (letter). Am J Clin Nutr 1979 Dec; 32 (12): 2374-5.

(391) Spiller GA, Gates JE. Effect of graded levels of four dietary fibers on fecal minerals in pig-tailed monkeys (abstract). Fed Proc 1979; 38 (3 Pt I): 548.

(392) Spiller GA, Shipley EA, Chernoff MC, Cooper WC. Bulk laxative efficacy of a psyllium seed hydrocolloid and of a mixture of cellulose and pectin. J Clin Pharmacol 1979 May-Jun; 19 (5-6): 313-20.

(393) Stasse-Wolthuis M, Hautvast JG, Hermus RJ, Katan MB, Bausch JE, Rietberg-Brussaard JH, Velema JP, Zondervan JH, Eastwood MA, Brydon WG. The effect of a natural high-fiber diet on serum lipids, fecal lipids, and colonic function. Am J Clin Nutr 1979 Sep; 32 (9): 1881-8.

(394) Stasse-Wolthuis M, Katan MB, Hermus RJ, Hautvast JG. Increase of serum cholesterol in man fed a bran diet. Atherosclerosis 1979 Sep; 34 (1): 87-91.

(395) Stasse-Wolthuis M. Effect of a natural high fibre diet on blood lipids and intestinal transit time in man. Qual Plant Plant Foods Hum Nutr 1979; 29 (1-2): 31-8.

(396) Stephen AM, Cummings JH. Effect of dietary fibre on faecal bacterial mass (abstract). Gut 1979 May; 20 (5): A457-8.

(397) Stephen AM, Cummings JH. Water-holding by dietary fibre in vitro and its relationship to faecal output in man. Gut 1979 Aug; 20 (8): 722-9.

(398) Stephen AM, Cummings JH. Water holding by dietary fibre in vitro and its relationship to faecal bulking in man (abstract). Proc Nutr Soc 1979 Sep; 38 (2): 55A.

(399) Stephen AM, Cummings JH. The influence of dietary fibre on faecal nitrogen excretion in man (abstract). Proc Nutr Soc 1979 Dec; 38 (3): 141A.

(400) Stokes J III. Dietary fiber and food flavoring (letter). Am J Clin Nutr 1979 Jan; 32 (1): 3.

(401) Story JA, Kritchevsky D, Eastwood MA. Dietary fiber — bile acid interactions. In: Inglett GE, Falkehag SI, eds. Dietary fibers: chemistry and nutrition. New York: Academic Press, 1979: 49-55.

(402) Susheelamma NS, Rao MV. Functional role of the arabinogalactan of black gram (Phaseolus mungo) in the texture of leavened foods (steamed puddings). J Food Sci 1979; 44 (5): 1309-12, 1316.

(403) Takeda H, Kiriyama S. Correlation between the physical properties of dietary fibers and their protective activity against amaranth toxicity in rats. J Nutr 1979 Jan; 109 (3): 388-96.

(404) Tashiro M, Maki Z. Purification and characterization of a trypsin inhibitor from rice bran. J Nutr Sci Vitaminol (Tokyo) 1979; 25 (3): 255-64.

(405) Taylor RH, Jenkins DJ, Nineham R, Sarson D, Bloom SR, Alberti KG. Synergism of dietary fibre and a glucosidehydrolase inhibitor in modification of carbohydrate absorption (abstract). Gastroenterology 1979 May; 76 (5 Pt 2): 1260.

(406) Taylor RH, Goff DV, Wolever TM, Fielden H. Dietary fibre and diabetes (letter). Lancet 1979 Apr 7; 1 (8119): 782-3.

(407) Taylor RH. Gastric emptying, fibre, and absorption (letter). Lancet 1979 Apr 21; 1 (8121): 872.

(408) Texter EC Jr, Mitchell C, Jordan HJ Jr, Hogue CJ. Large bowel cancer. J Arkansas Med Soc 1979 Apr; 75 (11): 415-8.

(409) Texter EC Jr. Epidemiology of carcinoma of the colon — with remarks on the cause, prevention and early detection. J Arkansas Med Soc 1979 Jul; 76 (2): 93-4.

(410) Tharanathan RN, Wankhede DB, Rao MR. Groundnut carbohydrates — a review. J Sci Food Agric 1979 Nov; 30 (11): 1077-84.

(411) Theander O, Aman P. The chemistry, morphology and analysis of dietary fiber components. In: Inglett GE, Falkehag SI, eds. Dietary fibers: chemistry and nutrition. New York: Academic Press, 1979: 215-44.

(412) Theander O, James P. European efforts in dietary fiber characterization. In: Inglett GE, Falkehag SI, eds. Dietary fibers: chemistry and nutrition. New York: Academic Press, 1979: 245-9.

(413) Theander O, Aman P. Studies on dietary fibres. 1. Analysis and chemical characterization of water-soluble and water-insoluble dietary fibres. Swed J Agric Res 1979; 9 (3): 97-106.

(414) Thompson SA, Weber CW, Hydrogen ion buffering capacities of fiber sources (abstract). Fed Proc 1979; 38 (3 Pt I): 768.

(415) Thompson SA, Weber CW. Influence of pH on the binding of copper, zinc and iron in six fiber sources. J Food Sci 1979; 44 (3): 752-4.

(416) Thorne MC. Bran and experimental colon cancer (letter). Lancet 1979 Jan 13; 1 (8107): 108.

(417) Thornton JR, Emmett PM, Heaton KW. Diet and Crohn's disease: characteristics of the pre-illness diet. Br Med J 1979 Sep 29; 2 (6193): 762-4.

(418) Thornton JR, Emmett PM, Heaton KW. Diet and Crohn's disease: characteristics of the pre-illness diet (abstract). Gut 1979 Oct; 20 (10): A941.

(419) Thorpe JA. Abdominal and thoracic pressures during defecation (letter). Br Med J 1979 Feb 3; 1 (6159): 344.

(420) Tjokroprawiro A, Beaven DW. The B-diet, the dietetic regimen for Indonesian patients with diabetes mellitus (abstract). Diabetes 1979; 28 (Program): 441.

(421) Toma RB, Orr PH, D'Appolonia B, Dintzis FR, Tabekhia MM. Physical and chemical properties of potato peel as a source of dietary fiber in bread. J Food Sci 1979; 44 (5): 1403-7, 1417.

(422) Tovey F. Progress report. Peptic ulcer in India and Bangladesh. Gut 1979 Apr; 20 (4): 329-47.

(423) Tredger J, Wright J, Marks V. The effect of guar gum on blood alcohol levels following gin and tonic consumption (abstract). Proc Nutr Soc 1979 Sep; 38 (2): 70A.

(424) Trimbo S, Kathman J, Kies C, Fox HM. Pantothenic acid nutritional status of adolescent humans as affected by dietary fiber and bran (abstract). Fed Proc 1979; 38 (3 Pt I): 556.

(425) Trowell H. Prescription for a better British diet (letter). Br Med J 1979 Mar 24; 1 (6166): 819.

(426) Trowell HC, Burkitt DP. Diverticular disease in urban Kenyans (letter). Br Med J 1979 Jun 30; 1 (6180): 1795.

(427) Trowell HC. Dietary fibre in human nutrition: a bibliography. London: John Libbey and Co Ltd, 1979.

(428) Trowell H. Western diseases and dietary changes with special reference to fibre. Trop Doct 1979 Jul; 9 (3): 133-42.

(429) Tsai RC, Lei KY. Dietary cellulose, zinc and copper: effects on tissue levels of trace minerals in the rat. J Nutr 1979 Jun; 109 (6): 1117-22.

(430) Tsuda M. Purification and characterization of a lectin from rice bran. J Biochem 1979 Nov; 86 (5): 1451-61.

(431) Tsujita J, Takeda H, Ebihara K, Kiriyama S. Comparison of protective activity of dietary fiber against the toxicities of various food colors in rats. Nutr Rep Int 1979 Nov; 20 (5): 635-42.

(432) van Beresteyn EC, van Schaik M, Mogot MF. Effect of bran and cellulose on lipid metabolism in obese female Zucker rats. J Nutr 1979 Dec; 109 (12): 2085-97.

(433) van Berge-Henegouwen GP, Huybregts AW, van de Werf S, Demacker P, Schade RW. Effect of a standardized wheat bran preparation on serum lipids in young healthy males. Am J Clin Nutr 1979 Apr; 32 (4): 794-8.

(434) van Berge Henegouwen GP, Huijbregts AW, Hectors M, van Schaik A, van de Werf S. Bran feeding and vegetarian diet do not alter biliary lipids and bile acid kinetics in young males (abstract). Gut 1979 Oct; 20 (10): A930.

(435) Van Ness MM, Wheby MS. High-fiber diet: its role in the treatment of diabetes mellitus reviewed. Va Med 1979 Nov; 106 (11): 852-5.

(436) Van Soest PJ. What is fiber? Med Times 1979 Jul; 107 (7): 69-71.

(437) Vinik AI, Smith C, Jackson WP. Effect of dietary fiber on serum glucose and insulin responses in diabetics with and without autonomic neuropathy and in healthy controls (abstract). Diabetes 1979; 28 (Program): 385.

(438) Vohra P, Shariff G, Kratzer FH. Growth inhibitory effect of some gums and pectin for Tribolium castaneum larvae, chickens and Japanese quail. Nutr Rep Int 1979 Apr; 19 (4): 463-9.

(439) Wahlqvist ML, Morris MJ, Littlejohn GO, Bond A, Jackson RV. The effects of dietary fibre on glucose tolerance in healthy males. Aust NZ J Med 1979 Apr; 9 (2): 154-8.

(440) Walker AR, Duvenhage A, Segal I. Comparison between communities (letter). Br Med J 1979 Jan 20; 1 (6157): 196-7.

(441) Walker AR, Segal I. Epidemiology of noninfective intestinal diseases in various ethnic groups in South Africa. Isr J Med Sci 1979 Apr; 15 (4): 309-13.

(442) Walker AR, Walker BF, Segal I. Faecal pH value and its modification by dietary means in South African black and white schoolchildren. S Afr Med J 1979 Mar 24; 55 (13): 495-8.

(443) Walker AR. Is appendicitis increasing in South African blacks? S Afr Med J 1979 Sep 22; 56 (13): 503-4.

(444) Waszczynskyj N, Rao CS, da Silva RS. Extraction of proteins from wheat bran: application of enzymes (abstract). Cereal Foods World 1979 Sep; 24 (9): 469.

(445) Watanabe A, Kimura S, Ohta Y, Randall JM, Kimura S. Nature of the deposit on reverse osmosis membranes during concentration of pectin/cellulose solutions. J Food Sci 1979; 44 (5): 1505-9.

(446) Watanabe K, Reddy BS, Weisburger JH, Kritchevsky D. Effect of dietary alfalfa, pectin, and wheat bran on azoxymethane- or methylnitrosourea-induced colon carcinogenesis in F344 rats. JNCI 1979 Jul; 63 (1): 141-5.

(447) Watt J, McLean C, Marcus R, Degradation of carrageenan for the experimental production of ulcers in the colon. J Pharm Pharmacol 1979 Sep; 31 (9): 645-6.

(448) Watts JC. Fibre optical illusion. World Med 1979 May 19; 14 (16): 14.

(449) Weingartner KE, Erdman JW Jr, Parker HM, Forbes RM. Effect of soybean hull upon the bioavailability of zinc and calcium from soy flour-based diets. Nutr Rep Int 1979 Feb; 19 (2): 223-31.

(450) Weiss FG, Scott ML. Effects of dietary fiber, fat and total energy upon plasma cholesterol and other parameters in chickens. J Nutr 1979 Apr; 109 (4): 693-701.

(451) Whitehead RG. A national policy for nutrition? Dietary goals: their scientific justification. R Soc Health J 1979 Oct: 99 (5): 181-4.

(452) Williams DR, James WP. Fibre and diabetes (letter). Lancet 1979 Feb 3; 1 (8110): 271-2.

(453) Williams DR, James WP. Guar and diabetes (letter). Lancet 1979 Mar 17; 1 (8116): 612.

(454) Williams JE, McLaren GA, Fahey GC Jr. Influence of acid-resistant hemicellulose degradation products on rat and microbial growth. Nutr Rep Int 1979 Apr; 19 (4): 491-8.

(455) Wolever TM, Jenkins DJ, Nineham R, Alberti KG. Guar gum and reduction of postprandial glycaemia: effect of incorporation into solid food, liquid food and both. Br J Nutr 1979 May; 43 (1): 505-10.

(456) Wolever TM, Taylor R, Goff DV, Ahern J. Fibre and diabetes (letter). Lancet 1979 Feb 24; 1 (8113): 435.

(457) Wong MA, Oace SM. Dietary fiber effects on gut segment transit time in the rat (abstract). Fed Proc 1979; 38 (3 Pt I): 389.

(458) Woods MN, Ingelfinger JA. Lack of effect of bran on digoxin absorption. Clin Pharmacol Ther 1979 Jul; 26 (1): 21-3.

(459) Wright A, Burstyn PG, Gibney MJ. Dietary fibre and blood pressure. Br Med J 1979 Dec 15; 2 (6204): 1541-3.

(460) Wursch P. Influence of tannin-rich carob pod fiber on the cholesterol metabolism in the rat. J Nutr 1979 Apr; 109 (4): 685-92.

(461) Wyse BW. I. Variation in nutrient levels. Nutrient analysis of exchange lists for meal planning. J Am Diet Assoc 1979 Sep; 75 (3): 238-42.

(462) Wyse BW, Hansen RG. II. Nutrient density food profiles. Nutrient analysis of exchange lists for meal planning. J Am Diet Assoc 1979 Sep; 75 (3): 242-9.

(463) Young VR, Richardson DP. Nutrients, vitamins and minerals in cancer prevention. Facts and fallacies. Cancer 1979 May; 43 (5 Suppl): 2125-36.

(464) Zilversmit DB. Dietary fiber. In: Levy RI, Rifkind BM, Dennis BH, Ernst N, eds. Nutrition, lipids and coronary heart disease. A global view. New York: Raven Press, 1979: 148-74. (Nutrition in health and disease; vol 1.)

CZECH

(465) Skapik M. New data on the diet therapy of chronic digestive tract diseases (English abstract). Vnitr Lek 1979 Jan; 25 (1): 19-28.

DANISH

(466) Bonnevie-Nielsen V. Drug information. Slocose. Ugeskr Laeger 1979 Jan 1: 141 (1): 32-3.

(467) Jensen KS, Sparsoe BH, Bonnevie O. Effect of an elemental diet on chronic abdominal pains occurring after surgery on the abdomen. A controlled clinical trial (English abstract). Ugeskr Laeger 1979 Oct 22; 141 (43): 2963-4.

(468) Nielsen JA. Prolonged treatment of constipation with wheat-bran with particular reference to the possible development of calcium and iron deficiencies (English abstract). Ugeskr Laeger 1979 Mar 26; 141 (13): 849-52.

(469) Petersen HD. Postprandial blood glucose increase following ingestion of various carbohydrates in stable diabetic patients (English abstract). Ugeskr Laeger 1979 Apr 16; 141 (16): 1062-4.

DUTCH

(470) Stasse-Wolthuis M, Jeveren JG, van Hermus RJ, Katan MB. Effect of high-fibre diets on cholesterol metabolism and intestinal function in healthy volunteers (English abstract). Voeding 1979; 40 (3): 107-12.

(471) van Staveren WA. Can the dietary fibre of a category of Dutch adults be estimated (English abstract). Voeding 1979; 40 (3): 113-21.

FINNISH

(472) Burton D. Dietary fiber. Duodecim 1979; 95 (14-15): 880-91.

FRENCH

(473) Alberti KG, Goulder TJ. Dietary fiber and diabetes mellitus, a British experience. Journ Annu Diabetol Hotel Dieu 1979;: 289-98.

(474) Audigier JC. Dietary fiber and biliary lipids. Med Chir Dig 1979; 8 (3): 215-7.

(475) Bernier JJ. Dietary fiber, intestinal motility and absorption. Effects of postprandial hyperglycaemia. Journ Annu Diabetol Hotel Dieu 1979;: 269-74.

(476) Berta JL. Boicherot AC, Rautureau J, Cubeau J, Guilloud-Bataille M. Dietary factors in constipation (letter). Nouv Presse Med 1979 Sep 17; 8 (35): 2837-8.

(477) Blery M, Bismuth V, Loiseau B, Chagnon S. Acute oesophageal obstruction from food or mucilage: a report on 15 cases (English abstract). J Radiol 1979 Jun-Jul; 60 (6-7): 395-40.

(478) Boyer L. Dietary fibre: the present position (English abstract). Can Home Econ J 1979; 29 (2): 65-7.

(479) Capdevielle P. Bran and stools in the tropics (letter). Nouv Presse Med 1979 Dec 24; 8 (50): 4114.

(480) Chaput JC, Labayle D, Poynard T, Rousseau C. Utilization of vegetable dietary fibers in therapeutic gastroenterology. Journ Annu Diabetol Hotel Dieu 1979;: 275-87.

(481) Coste T, Karsenti P, Berta JL, Cubeau J, Guilloud-Bataille M. Dietetic factors in cholelithiasis: comparison of food consumption of patients with gallstones with that of control subjects (English abstract). Gastroenterol Clin Biol 1979 May; 3 (5): 417-23.

(482) Courtois JE. Galactomannans from leguminosae in foods. Ann Nutr Aliment 1979; 33 (2): 189-98.

(1.15)   Miscellaneous gastrointestinal
3*, 10, 26*, 27*, 33, 58*, 83, 96, 97*, 106, 118*, 119*, 159*, 160*, 169, 175,
189*, 192*, 193*, 206*, 223, 247*, 252*, 253, 254, 288*, 300, 308, 314*,
316*, 321, 322, 328, 329*, 334*, 357*, 361*, 368, 377*, 420, 422*, 433*, 449,
454*

(2) CARDIOVASCULAR
(2.1)   Lipid metabolism, cholesterol, triglycerides
3*, 6, 7, 8*, 10*, 11, 12*, 17, 32*, 37*, 43*, 48, 49*, 50*, 83*, 90*, 98, 116,
132, 135, 136, 140, 144*, 152*, 154, 159, 163, 169*, 172, 177*, 178*, 179*,
182*, 186*, 187, 196*, 209, 217, 218, 219, 222, 231, 232, 254, 258*, 267, 285*,
289, 297*, 306*, 310*, 319, 352*, 353, 359*, 360*, 367, 374, 375*, 376, 378,
380*, 381*, 382*, 400*, 401*, 403, 424, 428, 434, 438*, 439, 449, 457*, 464*,
465*

(2.2)   Atherosclerosis, ischaemic heart disease
196*, 472

(2.3)   Venous thrombosis, varicose veins, haemorrhoids
No paper relevant

(2.4)   Hypertension
42, 43*, 73, 177, 274, 276, 332, 352*, 392, 399

(3) METABOLIC
(3.1)   Diabetes mellitus, carbohydrate metabolism
6*, 8*, 9, 10*, 11*, 12*, 19, 24, 32*, 45, 46*, 54*, 56*, 58*, 62, 63, 71, 74,
113*, 117, 126*, 153*, 154*, 155*, 156, 157*, 158*, 159*, 160*, 161*, 162,
166, 170, 172, 175*, 177, 180*, 190, 201, 206*, 207, 220, 221, 222, 232, 239,
264, 265, 268*, 280, 297*, 319, 321*, 327, 363, 364, 365, 374, 379, 391*, 400*,
401*, 403, 407*, 409*, 412, 414, 420*, 423*, 424, 427, 430, 438*, 439, 446*,
449, 450, 453*, 464*, 470*

(3.2)   Obesity
6, 12, 32, 38*, 53*, 56, 83*, 86, 126*, 177, 375*, 376, 383*, 386, 393*, 438

(4) FIBRE AND FOOD
(4.1)   Fibre: definition, terminology, composition, analysis
13*, 14*, 20*, 22, 31*, 52, 60*, 72, 75*, 95, 104, 105, 108*, 109, 129, 133*,
139, 151*, 168*, 169*, 225*, 230*, 245*, 246, 259*, 311*, 312*, 323*, 324*,
346*, 356*, 366*, 397, 398, 425*, 432*, 437*, 441*, 443*, 444*, 448, 462*,
466*, 471, 474*, 475, 477*

(4.2)   Fibre in the diet and food, except cereals
14*, 29*, 31*, 47, 51, 57, 61*, 66, 67, 68, 75*, 79, 81, 95, 101*, 134, 135, 137,
143, 149*, 151*, 164, 165*, 167, 169*, 171*, 176*, 177, 198, 207, 212*, 213,
225*, 229, 230*, 234, 240*, 245*, 256, 260, 262, 269, 287, 288, 315, 324*, 333*,
343, 347, 356*, 390*, 415*, 419, 432*, 437*, 443, 445, 448, 455*, 461*, 474*,
475, 477*

(4.3)   Fibre in cereal and cereal foods
4*, 13*, 14*, 29*, 38, 88, 151*, 171*, 176, 203*, 211*, 214, 225*, 282, 324*,
333*, 372*, 385*, 390*, 431, 441*, 456*, 475

(4.4)   Modern dietary change
29*, 66, 88, 416, 431

(5) MISCELLANEOUS
(5.1)   Antitoxic action
145*, 181*, 188*, 317*, 342*, 387, 395*, 463*

THE REFERENCES

(1) Aamodt RL, Rumble WF, Johnston GS, Markley EJ, Volpe T, Henkin RI. Effects of fiber on zinc metabolism in humans (abstract). Fed Proc 1980 Mar; 39 (3 Pt I): 651.

(2) Abraham R, Barbolt TA, Rodgers JB. Inhibition by bran of the colonic cocarcinogenicity of bile salts in rats given dimethylhydrazine. Exp Mol Pathol 1980 Oct; 33 (2): 133-43.

(3) Akiba Y, Matsumoto T. Effects of several types of dietary fibers on lipid content in liver and plasma, nutrient retentions and plasma transaminase activities in force-fed growing chicks. J Nutr 1980 Jun; 110 (6): 1112-21.

(4) Allen KG, Klevay LM. Copper and zinc in selected breakfast cereals. Nutr Rep Int 1980 Sep; 22 (3): 389-94.

(5) Almy TP, Howell DA. Medical progress. Diverticular disease of the colon. N Engl J Med 1980 Feb 7; 302 (6): 324-31.

(6) Anderson JW. The role of dietary carbohydrate and fiber in the control of diabetes. Adv Intern Med 1980; 26: 67-96.

(7) Anderson JW, Kirby RW, Rees ED. Oat-bran ingestion selectively lowers serum low-density lipoprotein cholesterol concentrations in men (abstract). Am J Clin Nutr 1980 Apr; 33 (4): 915.

(8) Anderson JW. High-fibre diets for diabetic and hypertriglyceridemic patients. Can Med Assoc J 1980 Nov 22; 123 (10): 975-9.

(9) Anderson JW, Ferguson SK, Karounos D, O'Malley L, Sieling B, Chen W-J. Mineral and vitamin status on high-fiber diets: long-term studies of diabetic patients. Diabetes Care 1980 Jan-Feb; 3 (1): 38-40.

(10) Anderson JW. Dietary fiber and diabetes. In: Spiller GA, Kay RM, eds. Medical aspects of dietary fiber. New York: Plenum Press, 1980: 193-221. (Spiro HM, ed. Topics in gastroenterology.)

(11) Anderson JW. Newer approaches to diabetic diets: high-fiber diet. Med Times 1980 May; 108 (5): 41-4.

(12) Anderson JW, Chen W-J, Sieling B. Hypolipidemic effects of high-carbohydrate, high-fiber diets. Metabolism 1980 Jun; 29 (6): 551-8.

(13) Anderson NE, Clydesdale FM. An analysis of the dietary fiber content of a standard wheat bran. J Food Sci 1980; 45 (2): 336-40.

(14) Anderson NE, Clydesdale FM. Effects of processing on the dietary fiber content of wheat bran, pureed green beans, and carrots. J Food Sci 1980; 45 (6): 1533-7.

(15) Andersson H, Bosaeus I, Falkheden T, Melkersson M. Transit time in constipated geriatric patients during treatment with a bulk laxative and bran - a comparison (abstract). In: Hambraeus L, ed. Nutrition in Europe. Education, policy and research activities. Proceedings of the third European Nutrition Conference. Stockholm: Almqvist and Wiksell International, 1980: 108-9.

(16) Anonymous. Dietary fiber. J Tenn Med Assoc 1980 Jan; 73 (1): 17-9, 21.

(17) Anonymous. Dietary fiber, exercise and selected blood lipid constituents. Nutr Rev 1980 Jun; 38 (6): 207-9.

(18) Arnold K. Gastro-intestinal diseases: the benefits of fibre. Geriatr Med 1980 Nov; 10 (11): 60-7.

(19) Aro A, Uusitupa M, Korhonen T, Siitonen O. Dietary fibre and calcium excretion in diabetes (letter). Br Med J 1980 Sep 27; 281 (6244): 871.

(20) Asp N-G. Evaluation of methods suggested for assay of dietary fibre. In: Santos W, Lopes N, Barbosa JJ, Chaves D, Valente JC, eds. Nutrition education and food science and technology. Proceedings of the eleventh International Congress on Nutrition. New York: Plenum Press, 1980: 741-4. (Nutrition and food science. Present knowledge and utilization; vol 2.)

(21) Awad M, Lewis LN. Avocado cellulase: extraction and purification. J Food Sci 1980; 45 (6): 1625-8.

(22) Baig MM, Burgin C, Cerda JJ. Fractionation and study of chemistry of pectic polysaccharides (abstract). Fed Proc 1980 Mar; 39 (3 Pt I): 784.

(23) Barbolt TA, Abraham R. Dose-response, sex difference, and the effect of bran in dimethylhydrazine-induced intestinal tumorigenesis in rats. Toxicol Appl Pharmacol 1980

Sep 30; 55 (3): 417-22.

(24) Barker HM, Jenkins DJ, Taylor RH, Wolever TM. Food factors determining postprandial glycaemia in man (abstract). J Physiol 1980 Jun; 303: 83P.

(25) Baron JH. Eating and ulcers (letter). Br Med J 1980 Mar 15; 280 (6216): 795.

(26) Bassett ML, Goulston KJ. False positive and negative hemoccult reactions on a normal diet and effect of diet restriction. Aust NZ J Med 1980 Feb; 10 (1): 1-4.

(27) Berman JI, Schultz MJ. Bulk laxative ileus. J Am Geriatr Soc 1980 May; 28 (5): 224-6.

(28) Bett NJ, Wells BW. Carcinoma of colon and appendix related to fecal stasis. Dis Colon Rectum 1980 Sep; 23 (6): 408-10.

(29) Bingham S, Cummings JH. Sources and intakes of dietary fiber in man. In: Spiller GA, Kay RM, eds. Medical aspects of dietary fiber. New York: Plenum Press, 1980: 261-84. (Spiro HM, ed. Topics in gastroenterology.)

(30) Blendis LM. Dietary fibre (editorial). Can Med Assoc J 1980 Dec 6; 123 (11): 1091-2.

(31) Boothby D. The pectic components of plum fruits. Phytochemistry 1980; 19 (9): 1949-53.

(32) Bosello O, Ostuzzi R, Armellini F, Micciolo R, Scuro LA. Glucose tolerance and blood lipids in bran-fed patients with impaired glucose tolerance. Diabetes Care 1980 Jan-Feb; 3 (1): 46-9.

(33) Braden GL, Masters JT, Onderdonk AB, Falchuk ZM. Lamina propria lymphocytes mediate mitogen-induced cellular cytotoxicity in guinea pigs with carrageenan-induced colitis (abstract). Gastroenterology 1980 May; 78 (5 Pt 2): 1144.

(34) Brodribb AJ. Dietary fiber in diverticular disease of the colon. In: Spiller GA, Kay RM, eds. Medical aspects of dietary fiber. New York: Plenum Press, 1980: 43-66. (Spiro HM, ed. Topics in gastroenterology.)

(35) Brodribb J, Condon RE, Cowles V, DeCosse JJ. Influence of dietary fiber on transit time, fecal composition, and myoelectrical activity of the primate right colon. Dig Dis Sci 1980 Apr; 25 (4): 260-6.

(36) Bruckstein AH. Laxatives and cathartics: uses and abuses. Indian J Med Sci 1980 May; 34 (5): 121-8.

(37) Brydon WG, Tadesse K, Eastwood MA, Lawson ME. The effect of dietary fibre on bile acid metabolism in rats. Br J Nutr 1980 Jan; 43 (1): 101-6.

(38) Bryson E, Dore C, Garrow JS. Wholemeal bread and satiety. J Hum Nutr 1980 Apr; 34 (2): 113-6.

(39) Burkitt D, Morley D, Walker A. Dietary fibre in under- and overnutrition in childhood. Arch Dis Child 1980 Oct; 55 (10): 803-7.

(40) Burkitt DP. Fiber in the etiology of colorectal cancer. In: Winawer SJ, Schottenfeld D, Sherlock P, eds. Colorectal cancer: prevention, epidemiology, and screening. New York: Raven Press, 1980: 13-8. (Progress in cancer research and therapy; vol 13.)

(41) Burkitt D. Colon cancer: the emergence of a concept. In: Spiller GA, Kay RM, eds. Medical aspects of dietary fiber. New York: Plenum Press, 1980: 75-81. (Spiro HM, ed. Topics in gastroenterology.)

(42) Burstyn P. Dietary fibre and blood pressure (letter). Br Med J 1980 Jan 19; 280 (6208): 182.

(43) Burstyn PG, Husbands DR. Fat induced hypertension in rabbits. Effects of dietary fibre on blood pressure and blood lipid concentration. Cardiovasc Res 1980 Apr; 14 (4): 185-91.

(44) Calder JF, Wachira MW, Van Sant T, Malik MS, Bowry RN. Diverticular disease, carcinoma of the colon and diet in urban and rural Kenyan Africans. Diagn Imaging 1980; 49 (1): 23-8.

(45) Canivet B, Creisson G, Freychet P, Dageville X. Fibre, diabetes, and risk of bezoar (letter). Lancet 1980 Oct 18; 2 (8199): 862.

(46) Cannon M, Flenniken A, Track NS. Demonstration of acute and chronic effects of dietary fibre upon carbohydrate metabolism. Life Sci 1980 Oct 13; 27 (15): 1397-401.

(47) Carlsson R, de Fremery D, Gumbmann MR, Kohler GO, Walker HG. Quality of leaf protein concentrates and fibre residues from various species grown in a hot temperate climate (abstract). In: Hambraeus L, ed. Nutrition in Europe. Education, policy and

242

research activities. Proceedings of the third European Nutrition Conference. Stockholm: Almqvist and Wiksell International, 1980: 134.

(48) Chang ML, Johnson MA. Effect of dietary pectin and fat on accumulation and removal of liver cholesterol in rats (abstract). Fed Proc 1980 Mar; 39 (3 Pt I): 658.

(49) Chang ML, Johnson MA. Effect of lignin versus cellulose on the absorption of taurocholate and lipid metabolism in rats fed cholesterol diet. Nutr Rep Int 1980 Apr; 21 (4): 513-8.

(50) Chang ML, Johnson MA. Effect of pectin and protein levels on cholesterol-4-^{14}C metabolism in rats. Nutr Rep Int 1980 Jul; 22 (1): 91-9.

(51) Chen ML. Bile acid binding capacity of food fibers (abstract). Sci Res Abstr Repub China 1980: 1: 94-5.

(52) Chen W-J, Anderson JW. Soluble plant fibers in selected cereals and vegetables (abstract). Fed Proc 1980 Mar; 39 (3 Pt I): 784.

(53) Cherry JA, Beane WL, Barbato GF. Temporal compensation of Japanese quail to changes in nutrient density. Nutr Rep Int 1980 Aug; 22 (2): 253-61.

(54) Christiansen JS, Bonnevie-Nielsen V, Svendsen PA, Rubin P, Ronn B, Nerup J. Effect of guar gum on 24-hour insulin requirements of insulin-dependent diabetic subjects as assessed by an artificial pancreas. Diabetes Care 1980 Nov-Dec; 3 (6): 659-62.

(55) Coe FJ. Unprocessed bran in idiopathic hypercalciuria (letter). Br Med J 1980 Sep 13; 281 (6242): 746-7.

(56) Cohen M, Leong VW, Salmon E, Martin FI. Role of guar and dietary fibre in the management of diabetes mellitus. Med J Aust 1980 Jan 26; 1 (2): 59-61.

(57) Colonna P, Gallant D, Mercier C. Pisum sativum and Vicia faba carbohydrates: studies of fractions obtained after dry and wet protein extraction processes. J Food Sci 1980; 45 (6): 1629-36.

(58) Connell AM, McCarroll AM, Chen MH. Effect of fibre from bran cereal on gastroenteropancreatic hormone responses of normal adults. Ir J Med Sci 1980 Feb; 149 (2): 49-52.

(59) Corley JR, Baker DH, Easter RA. Biological availability of phosphorus in rice bran and wheat bran as affected by pelleting. J Anim Sci 1980 Feb; 50 (2): 286-92.

(60) Cornelius JA. Rice bran oil for edible purposes: a review. Trop Sci 1980; 22 (1): 1-26.

(61) Cottrell JI, Pass G, Phillips GO. The effect of stabilisers on the viscosity of an ice cream mix. J Sci Food Agric 1980 Oct; 31 (10): 1066-70.

(62) Coulston A, Greenfield M, Kraemer F, Tobey T, Reaven G. Effect of source of dietary carbohydrate on plasma glucose and insulin responses to test meals in normal subjects. Am J Clin Nutr 1980 Jun; 33 (6): 1279-82.

(63) Crapo PA, Kolterman OG, Waldeck N, Reaven GM, Olefsky JM. Postprandial hormonal responses to different types of complex carbohydrate in individuals with impaired glucose tolerance. Am J Clin Nutr 1980 Aug; 33 (8): 1723-8.

(64) Cullen RW, Oace SM. Impact on B$_{12}$ status of pectin and six dietary fibers in rats (abstract). Fed Proc 1980 Mar; 39 (3 Pt I): 785.

(65) Cummings JH, Stephen AM. The role of dietary fibre in the human colon. Can Med Assoc J 1980 Dec 6; 123 (11): 1109-14.

(66) Cummings JH. Some aspects of dietary fibre metabolism in the human gut. In: Birch GG, Parker KJ, eds. Food and health; science and technology. London: Applied Science Publishers Ltd, 1980: 441-58.

(67) Daghir NJ, Mahmoud HK, EL-Zein A. Buffalo gourd (Cucurbita foetidissima) meal: nutritive value and detoxification. Nutr Rep Int 1980 Jun; 21 (6): 837-47.

(68) Daghir NJ, Sell JL. Buffalo gourd (Cucurbita foetidissima) seed and seed components for growing chickens. Nutr Rep Int 1980 Sep; 22 (3): 445-52.

(69) Day RM, Thomas OP. Growth depression of chicks fed a crude rye extract containing pectic substances. Poult Sci 1980 Dec; 59 (12): 2754-9.

(70) De Wilde R. Influence of supplementing citruspectins to a diet with and without antibiotics on the digestibility of the pectins and the other nutrients in pigs. Z Tierphysiol 1980 Feb; 43 (2): 109-16.

(71) Dilawari J B, Kamath PS, Batta RP, Mukewar S, Raghavan KS. Exceptionally low blood glucose response to dried beans (letter). Br Med J 1980 Oct 11; 281 (6246): 1007.

(72) Dintzis FR, Harris CC. Starch determination in some dietary fiber sources (abstract). Cereal Foods World 1980 Aug; 25 (8): 523.

(73) Dodson PM. Dietary fibre, sodium, and blood pressure (letter). Br Med J 1980 Feb 23; 280 (6213): 564. Correction. Br Med J 1980 Mar 8; 280 (6215): 720.

(74) Drury MI. Bran for diabetics (letter). Br Med J 1980 Jun 28; 280 (6231): 1622.

(75) Eaks IL, Sinclair WB. Cellulose-hemicellulose fractions in the alcohol-insoluble solids of Valencia orange peel. J Food Sci 1980; 45 (4): 985-8.

(76) Eastwood MA, Smith AN, Mitchell WD, Pritchard JL. Faecal characteristics and colonic intraluminal pressure in diverticular disease. Digestion 1980; 20 (6): 399-402.

(77) Eastwood MA, Brydon WG, Tadesse K. Effect of fiber on colon function. In: Spiller GA, Kay RM, eds. Medical aspects of dietary fiber. New York; Plenum Press, 1980: 1-26. (Spiro HM, ed. Topics in gastroenterology.)

(78) Eastwood MA. Fibre in human nutrition — present status. Proc Nutr Soc Aust 1980; 5: 112-8.

(79) Eggum BO, Kreft I, Javornik B. Chemical composition and protein quality of buckwheat (Fagopyrum esculentum Moench). Qual Plant Plant Foods Hum Nutr 1980; 30 (3-4): 175-9.

(80) Ellis R, Morris ER. The association of phytate with iron and zinc of wheat bran and soybeans and bioutilization of zinc (abstract). Fed Proc 1980 Mar; 39 (3 Pt II): 896.

(81) El-Nahry FI, Mourad FE, Abdel Khalik SM, Bassily NS. Chemical composition and protein quality of lentils (Lens) consumed in Egypt. Qual Plant Plant Foods Hum Nutr 1980; 30 (2): 87-95.

(82) Elsenhans B, Sufke U, Blume R, Caspary WF. The influence of carbohydrate gelling agents on rat intestinal transport of monosaccharides of neutral amino acids in vitro Clin Sci 1980 Nov; 59 (5): 373-80.

(83) Enzi G, Inelmen EM, Crepaldi G. Effect of a hydrophilic mucilage in the treatment of obese patients. Pharmatherapeutica 1980; 2 (7): 421-8.

(84) Ewerth S, Ahlberg J, Holmstrom B, Persson U, Uden R. Influence on symptoms and transit-time of Vi-Siblin[R] in diverticular disease. Acta Chir Scand (Suppl) 1980; Suppl 500: 49-50.

(85) Fahey GC Jr, Frank GR, Jensen AH, Masters SS. Influence of various purified and isolated cell wall fibers on the utilization of certain nutrients by swine and hamsters. J Food Sci 1980; 45 (6): 1675-80.

(86) Fielding J F, Kehoe M. A therapeutic trial of different dietary fibre intakes in the irritable bowel syndrome. Ir J Food Sci Technol 1980; 4 (2): 89-92.

(87) Fioramonti J, Bueno L. Motor activity in the large intestine of the pig related to dietary fibre and retention time. Br J Nutr 1980 Jan; 43 (1): 155-62.

(88) Fisher N. Cereal foods today and tomorrow. J Hum Nutr 1980 Feb; 34 (1): 27-40.

(89) Flaherty EV, O'Doherty J, Fielding JF. The palatability of colloidal bulk forming agents. J Int Med Res 1980; 8 (4): 262-4.

(90) Flanagan M, Little C, Milliken J, Wright E, McGill AR, Weir DG, O'Moore RR. The effects of diet on high density lipoprotein cholesterol. J Hum Nutr 1980 Feb; 34 (1): 43-5.

(91) Fleiss PM, Gordon J, Douglass JM. One more hazard (letter). West J Med 1980 Apr; 132(4): 365-6.

(92) Fleiszer DM, Murray D, Richards GK, Brown RA. Effects of diet on chemically induced bowel cancer. Can J Surg 1980 Jan; 23 (1): 67-73.

(93) Floch MH, Wolfman M, Doyle R. Fibre and gastrointestinal microecology. J Clin Gastroenterol 1980 Jun; 2 (2): 175-84.

(94) Flynn M, Hyland J, Hammond P, Darby C, Taylor I. Faecal bile acid excretion in diverticular disease. Br J Surg 1980 Sep; 67 (9): 629-32.

(95) Food and Agriculture Organisation. Carbohydrates in human nutrition. Rome: FAO, 1980.

(96) Forman LP, Schneeman BO. Effect of dietary pectin and fat on digestive enzyme activities in the rat (abstract). Fed Proc 1980 Mar; 39 (3 Pt I): 658.

(97) Forman LP, Schneeman BO. Effects of dietary pectin and fat on the small intestinal contents and exocrine pancreas of rats. J Nutr 1980 Oct; 110 (10): 1992-9.

(98) Forsythe WA, Miller ER, Bennink MR. Dietary fiber and exercise induced alterations in body composition, plasma cholesterol parameters and LCAT activity (abstract). Fed Proc 1980 Mar; 39 (3 Pt I): 649.

(99) Franz KB, Kennedy BM, Fellers DA. Relative bioavailability of zinc from selected cereals and legumes using rat growth. J Nutr 1980 Nov; 110 (11): 2272-83.

(100) Freeland-Graves JH, Lavone Ebangit M, Hendrikson PJ. Alterations in zinc absorption and salivary sediment zinc after a lacto-ovo-vegetarian diet. Am J Clin Nutr 1980 Aug; 33 (8): 1757-66.

(101) Freeland-Graves JH, Bodzy PW, Eppright MA. Zinc status of vegetarians. J Am Diet Assoc 1980 Dec; 77 (6): 655-61.

(102) Freeman HJ, Spiller GA, Young SK. A double-blind study on the effects of differing purified cellulose and pectin fiber diets on 1, 2-dimethylhydrazine-induced rat colonic neoplasia. Cancer Res 1980 Aug; 40 (8 Pt I): 2661-5.

(103) Freeman HJ. Experimental animal studies in colonic carcinogenesis and dietary fiber. In: Spiller GA, Kay RM, eds. Medical aspects of dietary fiber. New York: Plenum Press, 1980: 83-117. (Spiro HM, ed. Topics in gastroenterology.)

(104) Frolich W, Asp N-G. Mineral bioavailability and cereal fiber (letter). Am J Clin Nutr 1980 Nov; 33 (11): 2397-8.

(105) Fulcher RG, O'Brien TP. Fluorescence microchemistry of cereal bran constituents: methods for niacin, amines, lipids and proteins (abstract). Cereal Foods World 1980 Aug; 25 (8): 519.

(106) Gangolli S, Miller K, Hopkins J. Carrageenan (letter). Lancet 1980 Jul 12; 2 (8185): 87.

(107) Gargallo J, Zimmerman DR. Effects of dietary cellulose and neomycin on function of the cecum of pigs. J Anim Sci 1980 Jul; 51 (1): 121-6.

(108) Gaydou EM, Raonizafinimanana R, Bianchini JP. Quantitative analysis of fatty acids and sterols in Malagasy rice bran oils. J Am Oil Chem Soc 1980; 57 (4): 141-2.

(109) Gembicka D, Chrapkowska KF. Amino acid composition of proteins of endosperm fraction and aleuronic layer in barley and oats brans. Acta Aliment Pol 1980; 6 (1-2): 13-20.

(110) George JR, Harbers LH, Reeves RD. Digestive responses of rats to fiber type, level and particle size. Nutr Rep Int 1980 Mar; 21 (3): 313-22.

(111) Godding EW. Investigating constipation (letter). Br Med J 1980 Jun 21; 280 (6230): 1538.

(112) Godding EW. Physiological yardsticks for bowel function and the rehabilitation of the constipated bowel. Pharmacology 1980; 20 (Suppl 1): 88-103.

(113) Gold LA, McCourt JP, Merimee TJ. Pectin: an examination in normal subjects. Diabetes Care 1980 Jan-Feb; 3 (1): 50-2.

(114) Goldin B. The role of diet and intestinal flora in the etiology of large bowel cancer. In: Winawer SJ, Schottenfeld D, Sherlock P, eds. Colorectal cancer: prevention, epidemiology, and screening. New York: Raven Press, 1980: 43-50. (Progress in cancer research and therapy; vol 13.)

(115) Goldin BR, Swenson L, Dwyer J, Sexton M, Gorbach SL. Effect of diet and Lactobacillus acidophilus supplements on human fecal bacterial enzymes. JNCI 1980 Feb; 64 (2): 255-61.

(116) Guild R, Cerda JJ, Burgin CW. Binding of bile salts by dietary fibre (abstract). Gastroenterology 1980 May; 78 (5 Pt 2): 1176.

(117) Hall SE, Bolton TM, Hetenyi G Jr. The effect of bran on glucose kinetics and plasma insulin in non-insulin-dependent diabetes mellitus. Diabetes Care 1980 Jul-Aug; 3 (4): 520-5.

(118) Harbers LH, George JR, Reeves RD. Digestion of lettuce in rats observed by scanning electron microscope. Nutr Rep Int 1980 May; 21 (5): 681-8.

(119) Harbers LH, George JR, Reeves RD. Surface changes in wheat bran by the rat digestive tract. Nutr Rep Int 1980 Jun; 21 (6): 849-54.

(120) Harland BF, Spiller GA, Gates J. Altered trace mineral bioavailability in primates: fiber, phytate, or both (abstract). Fed Proc 1980 Mar; 39 (3 Pt I): 785.

(121) Harmuth-Hoene AE, Schelenz R. The effect of indigestible polysaccharides on absorption of minerals and trace elements in growing rats (abstract). In: Hambraeus L, ed. Nutrition in Europe. Education, policy and research activities. Proceedings of the third European Nutrition Conference. Stockholm: Almqvist and Wiksell International, 1980: 109-10.

(122) Harmuth-Hoene A-E, Schelenz R. Effect of dietary fiber on mineral absorption in growing rats. J Nutr 1980 Sep; 110 (9): 1774-84.

(123) Harrison RJ, Leeds AR, Bolster NR, Judd PA. Exercise and wheat bran: effect on whole-gut transit (abstract). Proc Nutr Soc 1980 Feb; 39 (1): 22A.

(124) Heath MJ. Intestinal obstruction due to ingestion of food bolus. Med Sci Law 1980 Apr; 20 (2): 108-9.

(125) Heaton KW. TL Cleave and the fibre story. J R Nav Med Serv 1980 Spring; 66 (1): 5-10.

(126) Heaton KW. Food intake regulation and fiber. In: Spiller GA, Kay RM, eds. Medical aspects of dietary fiber. New York: Plenum Press, 1980: 223-38. (Spiro HM, ed. Topics in gastroenterology.)

(127) Heaton KW. Gallstones. Nutr Bull 1980 May; 5 (5): 228-32.

(128) Heller SN, Hackler LR, Rivers JM, Van Soest PJ, Roe DA, Lewis BA, Robertson J. Dietary fiber: the effect of particle size of wheat bran on colonic function in young men. Am J Clin Nutr 1980 Aug; 33 (8): 1734-44.

(129) Holloway WD, Tasman-Jones C, Bell E. The hemicellulose component of dietary fiber. Am J Clin Nutr 1980 Feb; 33 (2): 260-3.

(130) Holloway WD, Lee SP, Nicholson GI. The composition and dissolution of phytobezoars. Arch Pathol Lab Med 1980 Mar; 104 (3): 150-61.

(131) Holt PR. Abuses of the digestive organs in 1860 (letter). Gastroenterology 1980 Nov; 79 (5 Pt 1): 967.

(132) Huang PC. Effects of high dietary fiber foods on blood and liver cholesterol and other lipids (abstract). Sci Res Abstr Repub China 1980 Nov; 1: 98-9.

(133) Hudson GJ, Bailey BS. Mutual interference effects in the colorimetric methods used to determine the sugar composition of dietary fibre. Food Chem 1980; 5 (3): 201-6.

(134) Hughes RE, Ellery P, Harry T, Jenkins V, Jones E. The dietary potential of the common nettle. J Sci Food Agric 1980 Dec; 31 (12): 1279-86.

(135) Huijbregts AW, Van Schaik A, Van Berge-Henegouwen GP, Van der Werf SD. Serum lipids, biliary lipid composition, and bile acid metabolism in vegetarians as compared to normal controls. Eur J Clin Invest 1980 Dec; 10 (6): 443-9.

(136) Huijbregts AW, Van Berge-Henegouwen GP, Hectors MP, Van Schaik A, Van der Werf SD. Effects of a standardized wheat bran preparation on biliary lipid composition and bile acid metabolism in young healthy males. Eur J Clin Invest 1980 Dec; 10 (6): 451-8.

(137) Hull C, Greco RS, Brooks DL. Alleviation of constipation in the elderly by dietary fiber supplementation. J Am Geriatr Soc 1980 Sep; 28 (9): 410-4.

(138) Hunter K, Linn MW, Harris R. Dietary patterns and cancer of the digestive tract in older patients. J Am Geriatr Soc 1980 Sep; 28 (9): 405-9.

(139) Hussain SS, Singh B. Properties of the phytase from triticale bran (abstract). Cereal Foods World 1980 Aug; 25 (8): 510.

(140) Hussain SS, Romani MZ, Lim JK. Effect of dietary fiber fractions on serum and liver cholesterol of rats at two feeding plants (abstract). Fed Proc 1980 Mar; 39 (3 Pt I): 784.

(141) Hyland JM, Taylor I. Does a high fibre diet prevent the complications of diverticular disease? Br J Surg 1980 Feb; 67 (2): 77-9.

(142) Hyland JM, Taylor I. High fibre diet (letter). Br J Surg 1980 Oct; 67 (10): 762-3.

(143) Ifon ET, Bassir O. The nutritive value of some Nigerian leafy green vegetables. 2. The distribution of protein, carbohydrates (including ethanol-soluble simple sugars), crude

fat, fibre and ash. Food Chem 1980; 5 (3): 231-5.

(144) Indira M, Vijayammal PL, Menon PV, Kurup PA. Effect of dietary fiber on intestinal bacterial β-glucuronidase activity in chicks fed a cholesterol-containing diet. Cancer 1980 Dec 1; 46 (11): 2430-2.

(145) Indira M, Kurup PA. Effect of blackgram fiber on toxic effects of organophosphorus insecticides. Indian J Exp Biol 1980 Dec; 18 (12): 1529-30.

(146) The Institute of Food Technologists' Expert Panel on Food Safety and Nutrition and the Committee on Public Information, Chicago. Dietary fiber. J Med Soc NJ 1980 Apr; 77 (4): 284-6.

(147) Jain M, Cook GM, Davis FG, Grace MG, Howe GR, Miller AB. A case-control study of diet and colo-rectal cancer. Int J Cancer 1980 Dec 15; 26 (6): 757-68.

(148) James WP. Dietary fiber and mineral absorption. In: Spiller GA, Kay RM, eds. Medical aspects of dietary fiber. New York: Plenum Press, 1980: 239-59. (Spiro HM, ed. Topics in gastroenterology.)

(149) Jansen GR. A consideration of allowable fibre levels in weaning foods. Food Nutr Bull 1980; 2 (4): 38-47.

(150) Jayaraj AP, Tovey FI, Clark CG. Possible dietary protective factors in relation to the distribution of duodenal ulcer in India and Bangladesh. Gut 1980 Dec; 21 (12): 1068-76.

(151) Jeltema MA, Zabik ME. Revised method for quantitating dietary fibre components. J Sci Food Agric 1980 Aug; 31 (8): 820-9.

(152) Jenkins DJ, Reynolds D, Slavin B, Leeds AR, Jenkins AL, Jepson EM. Dietary fiber and blood lipids: treatment of hypercholesterolemia with guar crispbread. Am J Clin Nutr 1980 Mar; 33 (3): 575-81.

(153) Jenkins DJ, Wolever TM, Bacon S, Nineham R, Lees R, Rowden R, Love M. Hockaday TD. Diabetic diets: high carbohydrate combined with high fiber. Am J Clin Nutr 1980 Aug; 33 (8): 1729-33.

(154) Jenkins DJ, Wolever TM, Taylor RH, Reynolds D, Nineham R, Hockaday TD. Diabetic glucose control, lipids, and trace elements on long-term guar. Br Med J 1980 Jun 7; 280 (6228): 1353-4.

(155) Jenkins DJ, Wolever TM, Taylor RH, Ghafari H, Jenkins AL, Barker H, Jenkins MJ. Rate of digestion of foods and postprandial glycaemia in normal and diabetic subjects. Br Med J 1980 Jul 5; 281 (6232): 14-7.

(156) Jenkins DJ, Taylor RH, Wolever TM, Bacon S, Hockaday TD, Reynolds DJ. Guar crispbread in the diabetic diet (letter). Br Med J 1980 Jul 5; 281 (6232): 62.

(157) Jenkins DJ, Wolever TM, Taylor RH, Barker HM, Fielden H. Exceptionally low blood responses to dried beans: comparison with other carbohydrate foods. Br Med J 1980 Aug 30; 281 (6240): 578-80.

(158) Jenkins DJ, Wolever TM, Taylor RH, Barker HM, Fielden H, Jenkins AL. Effect of guar crispbread with cereal products and leguminous seeds on blood glucose concentrations of diabetics. Br Med J 1980 Nov 8; 281 (6250): 1248-50.

(159) Jenkins DJ, Wolever TM, Nineham R, Sarson DL, Bloom SR, Ahern J, Alberti KG, Hockaday TD. Improved glucose tolerance four hours after taking guar with glucose. Diabetologia 1980 Jul; 19 (1): 21-4.

(160) Jenkins DJ, Bloom SR, Albuquerque RH, Leeds AR, Sarson DL, Metz GL, Alberti KG. Pectin and complications after gastric surgery: normalisation of postprandial glucose and endocrine responses. Gut 1980 Jul; 21 (7): 574-9.

(161) Jenkins DJ. Dietary fiber and carbohydrate metabolism. In: Spiller GA, Kay RM, eds. Medical aspects of dietary fiber. New York: Plenum Press, 1980: 175-92. (Spiro HM, ed. Topics in gastroenterology.)

(162) Jenkins DJ, Wolever TM, Taylor RH, Barker HM, Fielden H, Baldwin JM, Newman HC, Bowling AC, Goff DV. Bioavailability to man of carbohydrate in foods (abstract). Proc Nutr Soc 1980 Feb; 39 (1): 11A.

(163) Johanning GL, Knehans AW, O'Dell B. Effect of dietary fiber on growth rate and serum cholesterol in guinea pigs (abstract). Fed Proc 1980 Mar; 39 (3 Pt I): 785.

(164) Johansson C-G, Asp N-G, Carlstedt I, Dahlqvist A, Dencker I, Jagerstad M, Paulsson M,

Norden A, Akesson B, Ockerman P-A. Dietary fibre in normal and vegan diets (abstract). In: Hambraeus L, ed. Nutrition in Europe. Education, policy and research activities. Proceedings of the third European Nutrition Conference. Stockholm: Almqvist and Wiksell International, 1980: 108.

(165) Johnson CK, Kolasa K, Chenoweth W, Bennink M. Health, laxation, and food habit influences on fiber intake of older women. J Am Diet Assoc 1980 Nov; 77 (5): 551-7.

(166) Johnson IT, Gee JM. Inhibitory effect of guar gum on the intestinal absorption of glucose in vitro (abstract). Proc Nutr Soc 1980 May; 39 (2): 52A.

(167) Joint FAO/WHO Expert Committee on Food Additives. Thickening agents. In: Evaluation of certain food additives. Geneva: WHO, 1980: 23-5. (Technical report series; no 653.)

(168) Jones GP. The chemical analysis of dietary fibre and its implications for human nutrition. Proc Nutr Soc Aust 1980; 5: 126-32.

(169) Judd PA. The effect of dietary fibre on blood lipids — with special reference to pectin. London, England: University of London, 1980. Thesis.

(170) Juhlin-Dannfelt A, Bjorkman O, Felig P, Wahren J. Glucose lowering effects of dietary fiber: altered absorption rather than metabolism of carbohydrate (abstract). Acta Endocrinol [Suppl] (Copenh) 1980; Suppl 237: 40.

(171) Kamath MV, Belavady B. Unavailable carbohydrates of commonly consumed Indian foods. J Sci Food Agric 1980 Feb; 31 (2): 194-202.

(172) Kang SS, Leeds AR. Effect of guar gum on insulin degradation and ^{14}C-glucose incorporation into rat adipose lipids (abstract). In: Hambraeus L, ed. Nutrition in Europe. Education, policy and research activities. Proceedings of the third European Nutrition Conference. Stockholm: Almqvist and Wiksell International, 1980: 110.

(173) Kanter Y, Eitan N, Brook G, Barzilai D. Improved glucose tolerance and insulin response in obese and diabetic patients on a fiber-enriched diet. Isr J Med Sci 1980 Jan; 16 (1): 1-6.

(174) Kaplan LR. Hypothyroidism presenting as a gastric phytobezoar. Am J Gastroenterol 1980 Aug; 74 (2): 168-9.

(175) Kasper H, Reiners C, Rabast U. Influence of dietary fibre substances on D-xylose absorption and gastric emptying time in healthy subjects (abstract). In: Hambraeus L, ed. Nutrition in Europe. Education, policy and research activities. Proceedings of the third European Nutrition Conference. Stockholm: Almqvist and Wiksell International, 1980: 109.

(176) Kasper H, Rabast U, Ehl M. Studies on the extent of dietary fiber intake in West Germany. Nutr Metab 1980; 24 (2): 102-9.

(177) Kay RM, Sabry ZI, Csima A. Multivariate analysis of diet and serum lipids in normal men. Am J Clin Nutr 1980 Dec; 33 (12): 2566-72.

(178) Kay RM. Effects of dietary fibre on serum lipid levels and fecal bile acid excretion. Can Med Assoc J 1980 Dec 20; 123 (12): 1213-7.

(179) Kay RM, Truswell AS. Dietary fiber: effects on plasma and biliary lipids in man. In: Spiller GA, Kay RM, eds. Medical aspects of dietary fiber. New York: Plenum Press, 1980: 153-73. (Spiro HM, ed. Topics in gastroenterology.)

(180) Kay RM. Effects of dietary fiber on carbohydrate metabolism. In: Santos W, Lopes N, Barbosa JJ, Chaves D, Valente JC, eds. Nutritional biochemistry and pathology. Proceedings of the eleventh International Congress on Nutrition. New York: Plenum Press, 1980: 453-60. (Nutrition and food science. Present knowledge and utilization; vol 3.)

(181) Kestens L, Schoeters G, Van Puymbroeck S, Vanderborght O. Alginate treatment and decrease of ^{226}Ra retention in the mouse femur after an IP contamination with various radium doses. Health Phys 1980 Nov; 39 (5): 805-9.

(182) Khalsa N, Sharma PK. Effect of guar (Cyamopsis tetragonoloba) on serum lipids, uric acid and proteins. Indian J Nutr Diet 1980 Aug; 17 (8): 297-301.

(183) Kidder DE, Manners MJ. Carbohydrases in pig small intestine mucosa. In: Low AG, Partridge IG, eds. Current concepts of digestion and absorption in pigs. Reading: National Institute for Research in Dairying, 1980: 94-8. (Technical bulletin; no 3.)

(184) Kies C, Peterson T, Ladlie F, Fox HM. Fecal phytate, dietary phytate, and utilization

of selected minerals by human adults fed fiber/bran supplements (abstract). Cereal Foods World 1980 Aug; 25 (8): 528-9.

(185) Kies C, Westring ME, Fox HM. Fecal fiber excretion of humans as affected by selected bran intake (abstract). Fed Proc 1980 Mar; 39 (3 Pt I): 785.

(186) Kim DN, Rogers DH, Li JR, Lee KT, Reiner JM, Thomas WA. Some effects of a grain-based mash diet on cholesterol metabolism in swine. Exp Mol Pathol 1980 Apr; 32 (2): 143-53.

(187) Kim DN, Lee KT. Effects of fibers from mash, wheat bran cereal, and alphacel on cholesterol and bile acid excretions in swine (abstract). Fed Proc 1980 Mar; 39 (3 Pt I): 336.

(188) Kimura T, Furuta H, Matsumoto Y, Yoshida A. Ameliorating effect of dietary fiber on toxicities of chemicals added to a diet in the rat. J Nutr 1980 Mar; 110 (3): 513-21.

(189) Kimura T, Iwata E, Watanabe K, Yoshida A. Effect of several chemicals added to a diet on intestinal enzyme activities of rats. J Nutr Sci Vitaminol (Tokyo) 1980; 26 (5): 483-96.

(190) Kinmonth AL, Angus R, Baum JD. Blood glucose control of diabetic children eating unrefined (U) or refined (R), high carbohydrate diets (abstract). Pediatr Res 1980 Dec; 14 (12): 1417.

(191) Klevay LM, Reck SJ, Jacob RA, Logan GM Jr, Munoz JM, Sandstead HH. The human requirement for copper. 1. Healthy men fed conventional, American diets. Am J Clin Nutr 1980 Jan; 33 (1): 45-50.

(192) Knehans AW, O'Dell BL. Intestinal microflora in the guinea pig as observed by scanning electron microscopy. Effect of fibrous dietary supplements. J Nutr 1980 Aug; 110 (8): 1543-54.

(193) Komai M, Kimura S. Gastrointestinal responses to graded levels of cellulose feeding in conventional and germ-free mice. J Nutr Sci Vitaminol (Tokyo) 1980; 26 (4): 389-99.

(194) Korner B, Zimmermann G, Berk Z. Orange pectinesterase: purification, properties, and effect on cloud stability. J Food Sci 1980; 45 (5): 1203-6.

(195) Kritchevsky D. Steroids, fiber and related factors in carcinogenesis. J Environ Pathol Toxicol 1980 Mar; 3 (4): 305-13.

(196) Kritchevsky D, Story JA, Vahouny GV. Influence of fiber on lipid metabolism. In: Santos W, Lopes N, Barbosa JJ, Chaves D, Valente JC, eds. Nutritional biochemistry and pathology. Proceedings of the eleventh International Congress on Nutrition. New York: Plenum Press, 1980: 461-71. (Nutrition and food science. Present knowledge and utilization; vol 3).

(197) Kuritza A, Arthur RA, Salyers AA. Digestion of larch arabinogalactan by a strain of human colonic Bacteroides (abstract). Am J Clin Nutr 1980 Nov; 33 (11): 2541.

(198) Labaneiah ME, Luh BS. Changes of starch, crude fiber and oligosaccharides in germinating dry beans (abstract). Cereal Foods World 1980 Aug; 25(8): 533.

(199) Lazaridis HN, Rosenau JR. Effects of emulsifying salts and carrageenan on rheological properties of cheese-like products prepared by direct acidification. J Food Sci 1980; 45 (3): 595-7.

(200) Lee BA, Oace SM. Cecal bacteria modify the effect of fibers on gastrointestinal transit time in the rat (abstract). Fed Proc 1980 Mar; 39 (3 Pt I): 785.

(201) Leeds AR, Kang SS, Low AG, Sambrook IE. The pig as a model for studies on the mode of action of guar gum in normal and diabetic man (abstract). Proc Nutr Soc 1980 May; 39 (2): 44A.

(202) Lei KY, Davis MW, Fang MM, Young LC. Effect of pectin on zinc, copper and iron balances in humans. Nutr Rep Int 1980 Sep; 22 (3): 459-66.

(203) Leklem JE, Miller LT, Perera AD, Peffers DE. Bioavailability of vitamin B-6 from wheat bread in humans. J Nutr 1980; 110 (9): 1819-28.

(204) Levine AS, Salom IL, Silvis SE. The effect of mechanical breakdown of food and fiber content of the diet on fat absorption (abstract). Gastroenterology 1980 May; 78 (5 Pt 2): 1205.

(205) Levine AS, Silvis SE. Absorption of whole peanuts, peanut oil, and peanut butter. N

Engl J Med 1980 Oct 16; 303 (16): 917-8.

(206) Levitt NS, Vinik AI, Sive AA, Child PT, Jackson WP. The effect of dietary fiber on glucose and hormone responses to a mixed meal in normal subjects and in diabetic subjects with and without autonomic neuropathy. Diabetes Care 1980 Jul-Aug; 3 (4): 515-9.

(207) Lindgarde F, Rasmusson M, Wendt B. Energy and dietary fibre intake and glucose tolerance in middle-aged men (abstract). In: Hambraeus L, ed. Nutrition in Europe. Education, policy and research activities. Proceedings of the third European Nutrition Conference. Stockholm: Almqvist and Wiksell International, 1980: 119.

(208) Liu YK, Luh BS. Quantitative aspects of pectic acid hydrolysis by endo-polygalacturonase from Rhizopus arrhizus. J Food Sci 1980; 45 (3): 601-4.

(209) Lo GS, Settle SL, Steinke FH, Hopkins DT. Effects of soy polysaccharides fiber (SPF) on lipid metabolism in rats (abstract). Fed Proc 1980 Mar; 39 (3 Pt I): 784.

(210) Lock S, Bender AE. Measurement of chemically-available iron in foods by incubation with human gastric juice in vitro. Br J Nutr 1980 May; 43 (3): 413-20.

(211) Lockhart HB, Lee HS, O'Mahony SP, Hensley GW, Houlihan EJ. Caloric value of fiber-containing cereal fractions and breakfast cereals. J Food Sci 1980; 45 (2): 372-4.

(212) Longe OG. Carbohydrate composition of different varieties of cowpea (Vigna unguiculata). Food Chem 1980 Dec; 6 (2): 153-61.

(213) Longe OG. Effect of processing on the chemical composition and energy value of cassava. Nutr Rep Int 1980 Jun; 21 (6): 819-28.

(214) Lorenz K. Cereal sprouts: composition, nutritive value, food applications. CRC Crit Rev Food Sci Nutr 1980 Dec; 13 (4): 353-85.

(215) Low AG. Nutrient absorption in pigs. J Sci Food Agric 1980 Nov; 31 (11): 1087-1130.

(216) Malagelada J-R, Carter SE, Brown ML, Carlson GL. Radiolabeled fiber: a physiologic marker for gastric emptying and intestinal transit of solids. Dig Dis Sci 1980 Feb; 25 (2): 81-7.

(217) Malinow MR, Burns AK. In vitro removal of micellar cholesterol by dietary plants rich in fiber (abstract). Am J Clin Nutr 1980 Apr; 33 (4): 940.

(218) Malinow MR, McLaughlin P, Stafford C, Livingston AL, Kohler GO. Alfalfa saponins and alfalfa seeds. Dietary effects in cholesterol-fed rabbits. Atherosclerosis 1980 Nov; 37 (3): 433-8.

(219) Malinow MR, McLaughlin P, Stafford C. Alfalfa seeds: effects on cholesterol metabolism. Experientia 1980 May 15; 36 (5): 562-4.

(220) Mann JI. Diet and diabetes. Diabetologia 1980 Feb; 18 (2): 89-95.

(221) Mann JI, Simpson HC. Fibre, diabetes, and hyperlipidaemia (letter). Lancet 1980 Jan 5; 1 (8158): 44.

(222) Mann JI. Diets for diabetics in the 1980s. Nutr Bull 1980 May; 5 (5): 246-55.

(223) Manshande J-P, Ngalimbaya, Kabaya. Fibre and postoperative ileus (letter). Lancet 1980 Aug 30; 2 (8192): 476.

(224) Marcus R, Watt J. Potential hazards of carrageenan (letter). Lancet 1980 Mar 15: 1 (8168): 602-3.

(225) Marlett JA, Lee SC. Dietary fiber, lignocellulose and hemicellulose contents of selected foods determined by modified and unmodified Van Soest procedures. J Food Sci 1980; 45 (6): 1688-93.

(226) Martini GA, Stenner A, Brandes WJ. Diet and ulcerative colitis (letter). Br Med J 1980 May 31; 280 (6227): 1321.

(227) Marzio L, Lanfranchi GA, Trento L, Campieri M. Effect of high residue diet on recto-anal motility in patients affected by idiopathic constipation (abstract). Gastroenterology 1980 May; 78 (5 Pt 2): 1218.

(228) Mason VC. Role of the large intestine in the processes of digestion and absorption in the pig. In: Low AG, Partridge IG, eds. Current concepts of digestion and absorption in pigs. Reading: National Institute for Research in Dairying, 1980: 112-29. (Technical bulletin; no 3.)

(229) Mathai CK, Kumaran PM, Chandy KC. Evaluation of commercially important

chemical constituents in wild black pepper types. Qual Plant Plant Foods Hum Nutr 1980; 30 (3-4): 199-202.

(230) Matulewicz MC, Cerezo AS. The carrageenan from Iridaea undulosa B; analysis, fractionation and alkaline treatment. J Sci Food Agric 1980 Feb; 31 (2): 203-13.

(231) Meier-Ploeger A, Leitzmann C. Influence of carob on blood lipids in healthy young adults of different body weights (abstract). In: Hambraeus L, ed. Nutrition in Europe. Education, policy and research activities. Proceedings of the third European Nutrition Conference. Stockholm: Almqvist and Wiksell International, 1980: 111.

(232) Michaelis OE IV, Reiser S, Trout DL, Hallfrisch J, Ellwood KC. Effects of fibers on metabolic parameters of rats meal-fed sugar diets (abstract). Fed Proc 1980 Mar; 39 (3 Pt I): 658.

(233) Miller LT, Shultz TD, Leklem JE. Influence of citrus pectin on the bioavailability of vitamin B6 in men (abstract). Fed Proc 1980 Mar; 39 (3 Pt I): 797.

(234) Modan B, Lubin F. Epidemiology of colon cancer: fiber, fats, fallacies, and facts. In: Spiller GA, Kay RM, eds. Medical aspects of dietary fiber. New York: Plenum Press, 1980: 119-35. (Spiro HM, ed. Topics in gastroenterology.)

(235) Modan B. Protective role of fiber in carcinogenesis. In: Santos W, Lopes N, Barbosa JJ, Chaves D, Valente JC, eds. Nutritional biochemistry and pathology. Proceedings of the eleventh International Congress on Nutrition. New York: Plenum Press, 1980: 487-94. (Nutrition and food science. Present knowledge and utilization; vol 3.)

(236) Mondal BK, Armitage B. Are laxatives necessary? Geriatr Med 1980 Jul; 10 (7): 9.

(237) Mongeau R, Brassard R. Neutral detergent fiber from breakfast cereals: mean particle size, water holding capacity and binding of bile salts in vitro (abstract). Cereal Foods World 1980 Aug; 25 (8): 529.

(238) Monnier L, Colette C, Aguirre L, Mirouze J. Evidence and mechanism for pectin-reduced intestinal inorganic iron absorption in idiopathic hemochromatosis. Am J Clin Nutr 1980 Jun; 33 (6): 1225-32.

(239) Monnier L, Blotman MJ, Cartry E, Vierne Y, Mirouze J. Influence of high fibre diets on diabetic control of insulin-requiring diabetic patients (abstract). In: Hambraeus L, ed. Nutrition in Europe. Education, policy and research activities. Proceedings of the third European Nutrition Conference. Stockholm: Almqvist and Wiksell International, 1980: 110.

(240) Monte WC, Maga JA. Extraction and isolation of soluble and insoluble fiber fractions from the pinto bean (Phaseolus vulgaris). J Agric Food Chem 1980 Nov-Dec; 28 (6): 1169-74.

(241) Moor D. Effects of dietary fibre on the absorption of digoxin (abstract). In: Hambraeus L, ed. Nutrition in Europe. Education, policy and research activities. Proceedings of the third European Nutrition Conference. Stockholm: Almqvist and Wiksell International, 1980: 110.

(242) Morris ER, Simpson KM, Cook JD. Dephytinized vs. nondephytinized wheat bran and iron absorption in man (abstract). Am J Clin Nutr 1980 Apr; 33 (4): 941.

(243) Morris ER, Ellis R, Steele P, Moser P. Inorganic nutrient balance of humans consuming whole wheat bran vs. dephytinized wheat bran (abstract). Fed Proc 1980 Mar; 39 (3 Pt I): 787.

(244) Morris ER, Ellis R. Bioavailability to rats of iron and zinc in wheat bran: response to low-phytate bran and effect of the phytate/zinc molar ratio. J Nutr 1980 Oct; 110 (10): 2000-10.

(245) Morrison IM. Hemicellulosic contamination of acid detergent residues and their replacement by cellulose residues in cell wall analysis. J Sci Food Agric 1980 Jul; 31 (7): 639-45.

(246) Morrison IM. Hemicellulosic contamination of acid-detergent residues and their replacement by cellulose residues in cell wall analysis (abstract). Proc Nutr Soc 1980 Sep; 39 (3): 70A.

(247) Murray D, Fleiszer D, McArdle AH, Brown RA. Effect of dietary fiber on intestinal mucosal sodium-potassium-activated ATPase. J Surg Res 1980 Aug; 29 (2): 135-40.

(248) Muztar AJ, Slinger SJ. The effect of fiber on metabolic and endogenous energy losses

Olefsky JM: 63
Olsen PS: 270
Olsson MS: 406
O'Malley L: 9
O'Mahony SP: 211
O'Moore RR: 90
Onderdonk AB: 33
O'Neill MA: 323
Ornstein MH: 271, 272
Ossenkopp K-P: 273
Oster P: 274
Ostuzzi R: 32
Owen GM: 374

Pacioni D: 297, 450
Paerregaard A: 406
Paganoni A: 322
Painter NS: 275
Parfrey P: 276
Parretta Zuccarini MG: 448
Parsons V: 392
Partridge IG: 277
Pass G: 61
Patel MB 278
Patil K: 304
Paul AA: 256, 390
Paulsson M: 164
Peffers DE: 203
Perera AD: 203
Perez M: 477
Perez-Lopez M: 474
Perrins EJ: 308
Persson U: 84
Peterson T: 184
Phillips GO: 61
Phillips SF: 279
Pilgaard S: 406
Pilnik W: 384
Pinilla I: 475
Plooy M: 411
Poulsen SS: 270
Powers P: 252
Poynard T: 280, 427
Prever F: 294
Pritchard JL: 76

Rabast U: 175, 176
Radrizzani D: 322
Raghavan KS: 71
Ramirez Varela A: 476
Rao BS: 281
Rao CN: 281
Raonizafinimanana R: 108
Rasmusson M: 207
Reaven GM: 62, 63

Reber M: 433
Reck SJ: 191
Reddick JE: 282
Reddy BS: 283, 284, 285,
    286, 388
Reddy NN: 287
Reddy NR: 288
Reddy PR: 289
Reed JP: 318
Rees ED: 7
Reeves RD: 110, 118, 119
Reid BL: 318
Reid RL: 378
Reiner JM: 186
Reiners C: 175
Reinhold JG: 290
Reiser R: 267
Reiser S: 232
Reizenstein P: 291
Renan MJ: 292
Rendleman JA: 293
Reynolds DJ: 152, 154, 156
Riccardi G: 297, 450
Richards GK: 92
Rinaudo M: 425
Rinetti M: 294
Ring SG: 323
Ritchie JA: 295, 296
Rivellese A: 297, 450
Rivers JM: 128
Robertson J: 128
Robertson JA: 298, 299
Rodgers JB: 2
Roe DA: 128
Roe FJ: 300
Rogers DH: 186
Rojas-Hidalgo E: 474, 477,
    478
Romani MZ: 140
Rombouts FM: 384
Ronn B: 54
Rosenau JR: 199
Rossi Corvi R: 448
Roth NJ: 282
Rotstein OD: 301, 302
Rousseau C: 420
Rowden R: 153
Rowe MJ: 341
Roy T: 380
Rubin P: 54
Rumble WF: 1
Russell RM: 290
Rustenmeyer C: 411
Rustia M: 304

Sabry ZI: 177
Sachar DB: 305

St Leger AS: 389
Salati R: 306
Salmon E: 56
Salom IL: 204
Salunkhe DK: 288
Salvioli G: 306
Salyers AA: 197
Sambrook IE: 201, 307
Sandeman DR: 308
Sandstead HH: 191, 309
Saraswathi G: 310
Sarson DL: 159, 160
Saunders RM: 311
Schaller DR: 312
Scheibel MS: 313
Schel JH: 314
Schelenz R: 121, 122
Schellenberg B: 274
Schelstraete M: 315
Scherz H: 443
Schlierf G: 274
Schneeman BO: 96, 97,
    316, 328, 329
Schoeters G: 181, 317
Schonhauser R: 445
Schulerud A: 456
Schultz MJ: 27
Schurg WA: 318
Schwartz SE: 319, 320, 321
Schweizer TF: 444
Sculati O: 322, 451
Scuro LA: 32
Segal I: 386
Sell JL: 68
Selvendran RR: 323, 324,
    356
Sestoft L: 409
Setti M: 451
Settle SL: 209
Sexton M: 115
Shah PJ: 325, 326
Sharma BB: 327
Sharma C: 286
Sharma PK: 182
Sharma RK: 327
Sharma RP: 288
Sharma S: 327
Sheard NF: 328, 329
Sheinfil A: 285
Shipley EA: 348
Shubik P: 304
Shultz TD: 233
Shurpalekar KS: 310
Sibbald IR: 330, 331
Sieling B: 9, 12
Siitonen O: 19
Silman AJ: 332, 333

(1) *GASTROINTESTINAL*

    (1.1)   Colonic function, faecal weight, transit time, constipation
6, 8, 23, 33, 47, 48, 54, 61*, 63*, 68*, 79*, 84*, 99*, 109, 111*, 119*, 140,
145, 154, 160*, 166, 187*, 192, 203, 207*, 208, 224, 225, 226*, 240*, 244,
245*, 256*, 257*, 260, 262, 265, 267, 268, 270, 281, 288, 289, 311, 312*, 319,
332*, 340, 342*, 346*, 355, 363, 369*, 385, 386, 387, 403*, 405*, 406, 413,
424, 430, 442, 443, 460, 467*, 485, 507*, 509, 510*, 511*, 512*, 514*, 516*,
525*, 529*, 531*, 532, 533, 534, 535, 536*, 545*, 551, 579*, 582, 600, 612*,
621, 626*, 627*, 628*, 629*, 630, 631*, 633*, 635, 639, 641, 657*

    (1.2)   Diverticular disease
23, 36, 37*, 82, 83, 89, 93, 94, 97, 121, 187*, 211*, 297, 311*, 340, 390, 402,
403*, 404, 405*, 409, 410, 492, 511*, 512*, 524*, 546, 563, 592, 600, 652*

    (1.3)   Irritable bowel syndrome
23, 37, 200, 317*, 318, 319, 340, 393, 625*, 628*, 629*, 630, 631*, 652*

    (1.4)   Large bowel cancer, colonic and faecal bacteria
4*, 25, 48, 54*, 62, 65, 68*, 93, 99*, 112, 117*, 119*, 120*, 127*, 138*, 140,
141, 172, 191, 192*, 198, 204, 218*, 221*, 224, 225, 236, 243, 250, 281*,
294*, 313*, 324, 325, 346*, 369*, 370, 374, 379, 384, 401*, 414, 424, 425,
441*, 442*, 443*, 473, 476*, 477*, 484, 491, 514*, 515*, 516*, 518, 524*,
531*, 532, 533, 534, 535, 538*, 544, 546*, 551, 555, 556, 564*, 566*, 582*,
587*, 591, 601, 614, 617, 637, 646*

    (1.5)   Appendicitis
50, 72, 93*, 179*, 261, 375*

    (1.6)   Ulcerative colitis, Crohn's disease
37, 212*, 330, 338, 389*, 480, 524, 645*

    (1.7)   The group of large bowel disorders
93, 212, 524

    (1.8)   Hiatus hernia
89*

    (1.9)   Stomach, gastric ulcer, small intestine, duodenal ulcer
8, 49, 69*, 74, 87*, 93, 99*, 122, 151, 153*, 154*, 160, 161*, 175, 204, 219,
220, 225, 233*, 235, 238*, 245*, 247, 270*, 296*, 299*, 302*, 303, 304, 342*,
346, 350, 373, 374, 399, 417, 439, 442*, 443*, 453*, 483, 489, 499, 514*, 516*,
523, 545, 551, 561, 570, 577, 589, 603*, 653

    (1.10) Dumping syndrome
71, 299*, 523

    (1.11) Digestibility, and digestion of fibre; absorption of nutrients, minerals and drugs
2, 4*, 8*, 9, 13*, 27*, 29, 33, 38, 39, 40*, 47*, 53, 54, 55*, 59, 61*, 62, 63*,
67, 68*, 70*, 79*, 96*, 101, 106, 110, 111*, 114*, 116, 117*, 118*, 119*, 122,
125, 127*, 128*, 129, 141, 146, 153*, 154, 159, 160*, 161, 165*, 167, 168*,
169*, 170*, 172, 180, 184, 185, 186, 189, 194*, 196, 199*, 201, 203, 204, 219,
223, 226, 229*, 233, 235, 240*, 241, 243, 245, 253, 256*, 257*, 258, 259,
260*, 265, 266, 267, 270, 271, 274, 275*, 276, 277, 278*, 281, 284, 285, 288,
289, 290, 294*, 295*, 301, 302, 320, 331, 334, 342*, 344, 349, 350*, 353,
354*, 364, 365, 366, 370, 374, 377, 379, 381, 382*, 383*, 385, 391*, 394,
398*, 399, 400, 411, 412*, 417, 428, 429, 430, 431*, 437*, 438*, 442, 443,
445*, 446*, 447, 449, 452, 453*, 454, 457, 464*, 467*, 468, 471, 474, 476*,
477*, 478*, 484*, 485, 488, 489, 495, 496*, 499, 503*, 509*, 525*, 531*, 532,
534, 535, 540, 542, 544*, 552*, 553*, 560*, 567, 585, 588*, 590, 598, 603*,
605*, 606*, 608, 612*, 635, 636*

(1.12)   Ileostomy
66, 478*, 484*

(1.13)   Gallstones, bile salt metabolism
8, 25, 37*, 42, 54, 56*, 60, 89, 97, 103, 149, 192*, 214*, 240*, 241, 250, 254, 268*, 269, 272*, 284*, 285, 313, 325, 336*, 339, 384, 386, 388*, 416*, 441*, 460, 467*, 470, 471*, 472*, 475*, 527, 529*, 538*, 539, 564*, 565, 566*, 568, 582*, 587*, 640

(1.14)   Phytobezoars
530, 615, 654

(1.15)   Miscellaneous gastrointestinal
37, 49, 51, 53, 69*, 85*, 92, 99*, 106, 116, 143*, 144, 146, 154*, 160*, 177, 180, 202, 225, 233*, 235, 246, 251, 276, 277, 281, 285, 288, 289, 294, 296*, 303, 310, 322*, 323, 334, 350, 369*, 370, 374, 389*, 396, 417, 426*, 432, 32, 445*, 446, 453*, 459*, 485, 488, 514*, 516*, 517, 524, 533, 540, 570, 579*, 626*, 627*, 628*, 631, 635

(2) *CARDIOVASCULAR*
(2.1)   Lipid metabolism, cholesterol, triglycerides
2, 14, 16, 17, 18, 28, 29*, 33*, 41*, 42, 43, 47*, 60, 67, 76*, 77, 98*, 99*, 101, 105, 106*, 116, 125, 129, 132, 135*, 149, 156*, 178, 185, 189, 192, 214, 220, 235, 237*, 239, 240*, 241, 249*, 250, 264*, 268*, 269, 272*, 275*, 276*, 277*, 278*, 280*, 284*, 285*, 290, 294, 298, 300*, 301, 306*, 309, 326, 327, 329*, 335*, 339, 344, 364, 378, 385*, 386, 387, 397, 407, 411*, 421*, 426*, 438, 440, 452, 455*, 466, 467*, 468, 470, 471*, 472*, 475*, 487, 500, 501*, 513, 516*, 527, 529*, 538*, 540*, 542*, 547, 556, 565, 567, 570, 582*, 583, 616, 622*, 635*, 638*, 639*, 642*, 643*, 648*

(2.2)   Atherosclerosis, ischaemic heart disease
132*, 137, 274, 284*, 333, 547, 574

(2.3)   Venous thrombosis, varicose veins, haemorrhoids
93, 222, 244, 279, 297, 627*, 632

(2.4)   Hypertension
86*, 93, 95, 136, 574*

(3) *METABOLIC*
(3.1)   Diabetes mellitus, carbohydrate metabolism
16*, 17, 18*, 24, 28, 29*, 31*, 63, 69*, 75*, 76*, 77, 95, 98*, 113, 115*, 116, 125, 133*, 135*, 142, 150*, 151*, 153*, 157*, 158, 161, 175, 199, 206, 213, 231*, 232*, 233*, 234*, 235*, 237*, 238*, 251*, 272, 273*, 279*, 283, 298*, 299*, 302, 303, 305, 326*, 327, 328, 329*, 348, 357*, 373*, 380, 391*, 392, 395*, 396, 407, 421*, 440, 447, 455*, 466, 481*, 489, 501*, 502*, 504*, 505, 517, 523, 537*, 569*, 570, 574*, 577*, 583, 619, 622*, 623*, 647*, 654

(3.2)   Obesity
37*, 75*, 135, 157*, 158, 364, 373, 413, 420, 565, 574*, 589*, 635*, 641*

(4) *FIBRE AND FOOD*
(4.1)   Fibre: definition, terminology, composition, analysis
1*, 7, 27, 32*, 34, 35, 44*, 45, 57*, 61, 68*, 81*, 88, 104*, 110, 123, 124*, 134*, 139*, 141, 147*, 159*, 162*, 163*, 164*, 174*, 176*, 180, 182*, 183*, 209, 215*, 216*, 217*, 227*, 228*, 242, 248*, 252, 263*, 292*, 295*, 307, 308, 316*, 321*, 341*, 343*, 353, 367*, 368, 418*, 420, 422*, 427, 435*, 436*, 437*, 444, 446, 458*, 461*, 465*, 469*, 478*, 479*, 482, 486, 490*, 493*, 508, 520*, 521*, 522, 525, 543, 546, 549, 557*, 558*, 571*, 580, 584*, 586*, 590*, 595*, 596*, 609, 610, 634, 651*

270

(4.2)   Fibre in the diet and food, except cereals
2, 13*, 20, 21, 22, 30, 32*, 44, 52, 57*, 64, 73, 78*, 80*, 95, 102, 103, 104*,
110*, 124*, 126, 127, 141, 155, 157, 163*, 172, 174, 176*, 183*, 187, 189,
190*, 195, 196, 197, 202, 209, 210, 217*, 230*, 248*, 252*, 263, 271, 287,
291*, 314, 315*, 316, 331*, 341, 343, 347, 353, 360, 361, 406, 408, 420, 433,
436, 444*, 456, 461*, 463, 465, 479, 482, 490*, 493*, 497, 519*, 521*, 526,
527, 541, 543, 554, 557*, 558*, 559, 584*, 585, 593, 604, 620, 650*, 655*

(4.3)   Fibre in cereal and cereal foods
1, 7, 15*, 19*, 20, 27, 32, 44, 46*, 57, 81*, 104*, 107, 108*, 123, 131, 139,
147*, 157, 162*, 163*, 176*, 181*, 182*, 183*, 242, 248*, 274, 337, 341*,
345, 350, 351*, 365, 368, 376, 408, 418, 419*, 420, 422*, 433, 435*, 436,
461*, 469*, 479, 490*, 493*, 498*, 519*, 521*, 548, 557*, 558*, 590, 610,
624

(4.4)   Modern dietary change
590, 624

(5) MISCELLANEOUS

(5.1)   Antitoxic action
85*, 152*, 177*, 185, 270*, 354*, 442*, 468*, 545*, 555, 591*, 646*

(5.2)   Ill-effects
27*, 85*, 92, 130*, 172*, 195*, 199*, 218*, 221*, 245, 262, 310*, 330*, 334,
356*, 365, 383, 389*, 426, 432*, 480*, 515*, 555, 562, 629, 630, 631

(5.3)   Early views on whole foods and dietary fibre before 1940
380

(5.4)   Experimental methods
134*, 182*, 207*, 208, 332*, 414, 448, 459*, 478*, 488*, 507*, 581, 590*,
617

(5.5)   Other
2, 5*, 30*, 70*, 73, 80*, 96*, 100*, 107, 108*, 110, 123, 151, 152, 160, 171,
176, 180, 196*, 201*, 247, 279*, 294*, 309, 321*, 350*, 351*, 353*, 356*,
362*, 367*, 376, 382*, 395*, 400, 411, 415*, 416*, 417, 434*, 444, 445*, 446,
451*, 452, 456*, 458*, 459*, 460*, 462*, 463*, 465*, 468*, 475*, 482, 496*,
497, 517, 541*, 542, 548*, 550*, 554*, 555, 559, 572, 578, 579*, 581, 588*,
590, 595*, 596*, 597*, 599*

(6) DIETARY FIBRE HYPOTHESES, GENERAL PRESENTATION
8, 10, 11, 12, 26, 58, 90, 91, 131, 148, 173, 188, 193, 205, 286, 293, 294*, 352,
358, 359, 372, 423, 433, 506, 529, 536*, 572, 574*, 575, 576, 594, 602, 607,
611, 613*, 618, 634, 644*, 649, 656

(7) BOOKS, SYMPOSIA, THESES
(7.1)   Books for the public
3, 282*, 450, 494*, 528*

(7.2)   Books for the scientist
227*, 255*, 371*, 519*, 573*

THE REFERENCES

(1) AACC Committee on Dietary Fiber. Collaborative study of an analytical method for insoluble dietary fiber in cereals. Cereal Foods World 1981 Jun; 26 (6): 295-7.

(2) Abdulla M, Andersson I, Asp N-G, Berthelsen K, Birkhed D, Dencker I, Johansson C-G, Jagerstad M, Kolar K, Nair BM, Nilsson-Ehle P, Norden A, Rassner S, Akesson B, Ockerman P-A. Nutrient intake and health status of vegans. Chemical analyses of diets using the duplicate portion sampling technique. Am J Clin Nutr 1981 Nov; 34 (11): 2464-77.

(3) Adams R, Murray F. High-fiber approach relieving constipation. Cancer Book House.

(4) Adlercreutz H, Fotsis T, Heikkinen R, Dwyer JT, Goldin BR, Gorbach SL, Lawson AM, Setchell KD. Diet and urinary excretion of lignans in female subjects. Med Biol 1981 Aug; 59 (4): 259-61.

(5) Akintunde EA. Seasonal variations in the quantity of carbohydrate, protein, lipid and crude fibre components of the food of Sarotherodon galilaeus (Syn Tilapia galilaea) (Fam: Cichlidae) of Lake Kainji, Nigeria. Nutr Rep Int 1981 Dec; 24 (6): 1109-21.

(6) Aktan H, Ozden A, Kesim E, Smith AN. Colon function in rural and urban populations of Turkey (abstract). Gut 1981 Oct; 22 (10): A865.

(7) Al-Bayati SH, Al-Rayess H. The chemical composition of Iraqi rice and rice by-products. J Food Sci Technol India 1981 Mar-Apr; 18 (2): 40-4.

(8) Ali R, Staub H, Coccodrilli G Jr, Schanbacher L. Nutritional significance of dietary fiber: effect on nutrient bioavailability and selected gastrointestinal functions. J Agric Food Chem 1981 May-Jun; 29 (3): 465-72.

(9) Allen MD, Greenblatt DJ, Harmatz JS, Smith TW. Effect of magnesium-aluminium hydroxide and kaolin-pectin on absorption of digoxin from tablets and capsules. J Clin Pharmacol 1981 Jan; 21 (1): 26-30.

(10) Almy TP. The dietary fiber hypothesis. Am J Clin Nutr 1981 Mar; 34 (3): 432-3.

(11) Almy TP. Fiber and the gut. Am J Med 1981 Aug; 71 (2): 193-5.

(12) American Academy of Pediatrics: Committee on Nutrition. Plant fiber intake in the pediatric diet. Pediatrics 1981 Apr; 67 (4): 572-5.

(13) Anderson BM, Gibson RS, Sabry JH. The iron and zinc status of long-term vegetarian women. Am J Clin Nutr 1981 Jun; 34 (6): 1042-8.

(14) Anderson JW, Chen W-J. Cholesterol-lowering properties of oat gum (abstract). Cereal Foods World 1981 Sep; 26 (9): 498.

(15) Anderson JW, Story L, Sieling B, Chen W-J. Plant fiber content of selected breakfast cereals. Diabetes Care 1981 Jul-Aug; 4 (4): 490-2.

(16) Anderson JW, Sieling B. High-fiber diets for diabetics: unconventional but effective. Geriatrics 1981 May; 36 (5): 64-72.

(17) Anderson JW. Fiber: diabetes and hyperlipidemia. In: Garry PJ, ed. Human nutrition. Clinical and biochemical aspects. Proceedings of the fourth Arnold O. Beckman conference in clinical chemistry. Washington, DC: American Society for Clinical Chemistry, 1981: 132-47.

(18) Anderson JW. Part VII. Regression of certain Western diseases. Diabetes Mellitus. In: Trowell HC, Burkitt DP, eds. Western diseases: their emergence and prevention. London: Edward Arnold, 1981: 373-91.

(19) Andersson Y, Hedlund B, Jonsson L, Svensson S. Extrusion cooking of a high-fiber cereal product with crispbread character. Cereal Chem 1981 Sep-Oct; 58 (5): 370-4.

(20) Angus R, Sutherland TM, Farrell DJ. Insoluble dietary fibre content of some local foods (abstract). Proc Nutr Soc Aust 1981; 6: 161.

(21) Angus R, Sutherland TM, Farrell DJ. A survey of fibre consumption by various age groups in two Australian communities (abstract). Proc Nutr Soc Aust 1981; 6: 162.

(22) Anonymous. Review of bulking aids. Br Food J 1981 Jan-Feb; 83 (900): 9-10.

(23) Anonymous. Wheat bran for bowel disorders. Drug Ther Bull 1981 Apr 10; 19 (8): 29-31.

(24) Anonymous. High-fibre diets and diabetes (editorial). Lancet 1981 Feb 21; 1 (8217): 423-4.

(25) Anonymous. Large-bowel cancer after cholecystectomy (editorial). Lancet 1981 Sep 12; 2 (8246): 562-3.

(26) Anonymous. Facts behind the headlines. 1: We should eat more dietary fibre. Nutr Bull 1981 Jan; 6 (1): 5-7.

(27) Antoniou T, Marquardt RR, Cansfield PE. Isolation, partial characterization, and antinutritional activity of a factor (pentosans) in rye grain. J Agric Food Chem 1981 Nov-Dec; 29 (6): 1240-7.

(28) Aro A, Uusitupa M, Voutilainen E, Hersio K, Korhonen T, Siitonen O. Long-term effects of guar gum in maturity-onset diabetes (abstract). Acta Endocrinol (Copenh) 1981; Suppl 245: 8.

(29) Aro A, Uusitupa M, Voutilainen E, Hersio K, Korhonen T, Siitonen O. Improved diabetic control and hypocholesterolaemic effect induced by long-term dietary supplementation with guar gum in type 2 (insulin-independent) diabetes. Diabetologia 1981 Jul; 21 (1): 29-33.

(30) Ashraf M, Khan N, Ahmad M, Elahi M. Studies on the pectinesterase activity and some chemical constituents of some Pakistani mango varieties during storage ripening. J Agric Food Chem 1981 May-Jun; 29 (3): 526-8.

(31) Asp N-G, Agardh C-D, Ahren B, Dencker I, Johansson C-G, Lundquist I, Nyman M, Sartor G, Schersten B. Dietary fibre in type II diabetes. Acta Med Scand (Suppl) 1981; 656: 47-50.

(32) Asp N-G, Johansson C-G. Techniques for measuring dietary fiber: principal aims of methods and a comparison of results obtained by different techniques. In: James WP, Theander O, eds. The analysis of dietary fiber in food. New York and Basel: Marcel Dekker Inc, 1981: 173-89. (Basic and clinical nutrition; vol 3.)

(33) Asp N-G, Bauer HG, Nilsson-Ehle P, Nyman M, Oste R. Wheat bran increases high-density-lipoprotein cholesterol in the rat. Br J Nutr 1981 Nov; 46 (3): 385-93.

(34) Asp N-G, Johansson C-G, Hallmer H, Siljestrom M. A rapid enzymatic gravimetric method for assay of dietary fiber (abstract). XII International Congress of Nutrition. San Diego, California: 1981: 47.

(35) Atkins E. Molecular structures of polysaccharides and their effect on gelation behaviour (abstract). Cereal Foods World 1981 Sep; 26 (9): 503-4.

(36) Avery Jones F. Are fibre supplements really necessary in diverticular disease of the colon (letter). Br Med J 1981 May 30; 282 (6278): 1792.

(37) Avery Jones F, Heaton KW, Eastwood MA, Parks TG, Burkitt DP, Howard A, Thornton JR, Plumley P, Van Itallie TB, Bushnell L, Southgate DA, Godding E, Ornstein MH, Brodribb AJ, Mitchell KG, Hill M, Jenkins DJ. Discussion. In: McLean Baird I, Ornstein MH, eds. Dietary fibre: progress towards the future. Proceedings of a symposium held at the Royal College of Physicians, London. Manchester, England: Kellogg Company of Great Britain Ltd, 1981: 81-8.

(38) Aykut M, Baysal A. Evaluation of protein requirements for women consuming usual Turkish diets (abstract). XII International Congress of Nutrition. San Diego, California: 1981: 112.

(39) Baekey P, Baig MM, Burgin CW, Cerda JJ. The effect of pectin on zinc and calcium absorption and turnover in rat (abstract). Am J Clin Nutr 1981 Apr; 34 (4): 632.

(40) Bagheri SM, Gueguen L. Influence of wheat bran diets containing unequal amounts of calcium, magnesium, phosphorus and zinc upon the absorption of these minerals in rats. Nutr Rep Int 1981 Jul; 24 (1): 47-56.

(41) Baig MM, Cerda JJ. Pectin: its interaction with serum lipoproteins. Am J Clin Nutr 1981 Jan; 34 (1): 50-3.

(42) Baig MM, Cerda JJ. Reply to letter by Judd and Leeds (letter). Am J Clin Nutr 1981 Nov; 34 (11): 2602.

(43) Baig MM, Burgin CW, Cerda JJ. Selective in vitro interaction of rhamnose rich citrus pectic polysaccharide with low density lipoprotein (abstract). Fed Proc 1981 Mar 1; 40 (3 Pt II): 846.

(44) Baker D. Notes on the neutral detergent fiber method. In: James WP, Theander O, eds. The analysis of dietary fiber in food. New York and Basel: Marcel Dekker Inc, 1981: 159-62. (Basic and clinical nutrition; vol 3.)

(45) Baker D. Rapid determination of fiber in cereals (abstract). Cereal Foods World 1981 Sep; 26 (9): 492.

(46) Baker D, Holden JM. Fiber in breakfast cereals. J Food Sci 1981 Mar-Apr; 46 (2): 396-8.

(47) Balters SK, Kies C, Fox HM. Lipid utilization of human adults as affected by dietary bran supplementation. Nutr Res 1981; 1 (4): 339-47.

(48) Banwell JG, Branch W, Cummings JH. The microbial mass in the human large intestine (abstract). Gastroenterology 1981 May; 80 (5 Pt 2): 1104.

(49) Barbosa CF, Jokl L. Effect of fiber-rich diet formulation on intestinal alkaline phosphatase and on cecum weight of growing rat (abstract). XII International Congress of Nutrition. San Diego, California: 1981: 48.

(50) Barker DJ, Liggins A. Acute appendicitis in nine British towns. Br Med J 1981 Oct 24; 283 (6299): 1083-5.

(51) Barker P, Black M, Arthur J, Farrell D. Effects of fluoride, dietary phosphate, wholemeal and white flour on the incidence of dental caries in growing rats (abstract). Proc Nutr Soc Aust 1981; 6: 103.

(52) Barta ES, Branern AL, Leung HK. Nutritional analysis of Puget Sound kelp (Nereocystis luetkeana). J Food Sci 1981 Mar-Apr; 46 (2): 494-7.

(53) Batchelor AJ, Compston JE. Effects of high fibre diet and intestinal malabsorption on the plasma half-life of 25-hydroxyvitamin D3 (abstract). Gut 1981 Oct; 22 (10): A867-8.

(54) Bauer HG, Asp N-G, Dahlqvist A, Fredlund PE, Nyman M, Oste R. Effects of two kinds of pectin and guar gum on 1,2-dimethylhydrazine initiation of colon tumors and on fecal β-glucuronidase activity in the rat. Cancer Res 1981 Jun; 41 (6): 2518-23.

(55) Beames RM, Eggum BO. The effect of type and level of protein, fibre and starch on nitrogen excretion patterns in rats. Br J Nutr 1981 Sep; 46 (2): 301-13.

(56) Bell EW, Emken EA, Klevay LM, Sandstead HH. Effects of dietary fiber from wheat, corn, and soyhull bran on excretion of fecal bile acids in humans. Am J Clin Nutr 1981 Jun; 34 (6): 1071-6.

(57) Belo PS Jr, de Lumen BO, Pectic substance content of detergent-extracted dietary fibers. J Agric Food Chem 1981 Mar-Apr; 29 (2): 370-3.

(58) Bender AE, Refined foods. Bibl Nutr Dieta 1981; (30): 160-5.

(59) Bender AE. Low digestibility of legumes in rats (abstract). XII International Congress of Nutrition. San Diego, California: 1981:70.

(60) Berry-Lortsch E, Sable-Amplis R. Qualitative and quantitative changes in biliary secretion induced by apple consumption in hamsters. Nutr Rep Int 1981 Mar; 23 (3): 505-16.

(61) Bertrand D, Brillouet JM, Rasper VF, Bouchet B, Mercier C. Effects of rat digestion upon native, enzymically or chemically modified wheat brans and native oat bran. Cereal Chem 1981 Sep-Oct; 58 (5): 375-80.

(62) Betschart AA, Saunders RM, Gumbmann MR, Hudson CA, Fleming S. Gnotobiotic studies on protein and total digestibility of wheat brans (abstract). XII International Congress of Nutrition. San Diego, California: 1981: 51.

(63) Bhat CM, Godara RB, Kaur AP. Effect of cellulose supplementation on bowel behaviour, blood glucose and serum protein levels. Indian J Nutr Diet 1981 May; 18 (5): 171-7.

(64) Bingham S, McNeil NI, Cummings JH. The diet of individuals: a study of a randomly-chosen cross section of British adults in a Cambridgeshire village. Br J Nutr 1981 Jan; 45 (1): 23-35.

(65) Bingham S, Cummings JH, Englyst H, James WP, Wiggins HS, Seppanen R, Helms
      P, Jensen O. Dietary fibre intake in relation to colon cancer incidence (abstract).
      XII International Congress of Nutrition. San Diego, California: 1981:11

(66) Bingham S, Cummings JH, McNeil NI. Diet for the ileostomist (abstract). XII
      International Congress of Nutrition. San Diego, California: 1981: 162.

(67) Bishawi K, Pubols MH, McGinnis J. Effects of guar gum on chick growth, carcass
      analysis and nutrient retention (abstract). XII International Congress of Nutrition.
      San Diego, California: 1981: 49.

(68) Black D, Tadesse K, Heaton KW, Stephen AM, Eastwood MA, Cole J, Brodribb
      AJ, Mann J, McLean Baird I, Englyst H, Turner M, Godding EW, Fisher N, Southgate
      D, Littlewood ER, Reinstein J, Hamilton WD, Avery-Jones F. Discussion. In:
      McLean Baird I, Ornstein MH, eds. Dietary fibre: progress towards the future.
      Proceedings of a symposium held at the Royal College of Physicians, London.
      Manchester, England: Kellogg Company of Great Britain Ltd, 1981: 25-32.

(69) Blackburn NA, Johnson IT. The effect of a guar gum on the viscosity of the gastrointestinal
      contents and on glucose uptake from the perfused jejunum in the rat. Br J Nutr
      1981 Sep; 46 (2): 239-46.

(70) Blacklock N. Part II. Environmental factors of certain diseases. Renal stone. In:
      Trowell HC, Burkitt DP, eds. Western diseases: their emergence and prevention.
      London: Edward Arnold, 1981: 60-70.

(71) Bloom SR. Treatment of dumping (letter). Lancet 1981 May 30; 1 (8231): 1209.

(72) Blumberg L. Acute appendicitis and diet (letter). S Afr Med J 1981 Oct 24; 60
      (17): 648.

(73) Bolin HR. Rheological properties of prune juice. J Food Sci 1981 May-Jun; 46 (3):
      886-8.

(74) Bollard J, Tasman-Jones C. The effect of dietary fiber on rat small intestine
      morphology (abstract). XII International Congress of Nutrition. San Diego,
      California: 1981: 51.

(75) Bolton RP, Heaton KW, Burroughs LF. The role of dietary fibre in satiety, glucose,
      and insulin: studies with fruit and fruit juice. Am J Clin Nutr 1981 Feb; 34 (2):
      211-7.

(76) Botha AP, Steyn AF, Esterhuysen AJ, Slabbert M. Glycosylated haemoglobin, blood
      glucose and serum cholesterol levels in diabetics treated with guar gum. S Afr Med J
      1981 Mar 7; 59 (10): 333-4.

(77) Botha AP. Glycosylated haemoglobin, blood glucose and serum cholesterol levels
      in diabetics treated with guar gum (letter). S Afr Med J 1981 May 16; 59 (21): 740.

(78) Braddock RJ, Crandall PG. A research note. Carboyhydrate fiber from orange
      albedo. J Food Sci 1981 Mar-Apr; 46 (2): 651-2, 654.

(79) Brauer PM, Slavin JL, Marlett JA. Apparent digestibility of neutral detergent fiber
      in elderly and young adults. Am J Clin Nutr 1981 Jun; 34 (6): 1061-70.

(80) Brillouet J-M, Treche S, Sealy L. Alterations in cell wall constituents of yams
      Dioscorea dumetorum and D. rotundata with maturation and storage conditions.
      Relation with post-harvest hardening of D. dumetorum yam tubers. J Food Sci
      1981 Nov-Dec; 46 (6): 1964-5, 1967.

(81) Brillouet J-M, Mercier C. Fractionation of wheat bran carbohydrates. J Sci Food
      Agric 1981 Mar; 32 (3): 243-51.

(82) Brodribb J. Are fibre supplements really necessary in diverticular disease of the
      colon (letter). Br Med J 1981 May 30; 282 (6278): 1792.

(83) Brodribb J. Are fibre supplements really necessary in diverticular disease of the
      colon (letter). Br Med J 1981 Aug 8; 283 (6288): 438.

(84) Brodribb AJ. Does fibre affect the colon? Recent primate experimental research.
      In: McLean Baird I, Ornstein MH, eds. Dietary fibre: progress towards the future.
      Proceedings of a symposium held at the Royal College of Physicians, London.
      Manchester, England: Kellogg Company of Great Britain Ltd, 1981: 21-4.

(85) Brooks RR, Fang Pong S. Effects of fasting, body weight, methylcellulose, and carboxymethylcellulose on hepatic glutathione levels in mice and hamsters. Biochem Pharmacol 1981 Mar 15; 30 (6): 589-94.

(86) Brussaard JH, van Raaij JM, Stasse-Wolthuis M, Katan MB, Hautvast JG. Blood pressure and diet in normotensive volunteers: absence of an effect of dietary fiber, protein or fat. Am J Clin Nutr 1981 Oct; 34 (10): 2023-9.

(87) Bueno L, Praddaude F, Fioramonti J, Ruckebusch Y. Effect of dietary fiber on gastrointestinal motility and jejunal transit time in dogs. Gastroenterology 1981 Apr; 80 (4): 701-7.

(88) Burdaspal PA, Legarda TM, Velez F, Pinilla I. Chemical methods in routine control of fiber content in foods crude fiber — dietary fiber value and its significance (abstract). XII International Congress of Nutrition. San Diego, California: 1981: 48.

(89) Burkitt DP. Hiatus hernia: is it preventable? Am J Clin Nutr 1981 Mar; 34 (3): 428-31.

(90) Burkitt D. Diet and disease. Ir Med J 1981 Feb; 74 (2): 36-8.

(91) Burkitt DP. The protective properties of dietary fiber. NC Med J 1981 Jul; 42 (7): 467-71.

(92) Burkitt D. No relation of sigmoid volvulus to fiber content of African diet (letter). N Engl J Med 1981 Apr 9; 304 (15): 914.

(93) Burkitt D. Part I. Emergence of Western diseases in Sub-Saharal Africans. Surgical diseases of the large bowel and other related diseases. In: Trowell HC, Burkitt DP, eds. Western diseases: their emergence and prevention. London: Edward Arnold, 1981: 33-43.

(94) Burkitt R. Are fibre supplements really necessary in diverticular disease of the colon (letter). Br Med J 1981 May 9; 282 (6275): 1546.

(95) Burr ML, Bates CJ, Fehily AM, St Leger AS. Plasma cholesterol and blood pressure in vegetarians. J Hum Nutr 1981 Dec; 35 (6): 437-41.

(96) Camire AL, Clydesdale FM. Effect of pH and heat treatment on the binding of calcium, magnesium, zinc, and iron to wheat bran and fractions of dietary fiber. J Food Sci 1981 Mar-Apr; 46 (2): 548-51.

(97) Capron J-P, Piperaud R, Dupas J-L, Delamarre J, Lorriaux A. Evidence for an association between cholelithiasis and diverticular disease of the colon. A case-controlled study. Dig Dis Sci 1981 Jun; 26 (6): 523-7.

(98) Carroll DG, Dykes V, Hodgson W. Guar gum is not a panacea in diabetes management. NZ Med J 1981 May 13; 93 (683): 292-4.

(99) Cassidy MM, Lightfoot FG, Grau LE, Story JA, Kritchevsky D, Vahouny GV. Effect of chronic intake of dietary fibers on the ultrastructural topography of rat jejunum and colon: a scanning electron microscopy study. Am J Clin Nutr 1981 Feb; 34 (2): 218-28.

(100) Chan HT Jr, Tam SY, Seo ST. Papaya polygalacturonase and its role in thermally injured ripening fruit. J Food Sci 1981 Jan-Feb; 46 (1): 190-1, 197.

(101) Chang ML. Dietary pectin and fecal excretion of cholesterol esters in rats fed cholesterol diet (abstract). Fed Proc 1981 Mar 1; 40 (3 Pt II): 845.

(102) Chavan JK, Kadam SS, Salunkhe DK. A research note. Changes in tannin, free amino acids, reducing sugars, and starch during seed germination of low and high tannin cultivars of sorghum. J Food Sci 1981 Mar-Apr; 46 (2): 638-9.

(103) Chen ML, Chang SC, Guoo JY. Fiber contents of Chinese vegetables and their in vitro binding capacity of bile acids (abstract). XII International Congress of Nutrition. San Diego, California: 1981: 50.

(104) Chen W-J, Anderson JW. Soluble and insoluble plant fiber in selected cereals and vegetables. Am J Clin Nutr 1981 Jun; 34 (6): 1077-82.

(105) Chen W-J, Anderson JW, Gould MR. Cholesterol-lowering effects of oat bran and oat gum (abstract). Fed Proc 1981 Mar 1; 40 (3 Pt II): 853.

(106) Chen W-J, Anderson JW, Gould MR. Effects of oat bran, oat gum and pectin on lipid metabolism of cholesterol-fed rats. Nutr Rep Int 1981 Dec; 24 (6): 1093-8.

(107) Cherry JP. Protein-polysaccharide interactions in functionally (abstract). Cereal Foods World 1981 Sep; 26 (9): 504.

(108) Christianson DD, Hodge JE, Osborne D, Detroy RW. Gelatinization of wheat starch as modified by xanthan gum, guar gum, and cellulose gum. Cereal Chem 1981 Nov-Dec; 58 (6): 513-7.

(109) Clark CG, Godfrey J. Constipation — a simple approach to treatment. J R Coll Gen Pract 1981 Jan; 31 (222): 38-40.

(110) Collins JL, Post AR. Peanut hull flour as a potential source of dietary fiber. J Food Sci 1981 Mar-Apr; 46 (2): 445-8, 451.

(111) Cornu A, Delpeuch F. Effect of fiber in sorghum on nitrogen digestibility. Am J Clin Nutr 1981 Nov; 34 (11): 2454-9.

(112) Correa P. Epidemiological correlations between diet and cancer frequency. Cancer Res 1981 Sep; 41 (9 Pt 2): 3685-90.

(113) Coulston A, Greenfield MS, Kraemer FB, Tobey TA, Reaven GM. Effect of differences in source of dietary carbohydrate on plasma glucose and insulin responses to meals in patients with impaired carbohydrate tolerance. Am J Clin Nutr 1981 Dec; 34 (12): 2716-20.

(114) Cousins BW, Tanksley TD Jr, Knabe DA, Zebrowska T. Nutrient digestibility and performance of pigs fed sorghums varying in tannin concentration. J Anim Sci 1981 Dec; 53 (6): 1524-37.

(115) Crapo PA, Insel J, Sperling M, Kolterman OG. Comparison of serum glucose, insulin, and glucagon responses to different types of complex carbohydrate in noninsulin-dependent diabetic patients. Am J Clin Nutr 1981 Feb; 34 (2): 184-90.

(116) Cruz AF, Jokl L. Effect of feeding a wheat bran-rich diet to alloxan diabetic and normal adult rats (abstract). XII International Congress of Nutrition. San Diego, California: 1981: 47.

(117) Cummings JH. Dietary fibre. Br Med Bull 1981 Jan; 37 (1): 65-70.

(118) Cummings JH. Mineral metabolism — how does dietary fibre affect it? In: McLean Baird I, Ornstein MH, eds. Dietary fibre: progress towards the future. Proceedings of a symposium held at the Royal College of Physicians, London. Manchester, England: Kellogg Company of Great Britain Ltd, 1981: 45-6.

(119) Cummings JH. Progress report. Short chain fatty acids in the human colon. Gut 1981 Sep; 22 (9): 763-79.

(120) Cummings JH. Dietary fibre and large bowel cancer. Proc Nutr Soc 1981 Jan; 40 (1): 7-14.

(121) Dabestani A, Aliabadi P, Dehdashti Shah-Rookh F, Borhanmanesh FA. Prevalence of colonic diverticular disease in Southern Iran. Dis Colon Rectum 1981 Jul-Aug; 24 (5): 385-7.

(122) Daley JM, Leeds AR. Effects of dietary fiber (letter). Gastroenterology 1981 Jun; 80 (6): 1611.

(123) D'Appolonia BL, Ciacco C. Structure and function of wheat pentosans (abstract). Cereal Foods World 1981 Sep; 26 (9): 504.

(124) Davies JN, Hobson GE. The constituents of tomato fruit — the influence of environment, nutrition and genotype. CRC Crit Rev Food Sci Nutr 1981 Nov; 15 (3): 205-280.

(125) Davis V, Matthews J, Reeves RD. Effect of dietary fiber and carbohydrate source on glucose tolerance, serum insulin and hepatic lipogenic enzyme activity (abstract). Fed Proc 1981 Mar 1; 40 (3 Pt II): 846.

(126) DeFouw CL, Zabik ME, Uebersax MA. Effect of heat treatment and level of navy bean hulls in sugar-snap cookies (abstract). Cereal Foods World 1981 Sep; 26 (9): 485.

(127) Dekker J, Palmer JK. Enzymatic degradation of the plant cell wall by a Bacteroides of human fecal origin. J Agric Food Chem 1981 May-Jun; 29 (3): 480-4.

(128) Delorme CB, Wojcik J, Gordon C. Method of addition of cellulose to experimental diets and its effect on rat growth and protein utilization. J Nutr 1981 Sep; 111 (9): 1522-7.

(129) deLumen BO, Reyes PS, Chiu D, Lubin B, Omaye ST. Effect of dietary pectin on the bioavailability of vitamin E in rats (abstract). Fed Proc 1981 Mar 1; 40 (3 Pt II): 893.

(130) Dempster JG. Contact dermatitis from bran and oats. Contact Dermatitis 1981 Mar; 7 (2): 122.

(131) DHSS. Nutritional aspects of bread and flour. Report of the panel on bread, flour and other cereal products. Committee on medical aspects of food policy. London: HMSO, 1981. (Report on health and social subjects; no 23.)

(132) Diehl HA, Mannerburg D. Part VII. Regression of certain Western diseases. Hypertension, hyperlipidaemia, angina and coronary heart disease. In: Trowell HC, Burkitt DP, eds. Western diseases: their emergence and prevention. London: Edward Arnold, 1981: 392-410.

(133) Dilawari JB, Kamath PS, Batta RP, Mukewar S, Raghavan S. Reduction of post-prandial plasma glucose by Bengal gram dal (Cicer arietinum) and Rajmah (Phaseolus vulgaris). Am J Clin Nutr 1981 Nov; 34 (11): 2450-3.

(134) Dintzis FR, Harris CC. Starch determination in some dietary fiber sources. Cereal Chem 1981 Sep-Oct; 58 (5): 467-70.

(135) Dodson PM, Stocks J, Holdsworth G, Galton DJ. High-fibre and low-fat diets in diabetes mellitus. Br J Nutr 1981 Sep; 46 (2): 289-94.

(136) Dodson PM, Humphreys DM, Patrick O, Cox EV. Dietary fibre, sodium, and blood pressure (abstract). Proc Nutr Soc 1981 May; 40 (3): 42A.

(137) Dodson PM, Humphreys DM. Part VII. Regression of certain Western diseases. Hypertension and angina. In: Trowell HC, Burkitt DP, eds. Western diseases: their emergence and prevention. London: Edward Arnold, 1981: 411-20.

(138) Doll R, Armstrong B. Part II. Environmental factors of certain diseases. Cancer. In: Trowell HC, Burkitt DP, eds. Western diseases: their emergence and prevention. London: Edward Arnold, 1981: 93-110.

(139) Douglas SG. A rapid method for the determination of pentosans in wheat flour. Food Chem 1981 Sep; 7 (2): 139-45.

(140) Doyle RB, Wolfman M, Vargo D, Floch MH. Alteration in bacterial flora induced by dietary pectin (abstract). Am J Clin Nutr 1981 Apr; 34 (4): 635.

(141) Dreyer JJ, Wehmeyer AS, de Klerk WA, van der Walt WH, Mahon EH. Indigestible dry matter (IDM) determination with caecectomized rats (abstract). XII International Congress of Nutrition. San Diego, California: 1981: 94.

(142) Dryden PA, Read RS, Kestin M, Jones GP, Burcher E, McLennan E. The effect of chronic ingestion of dietary fibre on the rate of absorption of glucose in rats (abstract). Proc Nutr Soc Aust 1981; 6: 160.

(143) Dunaif G, Schneeman BO. The effect of dietary fiber on human pancreatic enzyme activity in vitro. Am J Clin Nutr 1981 Jun; 34 (6): 1034-5.

(144) Dunaif G, Schneeman BO. Effects of several sources of dietary fiber on human pancreatic enzyme activity in vitro (abstract). Fed Proc 1981 Mar 1; 40 (3 Pt II): 846.

(145) Duncan SJ, Jones GP. Dietary fibre and constipation in pre-school children (abstract). Proc Nutr Soc Aust 1981; 5: 214.

(146) Dutta SK, Bustin M, Rubin J. Effect of dietary fiber on pancreatic enzymes and fat malabsorption in pancreatic insufficiency (abstract). Gastroenterology 1981 May; 80 (5 Pt 2): 1139.

(147) Earp CF, Akingbala JO, Ring SH, Rooney LW. Evaluation of several methods to determine tannins in sorghums with varying kernel characteristics. Cereal Chem 1981 May-Jun; 58 (3): 234-8.

(148) Eastwood MA. Uses and abuses of fibre. In: McLean Baird I, Ornstein MH, eds. Dietary fibre: progress towards the future. Proceedings of a symposium held at the Royal College of Physicians, London. Manchester, England: Kellogg Company of Great Britain Ltd, 1981: 77-80.

(149) Eastwood M. In vitro adsorption of bile acids by lignin or by charcoal (letter). Lancet 1981 Jul 18; 2 (8238): 150.

(150) Ebihara K, Masuhara R, Kiriyama S. Effect of konjac mannan, a water-soluble dietary fiber on plasma glucose and insulin responses in young men undergoing glucose tolerance test. Nutr Rep Int 1981 Apr; 23 (4): 577-83.

(151) Ebihara K, Masuhara R, Kiriyama S, Manabe M. Correlation between viscosity and plasma glucose- and insulin-flattening activities of pectins from vegetables and fruits in rats. Nutr Rep Int 1981 May; 23 (5): 985-92.

(152) Ebihara K, Kiriyama S. Increase in protective activity by delignification of cereal dietary fibers against amaranth toxicity in rats. Nutr Rep Int 1981 Jun; 23 (6): 1139-44.

(153) Ebihara K, Masuhara R, Kiriyama S. Major determinants of plasma glucose-flattening activity of a water-soluble dietary fiber: effects of konjac mannan on gastric emptying and intraluminal glucose-diffusion. Nutr Rep Int 1981 Jun; 23 (6): 1145-56.

(154) Ecknauer R, Sircar B, Johnson LR. Effect of dietary bulk on small intestinal morphology and cell renewal in the rat. Gastroenterology 1981 Oct; 81 (4): 781-6.

(155) Elhardallou SB. Carbohydrates of chickpea (Cicer arietinum) pigeon pea (Cajanus cajan) and Bonavist bean (Dolichos lablab) (abstract). XII International Congress of Nutrition. San Diego, California: 1981: 69.

(156) Elliott J, Mulvihill E, Duncan C, Forsythe R, Kritchevsky D. Effects of tomato pomace and mixed-vegetable pomace on serum and liver cholesterol in rats. J Nutr 1981 Dec; 111 (12): 2203-11.

(157) Ellis PR, Apling EC, Leeds AR, Bolster NR. Guar bread: acceptability and efficacy combined. Studies on blood glucose, serum insulin and satiety in normal subjects. Br J Nutr 1981 Sep; 46 (2): 267-76.

(158) Ellis PR, Apling EC, Leeds AR. The satiating effect of guar bread (abstract). XII International Congress of Nutrition. San Diego, California: 1981: 69.

(159) Ellis R, Morris ER. Relation between phytic acid and trace metals in wheat bran and soybean. Cereal Chem 1981 Sep-Oct; 58 (5): 367-70.

(160) Elsenhans B, Blume R, Caspary WF. Long-term feeding of unavailable carbohydrate gelling agents. Influence of dietary concentration and microbiological degradation on adaptive responses in the rat. Am J Clin Nutr 1981 Sep; 34 (9): 1837-48.

(161) Elsenhans B, Sufke U, Blume R, Caspary WF. In vitro inhibition of rat intestinal surface hydrolysis of disaccharides and dipeptides by guaran. Digestion 1981; 21 (2): 98-103.

(162) Emiola LO, de la Rosa LC. Characterization of pearl millet nonstarchy polysaccharides. J Food Sci 1981 May-Jun; 46 (3): 781-5.

(163) Englyst H. Determination of carbohydrate and its composition in plant materials. In: James WP, Theander O, eds. The analysis of dietary fiber in food. New York and Basel: Marcel Dekker Inc, 1981: 71-93. (Basic and clinical nutrition; vol 3.)

(164) Englyst H. What is dietary fibre? New methods of chemical analysis. In: McLean Baird I, Ornstein MH, eds. Dietary fibre: progress towards the future. Proceedings of a symposium held at the Royal College of Physicians, London. Manchester, England: Kellogg Company of Great Britain Ltd, 1981: 5-11.

(165) Erdman JW Jr. Bioavailability of trace minerals from cereals and legumes. Cereal Chem 1981 Jan-Feb; 58 (1): 21-6.

(166) Eshchar J, Cohen L. Re-education of constipated patients — a non-medicinal treatment. Am J Proctol Gastroenterol Colon Rectal Surg 1981 Sep; 32 (9): 16-7, 24.

(167) Fairweather-Tait S. The effect of different levels of wheat bran on iron absorption by rats from bread containing similar amounts of phytate (abstract). XII International Congress of Nutrition. San Diego, California: 1981: 55.

(168) Faraji B, Reinhold JG, Abadi P. Human studies of iron absorption from fiber-rich Iranian flat breads. Nutr Rep Int 1981 Feb; 23 (2): 267-78.

(169) Faturoti EO, Tewe OO, Ajayi SS. Performance of the African giant rat (Cricetomys gambianus Waterhouse) on varying dietary crude fibre levels. Nutr Rep Int 1981 Oct; 24 (4): 707-15.

(170) Faturoti EO, Tewe OO, Ajayi SS. Nutrient digestibility and utilization by the African giant rat (Cricetomys gambianus Waterhouse) on varying crude fibre levels. Nutr Rep Int 1981 Oct; 24 (4): 717-29.

(171) Faubion JM. A mechanism for the oxidative gelation of wheat flour water soluble pentosans (abstract). Cereal Foods World 1981 Sep; 26 (9): 495.

(172) Fleming SE. A study of relationships between flatus potential and carbohydrate distribution in legume seeds. J Food Sci 1981 May-Jun; 46 (3): 794-8, 803.

(173) Floch MH. Fiber and the intestinal microflora. In: Nutrition and diet therapy in gastrointestinal disease. New York: Plenum Press, 1981: 83-99.

(174) Foo LY, Porter LJ. The structure of tannins of some edible fruits. J Sci Food Agric 1981 Jul; 32 (7): 711-6.

(175) Forman LP, Schneeman BO. Dietary pectin's effect on starch absorpt:on and utilization (abstract). Fed Proc 1981 Mar 1; 40 (3 Pt II): 853.

(176) Foy WL Jr, Evans JL, Wohlt JE. Detergent fiber analyses on thirty foodstuffs ingested by man. Nutr Rep Int 1981 Sep; 24 (3): 575-80.

(177) Frape DL, Wayman BJ, Tuck MG. The effect of dietary fibre sources on aflatoxicosis in the weanling male rat. Br J Nutr 1981 Sep; 46 (2): 315-26.

(178) Fraser GE, Jacobs DR Jr, Anderson JT, Foster N, Palta M, Blackburn H. The effect of various vegetable supplements on serum cholesterol. Am J Clin Nutr 1981 Jul; 34 (7): 1272-7.

(179) Friedlander ML, Gelfand M. Acute appendicitis, an urban disease in Africans. Trop Doct 1981 Jan; 11 (1): 22-3.

(180) Frolich W, Asp N-G. Reply to letter by Reinhold (letter). Am J Clin Nutr 1981 Aug; 34 (8): 1630.

(181) Frolich W, Asp N-G. Dietary fiber content in cereals in Norway. Cereal Chem 1981 Nov-Dec; 58 (6): 524-7.

(182) Fulcher RG, O'Brien TP, Wong SI. Microchemical detection of niacin, aromatic amine, and phytin reserves in cereal bran. Cereal Chem 1981 Mar-Apr; 58 (2): 130-5.

(183) Furda I. Simultaneous analysis of soluble and insoluble dietary fiber. In: James WP, Theander O, eds. The analysis of dietary fiber in food. New York and Basel: Marcel Dekker Inc, 1981: 163-72. (Basic and clinical nutrition; vol 3.)

(184) Russell SI, Oace SM. Hemoglobin response to ferrous suplhate in rats fed pectin or cellulose (abstract). XII International Congress of Nutrition. San Diego, California: 1981: 49.

(185) Garcia E, Reyes PS, Briggs GM. The effects of a plant fiber mix on caffeine toxicity in weanling rats (abstract). Fed Proc 1981 Mar 1; 40 (3 Pt II): 846.

(186) Garcia-L SJ, Wyatt CJ. The effect of fiber on bioavailability of iron from corn tortillas and cooked beans (abstract). XII International Congress of Nutrition. San Diego, California: 1981: 111.

(187) Gear JS, Brodribb AJ, Ware A, Mann JI. Fibre and bowel transit times. Br J Nutr 1981 Jan; 45 (1): 77-82.

(188) Gelfand M. Part IV. Peasant agriculturalists. Zimbabwe. In: Trowell HC, Burkitt DP, eds. Western diseases: their emergence and prevention. London: Edward Arnold, 1981: 194-203.

(189) Gibson RS, Anderson BM. The trace element status of long-term vegetarian women (abstract). XII International Congress of Nutrition. San Diego, California: 1981: 152.

(190) Giri J, Parvatham R, Santhini K. Effect of germination on the levels of pectins, phytins and minerals in three selected legumes. Indian J Nutr Diet 1981 Mar; 18 (3): 87-91.

(191) Glauert HP, Bennink MR. Influence of diet, intrarectal bile acid injections, and 1, 2-dimethylhydrazine (DMH) on rat colon epithelial cell proliferation (abstract). Fed Proc 1981 Mar 1; 40 (3 Pt II): 929.

(192) Glauert HP, Bennink MR, Sander CH. Enhancement of 1, 2-dimethylhydrazine-induced colon carcinogenesis in mice by dietary agar. Food Cosmet Toxicol 1981 Jun; 19 (3): 281-6.

(193) Glober GA, Stemmermann GN. Part V. Migrants and mixed ethnic groups. Hawaii ethnic groups. In: Trowell HC, Burkitt DP, eds. Western diseases: their emergence and prevention. London: Edward Arnold, 1981: 319-333.

(194) Godara R, Kaur AP, Bhat CM. Effect of cellulose incorporation in a low fiber diet on fecal excretion and serum levels of calcium, phosphorus, and iron in adolescent girls. Am J Clin Nutr 1981 Jun; 34 (6): 1083-6.

(195) Goel R, Verma J. Removal of flatulence factor of some pulses by microbial fermentation. Indian J Nutr Diet 1981 Jun; 18 (6): 215-7.

(196) Gormley R. Dietary fibre — some properties of alcohol-insoluble solids residues from apples. J Sci Food Agric 1981 Apr; 32 (4): 392-8.

(197) Graham HD, Negron de Bravo E. Composition of the breadfruit. J Food Sci 1981 Mar-Apr; 46 (2): 535-9.

(198) Graham S, Mettlin C. Fiber and other constituents of vegetables in cancer epidemiology. In: Newell GR, Ellison NM, eds. Nutrition and cancer: etiology and treatment. New York: Raven Press, 1981: 189-215. (Progress in cancer research and therapy; vol 17.)

(199) Graham SL, Arnold A, Kasza L, Ruffin GE, Jackson RC, Watkins TL, Graham CH. Subchronic effects of guar gum in rats. Food Cosmet Toxicol 1981 Jun; 19 (3): 287-90.

(200) Greenbaum DS, Stein GE. Psyllium and the irritable bowel syndrome (letter). Ann Intern Med 1981 Nov; 95 (5): 660.

(201) Griffith HM, O'Shea B, Kevany JP, McCormick JS. A control study of dietary factors in renal stone formation. Br J Urol 1981 Oct; 53 (5): 416-20.

(202) Griffiths DW. The polyphenolic content and enzyme inhibitory activity of testas from bean (Vicia faba) and pea (Pisum spp.) varieties. J Sci Food Agric 1981 Aug; 32 (8): 797-804.

(203) Gueguen L, Bagheri S, Rerat A. Influence of wheat bran on the interstinal absorption of minerals in the growing pig. Role of the hind gut (abstract). XII International Congress of Nutrition. San Diego, California: 1981: 51.

(204) Guild R, Baig M, Burgin C, Cerda J. Absorption and distribution of orally administered radiolabeled pectin in the mouse (abstract). Gastroenterology 1981 May; 80 (5 Pt 2): 1165.

(205) Hallgren B. The role of dietary fibre in food. In: Aebi HE, Brubacher GB, Turner MR, eds. Problems in nutrition research today. London: Academic Press, 1981: 75-84.

(206) Hallmans G, Nygren C, Berglund O, Taljedal I-B. Effect of bran on the development of hereditary diabetes in mice (abstract). XII International Congress of Nutrition. San Diego, California: 1981: 51.

(207) Harbers LH, Arambel MJ, Bartley EE. Cohesive characteristics of cerium as an inert marker of fibrous feedstuffs. Nutr Rep Int 1981 Nov; 24 (5): 1029-35.

(208) Harbers LH, Arambel MJ, Bartley EE. Cohesive characteristics of dyprosium as an inert marker of feedstuffs. Nutr Rep Int 1981 Dec; 24 (6): 1271-7.

(209) Harland BF, Harwood JP, Prosky L. Nutritional assessment and biomedical importance of dietary fiber (abstract). Cereal Foods World 1981 Sep; 26 (9): 493.

(210) Harrison SL, Konishi F. Acceptability of foods containing a tofu (soy curd)-with-fiber product (abstract). XII International Congress of Nutrition. San Diego, California: 1981: 47.

(211) Heaton KW. Is bran useful in diverticular disease? Br Med J 1981 Dec 5; 283 (6305): 1523-4.

(212) Heaton KW. Inflammatory bowel disease — what is the place of refined carbohydrate and dietary fibre? In: McLean Baird I, Ornstein MH, eds. Dietary fibre: progress towards the future. Proceedings of a symposium held at the Royal College of Physicians, London. Manchester, England: Kellogg Company of Great Britain Ltd: 59-64.

(213) Heaton KW, Hartog M, Manhire A, Henry CL. Dietary fibre and diabetes (letter). Lancet 1981 May 23; 1 (8230): 1157.

(214) Heaton K. Part II. Environmental factors of certain diseases. Gallstones. In: Trowell HC, Burkitt DP, eds. Western diseases: their emergence and prevention. London: Edward Arnold, 1981: 47-59.

(215) Heckman MM, Lane SA. Comparison of dietary fiber methods for foods. J Assoc Off Anal Chem 1981 Nov; 64 (6): 1339-43.

(216) Hellendoorn EW. Dietary fiber or indigestible residue (letter). Am j Clin Nutr 1981 Jul; 34 (7): 1437-9.

(217) Herranz J, Vidal-Valverde C, Rojas-Hidalgo E. Cellulose, hemicellulose and lignin content of raw and cooked Spanish vegetables. J Food Sci 1981 Nov-Dec; 46 (6): 1927-33.

(218) Hirono I, Sumi Y, Kuhara K, Miyakawa M. Effect of degraded carrageenan on the intestine in germfree rats. Toxicol Lett 1981 Jun-Jul; 8 (4-5): 207-12.

(219) Holt S, Heading RC, Clements J. Effects of dietary fiber (letter). Gastroenterology 1981 Jun; 80 (6): 1611-2.

(220) Holtzapple PG, Schwartz SE, Starr CM, Bachman S. Effect of chronic pectin ingestion on intestinal cholesterol metabolism in rats (abstract). Gastroenterology 1981 May; 80 (5 Pt 2): 1179.

(221) Hopkins J. Carcinogenicity of carrageenan (news). Food Cosmet Toxicol 1981 Dec; 19 (6): 779-81.

(222) Hunt PS, Korman MG. Fybogel in haemorrhoid treatment (letter). Med J Aust 1981 Sep 5; 2 (5): 256, 258.

(223) Hunter JE. Iron availability and absorption in rats fed sodium phytate. J Nutr 1981 May; 111 (5): 841-7.

(224) Jacobs LR, White F, Schneeman BO. Stimulation of rat colonic mucosal cell growth by dietary wheat bran (abstract). Fed Proc 1981 Mar 1; 40 (3 Pt II): 854.

(225) Jacobs LR, White FA. Regulation of colonic mucosal cell exfoliation and synthesis by dietary wheat bran (abstract). Gastroenterology 1981 May; 80 (5 Pt 2): 1182.

(226) Jacobs LR, Schneeman BO. Effects of dietary wheat bran on rat colonic structure and mucosal cell growth. J Nutr 1981 May; 111 (5): 798-803.

(227) James WP, Theander O, eds. The analysis of dietary fiber in food. New York and Basel: Marcel Dekker Inc, 1981. (Basic and clinical nutrition; vol 3.)

(228) James WP, Southgate DA, Selvendran RR, Theander O, Van Soest P.J, Asp N-G, Schweizer TF, Koivistoinen PE, Rasper VF, Englyst H, Baker D, Menger A, Furda I, Katan MB, Fidanza F, Cummings JH. General discussion. In: James WP, Theander O, eds. The analysis of dietary fiber in food. New York and Basel: Marcel Dekker Inc, 1981: 241-62. (Basic and clinical nutrition; vol 3.)

(229) Jank J, Kies C, Fox HM. Protein nutritional status of human subjects fed wheat and rice bran supplemented diets. Nutr Rep Int 1981 Sep; 24 (3): 581-9.

(230) Jaya TV, Venkataraman LV. Changes in the carbohydrate constituents of chickpea and greengram during germination. Food Chem 1981 Sep; 7 (2): 95-104.

(231) Jenkins DJ, Wolever TM, Taylor RH, Barker H, Fielden H, Baldwin JM, Bowling AC, Newman HC, Jenkins AL, Goff DV. Glycemic index of foods: a physiological basis for carbohydrate exchange. Am J Clin Nutr 1981 Mar; 34 (3): 362-6.

(232) Jenkins DJ, Wolever TM, Taylor RH, Barker HM, Fielden H, Gassull MA. Lack of effect of refining on the glycemic response to cereals. Diabetes Care 1981 Sep-Oct; 4 (5): 509-13.

(233) Jenkins DJ. Can diabetes mellitus be treated with dietary fibre? In: McLean Baird I, Ornstein M, eds. Dietary fibre: progress towards the future. Proceedings of a symposium held at the Royal College of Physicians, London. Manchester, England: Kellogg Company of Great Britain Ltd, 1981: 36-44.

(234) Jenkins DJ. Gel-forming and other fibres in diabetes. In: Turner M, Thomas B, eds. Nutrition and diabetes. London: John Libbey, 1981: 33-40.

(235) Jenkins DJ, Wolever TM. Slow release carbohydrate and the treatment of diabetes. Proc Nutr Soc 1981 May; 40 (2): 227-35.

(236) Johanning GL, O'Dell BL. Inhibition of a cecal anaerobe by a dietary fiber component (abstract). Fed Proc 1981 Mar 1; 40 (3 Pt II): 854.

(237) Johansen K. Decreased urinary glucose excretion and plasma cholesterol level in non-insulin dependent diabetic patients with guar. Diabete Metab 1981; 7 (2): 87-90.

(238) Johnson IT, Gee JM. Effect of gel-forming gums on the intestinal unstirred layer and sugar transport in vitro. Gut 1981 May; 22 (5): 398-403.

(239) Johnson MA, Chang ML. The interaction of the dietary effect of pectin or saponin and soy lecithin on lipid metabolism in rats (abstract). Fed Proc 1981 Mar 1; 40 (3 Pt II): 845.

(240) Judd PA, Truswell AS. The effect of rolled oats on blood lipids and fecal steroid excretion in man. Am J Clin Nutr 1981 Oct; 34 (10): 2061-7.

(241) Judd PA, Leeds AR. Pectin and serum cholesterol levels (letter). Am J Clin Nutr 1981 Nov; 34 (11): 2601.

(242) Juliano BO, Pascual CG, Maningat CC, Novenario VG. Nonstarch polysaccharides of milled rice and rice bran (abstract). Cereal Foods World 1981 Sep; 26 (9): 496.

(243) Just A, Jorgensen H, Fernandez JA. The digestive capacity of the caecum-colon and the value of the nitrogen absorbed from the hindgut for protein synthesis in pigs. Br J Nutr 1981 Jul; 46 (1): 209-19.

(244) Kakande I. Varicose veins in Africans as seen at Kenyatta National Hospital, Nairobi. East Afr Med J 1981 Sep; 58 (9): 667-76.

(245) Kamat AD, Kulkarni PR. Dietary effect of non starch polysaccharides of black gram (Phaseolus mungo). J Food Sci Technol India 1981 Sep-Oct; 18 (5): 216-7.

(246) Kanamori M, Maki Z, Tashiro M, Asao T. Inhibitory specificity of rice bran trypsin inhibitor (abstract). XII International Congress of Nutrition. San Diego, California: 1981: 56.

(247) Kasper H, Reiners C, Eilles C. The influence of dietary fiber on gastric emptying in man (abstract). XII International Congress of Nutrition. San Diego, California: 1981: 85.

(248) Katan MB, van de Bovenkamp P. Determination of total dietary fiber by difference and of pectin by colorimetry or copper titration. In: James WP, Theander O, eds. The analysis of dietary fiber in food. New York and Basel: Marcel Dekker Inc, 1981: 217-39. (Basic and clinical nutrition; vol 3.)

(249) Kaur AP, Bhat CM, Godara RB. Effect of cellulose on serum lipids in adolescent girls. J Hum Nutr 1981 Dec; 35 (6): 456-8.

(250) Kay RM. Effects of diet on the fecal excretion and bacterial modification of acidic and neutral steroids, and implications for colon carcinogenesis. Cancer Res 1981 Sep; 41 (9 Pt 2): 3774-7.

(251) Kay RM, Grobin W, Track NS. Diets rich in natural fibre improve carbohydrate tolerance in maturity-onset, non-insulin dependent diabetics. Diabetologia 1981; 20 (1): 18-21.

(252) Kayisu K, Hood LF, Van Soest PJ. Characterization of starch and fiber of banana fruit. J Food Sci 1981 Nov-Dec; 46 (6): 1885-90.

(253) Keagy PM, Oace SM. Folacin bioavailability from high fiber diets in rats (abstract). Cereal Foods World 1981 Sep; 26 (9): 513.

(254) Kelley MJ, Thomas JN, Story JA. Modification of spectrum of fecal bile acids in rats by dietary fiber (abstract). Fed Proc 1981 Mar 1; 40 (3 Pt II): 845.

(255) Kellogg Company. Dietary fiber bibliography. Battle Creek M1 49016: Kellogg Company. (1981 Mar; 1 (1): 1-39.)

(256) Kelsay JL, Goering HK, Behall KM, Prather ES. Effect of fiber from fruits and vegetables on metabolic responses of human subjects: fiber intakes, fecal excretions, and apparent digestibilities. Am J Clin Nutr 1981 Sep; 34 (9): 1849-52.

(257) Kelsay JL. Effect of diet fiber level on bowel function and trace mineral balances of human subjects. Cereal Chem 1981 Jan-Feb; 58 (1): 2-5.

(258) Kelsay JL, Prather ES. Effect of fiber and oxalic acid on mineral balances of adult human subjects (abstract). Fed Proc 1981 Mar 1; 40 (3 Pt II): 854.

(259) Kelsay JL, Prather ES. Effect of length of study period on mineral balances of men consuming diets containing oxalic acid and fiber (abstract). XII International Congress of Nutrition. San Diego, California: 1981: 46.

(260) Kelsay JL, Clark WM, Herbst BJ, Prather ES. Nutrient utilization by human subjects consuming fruits and vegetables as sources of fiber. J Agric Food Chem 1981 May-Jun; 29 (3): 461-5.

(307) Lewis BA, Horvath PJ, Robertson JB, Van Soest PJ. Analysis and characterization of fiber and associated polysaccharides (abstract). Cereal Foods World 1981 Sep; 26 (9): 492.

(308) Li BW, Schuhmann PJ. GLC analysis of water soluble polysaccharides in foods (abstract). Cereal Foods World 1981 Sep; 26 (9): 492.

(309) Lindgarde F, Larsson L, Lithell H, Mattiasson I. Effect of bran on plasma lipids and release of platelet a-granule components (abstract). XII International Congress of Nutrition. San Diego, California: 1981: 112.

(310) Lindtjorn B, Breivik K, Lende S. Intestinal volvulus in Sidamo, South Ethiopia. East Afr Med J 1981 Mar; 58 (3): 208-11.

(311) Littlewood ER, Ornstein MH, McLean Baird I, Cox AG. Doubts about diverticular disease. Br Med J 1981 Dec 5; 283 (6305): 1524-6.

(312) Littlewood ER, McLean Baird I, Ornstein MH, Bartlett SM, Cox AG. How does dietary fibre produce faecal bulking? A long-term study. In: Howard AN, McLean Baird I, eds. Recent advances in clinical nutrition: I. Proceedings of the first international symposium on clinical nutrition. London: John Libbey, 1981: 104-5.

(313) London JF, Clapp NK, Henke MA. Effects of dietary bran and the colon carcinogen 1,2-dimethylhydrazine on faecal β-glucuronidase activity in mice. Food Cosmet Toxicol 1981 Dec; 19 (6): 707-11.

(314) Lonergan ME, Milne JS, Fogo M. Intakes of dietary fiber in older people in Edinburgh, Scotland (abstract). XII International Congress of Nutrition. San Diego, California: 1981: 112.

(315) Longe OG. Effect of boiling on the carbohydrate constituents of some non-leafy vegetables. Food Chem 1981 Jul; 7 (1): 1-6.

(316) Longe OG, Norton G, Lewis D. Fractionation and determination of the carbohydrate components from microbial products. J Sci Food Agric 1981 Aug; 32 (8): 813-8.

(317) Longstreth GF, Fox DB, Youkeles L, Forsythe AB, Wolochow DA. Psyllium therapy in the irritable bowel syndrome. A double-blind trial. Ann Intern Med 1981 Jul; 95 (1): 53-6.

(318) Longstreth GF. Psyllium and the irritable bowel syndrome (letter). Ann Intern Med 1981 Nov; 95 (5): 660.

(319) Longstreth GF, Fox DB, Youkeles L, Forsythe AB, Wolochow DA. Psyllium therapy in the irritable bowel syndrome (IBS) (abstract). Gastroenterology 1981 May; 80 (5 Pt 2): 1217.

(320) Low AG, Keal HD. Absence of a harmful effect of guar gum on nitrogen digestibility and balance in pigs (abstract). XII International Congress of Nutrition. San Diego, California: 1981: 56.

(321) Luderitz T, Grisebach H. Enzymic synthesis of lignin precursors. Comparison of cinnamoyl-CoA reductase and cinnamoyl alcohol: $NADP^{+}$ dehydrogenase from spruce (Picea abies L.) and soybean (Glycine max L.). Eur J Biochem 1981 Sep; 119 (1): 115-24.

(322) Madsen KO. The anticaries potential of seeds. Cereal Foods World 1981 Jan; 26 (1): 19-25.

(323) Madsen KO, Miller A. The anticaries potential of certain dietary fiber sources (abstract). XII International Congress of Nutrition. San Diego, California: 1981: 112.

(324) Maisto OE, Bremner CG. Cancer of the colon and rectum in the coloured population of Johannesburg. Relationship to diet and bowel habits. S Afr Med J 1981 Oct 10; 60 (15): 571-3.

(325) Malhotra SL. Cholecystectomy and carcinoma of the colon (letter). Lancet 1981 Oct 24; 2 (8252): 931-2.

(326) Manhire A, Henry CL, Hartog M, Heaton KW. Unrefined carbohydrate and dietary fibre in treatment of diabetes mellitus. J Hum Nutr 1981 Apr; 35 (2): 99-101.

(327) Mann JI, Simpson HC, Hockaday TD. How much carbohydrate (letter). Diabetologia 1981 Apr; 20 (4): 508-9.

(328) Mann JI, Kinmonth AL, Todd E, Angus RM, Simpson HC, Hockaday TD. High fibre diets and diabetes (letter). Lancet 1981 Mar 28; 1 (8222): 731-2.

(329) Mann JI. Wholesome diets in the management of diabetes. In: Turner M, Thomas B, eds. Nutrition and diabetes. London: John Libbey, 1981: 41-3.

(330) Marcus R, Watt J. Danger of carrageenan in foods and slimming recipes (letter). Lancet 1981 Feb 7; 1 (8215): 338.

(331) Marlett JA, Bokram RL. Relationship between calculated dietary and crude fiber intakes of 200 college students. Am J Clin Nutr 1981 Mar; 34 (3): 335-42.

(332) Marlett JA, Slavin JL, Brauer PM. Comparison of dye and pellet gastrointestinal transit time during controlled diets differing in protein and fiber levels. Dig Dis Sci 1981 Mar; 26 (3): 208-13.

(333) Marr JW, Morris JN. Dietary intake and the risk of coronary heart disease in Japanese men living in Hawaii (letter). Am J Clin Nutr 1981 Jun; 34 (6): 1156-7.

(334) Marthinsen D, Fleming SE. Effect of dietary fiber on breath and flatus gas production in humans (abstract). XII International Congress of Nutrition. San Diego, California: 1981: 53.

(335) Martinez de Prado MT, Sanchez-Muniz FJ, Katan MB, Hermus RJ. The effect of different fiber sources on the neutral steroid excretions of hypercholesterolemic casein fed rabbits. Rev Esp Fisiol 1981 Dec; 37 (4): 407-12.

(336) Mathe D, Chevallier F. Effects of dietary cholesterol, L thyroxine, and various diets on the pools and fecal elimination of bile acids in the rat. Nutr Rep Int 1981 Apr; 23 (4): 689-95.

(337) Matthews J, Wadsworth JI, Spadaro JJ. Chemical composition of starbonnet variety rice fractionated by rough-rice kernel thickness. Cereal Chem 1981 Jul-Aug; 58 (4): 331-4.

(338) Mayberry JF, Rhodes J, Allan R, Newcombe RG, Regan GM, Chamberlain LM, Wragg KG. Diet in Crohn's disease. Two studies of current and previous habits in newly diagnosed patients. Dig Dis Sci 1981 May; 26 (5): 444-8.

(339) Meier-Ploeger A, Leitzmann. Influence of different dietary fibers on blood lipids in healthy young adults (abstract). XII International Congress of Nutrition. San Diego, California: 1981: 111.

(340) Mendeloff AI. Dietary fiber, diverticular disease and the irritable bowel syndrome. In: Howard AN, McLean Baird I, eds. Recent advances in clinical nutrition: I. Proceedings of the first international symposium on clinical nutrition. London: John Libbey, 1981: 93-8.

(341) Menger A. Some contributions to the analysis of dietary fiber. In: James WP, Theander O, eds. The analysis of dietary fiber in food. New York and Basel: Marcel Dekker Inc, 1981: 191-201. (Basic and clinical nutrition; vol 3.)

(342) Mercurio KC, Behm PA. Effects of fiber type and level on mineral excretion, transit time, and intestinal histology. J Food Sci 1981 Sep-Oct; 46 (5): 1462-3, 1477.

(343) Meyer MT, Phaff HJ. An enzymatic method for the determination of yeast cell wall glucan in foods. J Food Sci 1981 Sep-Oct; 46 (5): 1489-92, 1497.

(344) Miller JD. Absorption of peanuts (letter). N Engl J Med 1981 Feb 5; 304 (6): 359.

(345) Miller LL, Setser C. Xanthan gum in a reduced egg white angel food cake (abstract). Cereal Foods World 1981 Sep; 26 (9): 492.

(346) Mirvish SS, Ghadirian P, Wallcave L, Raha C, Bronczyk S, Sams JP. Effect of diet on fecal excretion and gastrointestinal tract distribution of unmetabolized benzo(a)pyrene and 3-methylcholanthrene when these compounds are administered orally to hamsters. Cancer Res 1981 Jun; 41 (6): 2289-93.

(347) Misaki A, Ohtani K. Characterization of lectin and cotyledon cell-wall polysaccharide of tora-bean (Phaseolus vulgaris) (abstract). XII International Congress of Nutrition. San Diego, California: 1981: 52.

(348) Miski AM, Kuraydiyyah S. Effects of dietary sucrose, starch, and wheat bran on glucose tolerance in growing broiler chicks (abstract). XII International Congress of Nutrition. San Diego, California: 1981: 48.

(349) Mod RR, Ory RL, Morris NM, Normand FL. In vitro interactions of rice hemicelluloses with trace minerals and their release by digestive enzymes (abstract). Cereal Foods World 1981 Sep; 26 (9): 501.

(350) Mod RR, Ory RL, Morris NM, Normand FL. Chemical properties and interactions of rice hemicellulose with trace minerals in vitro. J Agric Food Chem 1981 May-Jun; 29 (3): 449-54.

(351) Mod RR, Normand FL, Ory RL, Conkerton EJ. Effect of hemicellulose on viscosity of rice flour. J Food Sci 1981 Mar-Apr; 46 (2): 571-3, 578.

(352) Modan B. Part V. Migrants and mixed ethnic groups. Israeli migrants. In: Trowell HC, Burkitt DP, eds. Western diseases: their emergence and prevention. London: Edward Arnold, 1981: 268-84.

(353) Moledina KH, Haydar M, Ooraikul B, Hadziyev D. Pectin changes in the pre-cooking step of dehydrated mashed potato production. J Sci Food Agric 1981 Nov; 32 (11): 1091-1102.

(354) Momcilovic B, Gruden N. The effect of dietary fibre on ^{85}Sr and ^{47}Ca absorption in infant rats. Experientia 1981 May 15; 37 (5): 498-9.

(355) Mongeau R, Brassard R. Bran particle size and fecal density in the rat (abstract). Cereal Foods World 1981 Sep; 26 (9): 513.

(356) Monis B, Rovasio RA. Teratogenic effect of lambda-carrageenan on the chick embryo. Teratology 1981 Apr; 23 (2): 273-8.

(357) Monnier LH, Blotman MJ, Colette C, Monnier MP, Mirouze J. Effects of dietary fibre supplementation in stable and labile insulin-dependent diabetics. Diabetologia 1981; 20 (1): 12-7.

(358) Monte WC. Fiber: its nutritional impact. J Appl Nutr 1981 Spr; 33 (1): 63-103.

(359) Moodie PM. Part III. Hunter-gatherers. Australian Aborigines. In: Trowell HC, Burkitt DP, eds. Western diseases their emergence and prevention. London: Edward Arnold, 1981: 154-67.

(360) Morgan KJ, Zabik ME, Leveille GA. The role of breakfast in nutrient intake of 5- to 12-year-old children. Am J Clin Nutr 1981 Jul; 34 (7): 1418-27.

(361) Moron MJ, Elias LF, Bressani R, Navarrete D, Gomez Brenes R, Molina M. Biochemical and nutritional studies of germinating soybeans (abstract). XII International Congress of Nutrition. San Diego, California: 1981: 68.

(362) Morris VJ, Chilvers GR. Rheological studies on specific ion forms of ι-carrageenate gels. J Sci Food Agric 1981 Dec; 32 (12): 1235-41.

(363) Moser SE, Graham DY, Estes MK. Comparison of corn and wheat bran in constipated women (abstract). Gastroenterology 1981 May; 80 (5 Pt 2): 1362.

(364) Mueller MA, Cleary MP, Kritchevsky D. The effect of various types of dietary fiber on lipid storage in adipose tissue (abstract). Fed Proc 1981 Mar 1; 40 (3 Pt II): 853.

(365) Muindi PJ, Thomke S, Ekman R. Effect of Magadi soda treatment on the tannin content and in-vitro nutritive value of grain sorghums. J Sci Food Agric 1981 Jan; 32 (1): 25-34.

(366) Muindi PJ, Thomke S. The nutritive value for rats of high- and low-tannin sorghums treated with Magadi soda. J Sci Food Agric 1981 Feb; 32 (2): 139-45.

(367) Murray D, Cundall RB. Fluorimetric assay of polyanions in complex fluids: carrageenan stabilisers in diary products and heparin in hog mucosa extracts. Analyst 1981 Mar; 106 (1260): 335-43.

(368) MacArthur LA, D'Appolonia BL. The nonstarchy polysaccharides of oats (abstract). Cereal Foods World 1981 Sep; 26 (9): 497.

(369) McKay LF, Brydon WG, Eastwood MA, Smith JH. The influence of pentose on breath methane. Am J Clin Nutr 1981 Dec; 34 (12): 2728-33.

(370) McKay LF, Brydon WG, Eastwood MA, Smith JH. The influence of pentose on breath methane excretion (abstract). Proc Nutr Soc 1981 May; 40 (2): 74A.

(371) McLean Baird I, Ornstein MH. Dietary fibre: progress towards the future. Proceedings of a symposium held at the Royal College of Physicians, London. Manchester, England: Kellogg Company of Great Britain Ltd, 1981.

(372) McLean Baird I, Ornstein M. The future of dietary fibre. In: McLean Baird I, Ornstein MH, eds. Dietary fibre: progress towards the future. Proceedings of a symposium held at the Royal College of Physicians, London. Manchester, England: Kellogg Company of Great Britain Ltd, 1981: 1-4.

(373) McLean Baird I, Van Itallie TB, Heaton KW, Jenkins DJ, Southgate DA, Simpson H. Discussion. In: McLean Baird I, Ornstein MH, eds. Dietary fibre: progress towards the future. Proceedings of a symposium held at the Royal College of Physicians, London. Manchester, England: Kellogg Company of Great Britain Ltd, 1981: 52-7.

(374) McLean Ross AH, McKay LF, Busuttil A, Anderson DM, Brydon WG, Eastwood MA. Gum arabic metabolism in the rat colon (abstract). Proc Nutr Soc 1981 May; 40 (2): 73A.

(375) McLellan DR. Viscid faecal masses and acute appendicitis. Br J Surg 1981 Mar; 68 (3): 177-8.

(376) McMaster GJ, Rerie W, Bushuk W. Functional glutenin: a complex of protein and polysaccharide components (abstract). Cereal Foods World 1981 Sep; 26 (9): 499-500.

(377) MacPhail AP, Bothwell TH, Torrance JD, Derman DP, Bezwoda WR, Charlton RW, Mayet F. Factors affecting the absorption of iron from Fe (III) EDTA. Br J Nutr 1981 Mar, 45 (2): 215-27.

(378) Nakamura H, Tamura A, Baba Y, Hachida K, Matsushita C. Effects of various dietary fiber components on cholesterol levels in rats (abstract). XII International Congress of Nutrition. San Diego, California: 1981: 47.

(379) Nassos PS, Chang GW. Decrease in blood urea nitrogen levels in uremic rats by various dietary fibers (abstract). Fed Proc 1981 Mar 1; 40 (3 Pt II): 846.

(380) Ney D, Hollingsworth DR. Nutritional management of pregnancy complicated by diabetes: historical perspective. Diabetes Care 1981 Nov-Dec; 4 (6): 647-55.

(381) Nguyen KN, Welsh JD, Manion CV. Effect of dietary fiber on breath hydrogen response following oral lactose in lactose malabsorption (abstract). Gastroenterology 1981 May; 80 (5 Pt 2): 1239.

(382) Nguyen LB, Gregory JF III, Burgin CW, Cerda JJ. In vitro binding of vitamin B-6 by selected polysaccharides, lignin, and wheat bran. J Food Sci 1981 Nov-Dec; 46 (6): 1860-2.

(383) Nguyen LB, Gregory JF III, Damron BL. Effects of selected polysaccharides on the bioavailability of pyridoxine in rats and chicks. J Nutr 1981 Aug; 111 (8): 1403-10.

(384) Nigro ND. Animal studies implicating fat and fecal steroids in intestinal cancer. Cancer Res 1981 Sep; 41 (9 Pt 2): 3769-70.

(385) Nomani MZ, Hussain SS, Lim JK, Albrink MJ, Gunnells CK, Davis GK. Fecal bulk, energy intake, and serum cholesterol: regression response of serum cholesterol to apparent digestibility of dry matter and suboptimal energy intake in rats on fiber-fat diet. Am J Clin Nutr 1981 Oct; 34 (10): 2078-87.

(386) Nomani MZ, Rodriguez NR, Lim JK, Watne AL, Jamil R, Giaquinto CM. Regression response of serum cholesterol to energy intake, fecal bulk and steroids in the rat (abstract). Fed Proc 1981 Mar 1; 40 (3 Pt I): 352.

(387) Normand FL, Ory RL, Mod RR, Saunders RM, Gumbmann MR. Influence of rice hemicellulose on fecal sterol composition and water retention in rats (abstract). Cereal Foods World 1981 Sep; 26 (9): 513.

(388) Normand FL, Ory RL, Mod RR. Interactions of several bile acids with hemicelluloses from several varieties of rice. J Food Sci 1981 Jul-Aug; 46 (4): 1159-61.

(389) Norris AA, Lewis AJ, Zeitlin IJ. Inability of degraded carrageenan fractions to induce inflammatory bowel ulceration in the guinea-pig. J Pharm Pharmacol 1981 Sep 33 (9): 612-3.

(390) Northover J. Are fibre supplements really necessary in diverticular disease of the colon (letter). Br Med J 1981 May 30; 282 (6278): 1792.

(391) Nygren C, Hallmans G, Lithner F. Long term effects of dietary fibre in bread on weight, blood glucose, glucosuria and faecal fat excretion in alloxan diabetic rats. Diabete Metab 1981 Jun; 7 (2): 115-20.

(392) Nygren C, Hallmans G, Lithner F. The effects of a high bran bread on blood glucose levels in insulin- dependent diabetic patients (abstract). XII International Congress of Nutrition. San Diego, California: 1981: 51.

(393) Nyhlin H, Eastwood M. Comparison of various treatments for irritable bowel syndrome (letter). Br Med J 1981 Jan 3; 282 (6257): 74-5.

(394) Obizoba IC. Zinc and copper metabolism of human adults fed combinations of corn, wheat, beans, rice, and milk containing various levels of phytates. Nutr Rep Int 1981 Aug: 24 (2): 203-10.

(395) O'Connor N, Tredger J, Morgan L. Viscosity differences between various guar gums. Diabetologia 1981 Jun; 20 (6): 612-5.

(396) O'Dea K, Snow P, Nestel P. Rate of starch hydrolysis in vitro as a predictor of metabolic responses to complex carbohydrate in vivo. Am J Clin Nutr 1981 Oct; 34 (10): 1991-3.

(397) O'Donnell JA III, Lee HS, Hurt HD. Effect of plant fibers on plasma and liver lipids of adult male gerbils (abstract). Fed Proc 1981 Mar 1; 40 (3 Pt II): 853.

(398) Ohsima M, Tamai M, Ueda H. Supplementary effects of leaf protein concentrate and amino acids to a barley bran on nutritive value and plasma amino acid concentrations in growing pigs. Nutr Rep Int 1981 Dec; 24 (6): 1233-40.

(399) Oku T, Konishi F, Hosoya N. Inhibitory effect of unabsorbable and undigestible carbohydrate on intestinal calcium absorption (abstract). XII International Congress of Nutrition. San Diego, California: 1981: 48.

(400) Omaye ST, Chow FI, Betschart AA. Interaction of ascorbic acid with hard red spring and soft white winter wheat brans in vitro (abstract). XII International Congress of Nutrition. San Diego, California: 1981: 50.

(401) Oohashi Y, Ishioka T, Wakabayashi K, Kuwabara N. A study on carcinogenesis induced by degraded carrageenan arising from squamous metaplasia of the rat colorectum. Cancer Lett 1981 Dec; 14 (3): 267-72.

(402) Ornstein MH, Littlewood ER, McLean Baird I, Fowler J, Cox AG. Are fibre supplements really necessary in diverticular disease of the colon (letter). Br Med J 1981 May 16, 282 (6276). 1629-30.

(403) Ornstein MH, Littlewood ER, McLean Baird I, Fowler J, North WR, Cox AG. Are fibre supplements really necessary in diverticular disease of the colon. A controlled clinical trial. Br Med J 1981 Apr 25; 282 (6273): 1353-6.

(404) Ornstein MH, Littlewood ER, McLean Baird I. Are fibre supplements really necessary in diverticular disease (letter). Br Med J 1981 Jul 11; 283 (6248): 140.

(405) Ornstein MH. Diverticular disease of the colon — what is the place of dietary fibre? In: McLean Baird I, Ornstein MH, eds. Dietary fibre: progress towards the future. Proceedings of a symposium held at the Royal College of Physicians, London. Manchester, England: Kellogg Company of Great Britain Ltd, 1981: 71-6.

(406) Orraca-Tetteh R, Neequaye MA. Effects of fibre contents of foods and diets in Ghana (abstract). XII International Congress of Nutrition. San Diego, California: 1981: 49.

(407) Osilesi O, Trout DL, Knight E. Effect of viscous and non-viscous gums on hepatic lipogenesis in starved-refed rats (abstract). Fed Proc 1981 Mar 1; 40 (3 Pt II): 853.

(408) Oyebiodun GL. Carbohydrate fractions of cassava, maize and guinea corn wastes (abstract). XII International Congress of Nutrition. San Diego, California: 1981: 47.

(409) Painter NS. Are fibre supplements really necessary in diverticular disease (letter). Br Med J 1981 Jul 11; 283 (6248): 140.

(410) Painter NS. Diverticular disease of the colon. 7th ed. 59-62 High Holborn, London WC1V 6EB: Norgine Ltd, 1981. (The present state of knowledge; no 1.)

(411) Patel MB, McGinnis J, Pubols MH. Effect of dietary cereal grain, citrus pectin, and guar gum on liver fat in laying hens and young chicks. Poult Sci 1981 Mar; 60 (3): 631-6.

(412) Pathak V, Kwatra BL, Bajaj S. Effect of dietary fibre on the absorption of calcium and zinc by human beings. J Res Punjab Agric Univ 1981; 18 (2): 216-20.

(413) Pecora P, Suraci C, Antonelli M, De Maria S, Marrocco W. Constipation and obesity: a statistical analysis. Boll Soc Ital Biol Sper 1981 Dec 15; 57 (23): 2384-8.

(414) Peto R. Random diets (letter). Nature 1981 Sep 10; 293 (5828): 96.

(415) Petrakis NL, King EB. Cytological abnormalities in nipple aspirates of breast fluid from women with severe constipation. Lancet 1981 Nov 28; 2 (8257): 1203-5.

(416) Pfeffer PE, Doner LW, Hoagland PD, McDonald GG. Molecular interactions with dietary fiber components. Investigation of the possible association of pectin and bile acids. J Agric Food Chem 1981 May-Jun; 29 (3): 455-61. Correction. Sep-Oct 1981; 29 (5). 1104.

(417) Phillips SF, Fernandez R. Pectin and cellulose binding of iron in vitro. Am J Clin Nutr 1981 Oct; 34 (10): 2322-3.

(418) Pichl I, Lutonska P, Svobodova M, Teper I. Fibre analysis in the relation to the sample homogenization. In Focus 1981; 8: 7-8, 12.

290

(419) Pillaiyar P. Rice bran as feed and food. Indian J Nutr Diet 1981 Mar; 18 (3): 109-15.

(420) Porrini M, Bossi E, Vercesi P, Testolin G, Ciappellano S, Pozza G, Caviezel F. Determination of dietary fiber and its utilization in dietary management of obesity (abstract). XII International Congress of Nutrition. San Diego, California: 1981: 49.

(421) Potter JG, Coffman KP, Reid RL, Krall JM, Albrink MJ. Effect of test meals of varying dietary fiber content on plasma insulin and glucose response. Am J Clin Nutr 1981 Mar; 34 (3): 328-34.

(422) Prentice N, Faber S. Beta-D-glucan in developing and germinating barely kernels. Cereal Chem 1981 Mar-Apr; 58 (2): 77-9.

(423) Prior IA, Tasman-Jones C. Part V. Migrants and mixed ethnic groups. New Zealand Maori and Pacific Polynesians. In: Trowell HC, Burkitt DP, eds. Western diseases: their emergence and prevention. London: Edward Arnold, 1981: 227-67.

(424) Prizont R, Piatt K. Glycoprotein degrading glycosidases in experimental cancer of the colon (abstract). Gastroenterology 1981 May; 80 (5 Pt 2): 1255.

(425) Prizont R, Piatt K. High dietary cellulose: protection against large bowel carcinoma (abstract). Gastroenterology 1981 May; 80 (5 Pt 2): 1256.

(426) Proia AD, McNamara DJ, Edwards KD, Anderson KE. Effects of dietary pectin and cellulose on hepatic and intestinal mixed-function oxidations and hepatic 3-hydroxy-3-methylglutaryl-coenzyme A reductase in the rat. Biochem Pharmacol 1981 Sep 15; 30 (18): 2553-8.

(427) Pussayanawin V, Wetzel DL. Pentosan analytical HPLC as furfural in the presence of hydroxymethyl furfural (abstract). Cereal Foods World 1981 Sep; 26 (9): 506.

(428) Ranhotra GS, Gelroth JA, Torrence FA, Bock MA, Winterringer GL, Faridi HA, Finney PL. Iranian flat breads: relative bioavailability of iron. Cereal Chem 1981 Sep-Oct; 58 (5): 471-4.

(429) Ranhotra GS, Gelroth JA, Torrence FA, Bock MA, Winterringer GL, Faridi HA, Finney PL. Iranian flat breads: bioavailability of iron (abstract). Cereal Foods World 1981 Sep; 26 (9): 501.

(430) Ranhotra GS, Gelroth JA, Torrence FA, Winterringer GL, Bachman AL. Effect of high fiber breads on fecal density (abstract). Cereal Foods World 1981 Sep; 26 (9): 513.

(431) Ranhotra GS, Gelroth JA, Torrence FA, Bock MA, Winterringer GL. Bread (white and whole wheat) and nonfat dry milk as sources of bioavailable calcium for rats. J Nutr 1981 Dec; 111 (12): 2081-6.

(432) Rao AB, McCartney T, Fletcher P. Volvulus of the colon. Am J Proctol Gastrenterol Colon Rectal Surg 1981 Mar; 32 (3): 12, 17-8, 20, 28.

(433) Rao AR, Sagar V, Prasad D. Dietary fibre — update 1980. Indian Nutr Diet 1981 Nov; 18 (11): 397-410.

(434) Rao MA, Walter RH, Cooley HJ. Effect of heat treatment on the flow properties of aqueous guar gum and sodium carboxymethylcellulose (CMC) solutions. J Food Sci 1981 May-Jun; 46 (3): 896-9, 902.

(435) Rasper VF. Fractionation of the insoluble residue in dietary fiber analysis. In: James WP, Theander O, eds. The analysis of dietary fiber in food. New York and Basel: Marcel Dekker Inc, 1981: 29-36. (Basic and clinical nutrition; vol 3.)

(436) Rasper VF. Analysis and testing of nondigestible polysaccharides. Cereal Foods World 1981 May; 26 (5): 228-32.

(437) Rasper VF, Brillouet JM, Bertrand D, Mercier C. Analysis of dietary fiber in feces of rats fed with fiber supplemented diets. J Food Sci 1981 Mar-Apr; 46 (2): 559-63.

(438) Rattan J, Levin N, Graff E, Weizer N, Gilat T. A high-fiber diet does not cause mineral and nutrient deficiencies. J Clin Gastroenterol 1981 Dec; 3 (4): 389-93.

(439) Read NW, Brown C, Edwards C. Effect of the weight and the composition of a meal on its transit through the small intestine in man (abstract). Gut 1981 Oct; 22 (10): A862.

(440) Reaven GM. How much carbohydrate (letter). Diabetologia 1981 Apr; 20 (4): 508-9.

(441) Reddy BS. Diet and excretion of bile acids. Cancer Res 1981 Sep; 41 (9 Pt 2): 3766 8.

(442) Reddy BS, Mori H. Effect of dietary wheat bran and dehydrated citrus fiber on 3, 2'-dimethyl-4-aminobiphenyl-induced intestinal carcinogenesis in F344 rats. Carcinogenesis 1981; 2 (1): 21-5.

(443) Reddy BS, Mori H, Nicolais M. Effect of dietary wheat bran and dehydrated citrus fiber on azoxymethane-induced intestinal carcinogenesis in Fischer 344 rats. JNCI 1981 Mar; 66 (3): 553-7.

(444) Reichert RD. Quantitative isolation and estimation of cell wall material from dehulled pea (Pisum sativum) flours and concentrates. Cereal Chem 1981 Jul-Aug; 58 (4). 266-70.

(445) Reinhold JG, Garcia L. JS, Garzon P. Binding of iron by fiber of wheat and maize. Am J Clin Nutr 1981 Jul; 34 (7): 1384-91.

(446) Reinhold JG. Water-soluble fiber (letter). Am J Clin Nutr 1981 Aug; 34 (8): 1629.

(447) Remesy C, Demigne C. Effects of fermentable carbohydrates on glucose and volatile fatty acid absorption and insulin secretion (abstract). XII International Congress of Nutrition. San Diego, California: 1981: 51.

(448) Remington MM, Brown ML, Robertson JS, Fleming CR, Carlson G, Whatley J, Thomford G, Malagelada J-R Transit of solid and liquid components of a meal in the short bowel syndrome quantified by total gut scintiscanning: effect of loperamide (abstract). Gastroenterology 1981 May; 80 (5 Pt 2): 1260.

(449) Rerat AA. Digestion and absorption of nutrients in the pig. Some new data concerning protein and carbohydrates. World Rev Nutr Diet 1981; 37: 229-87.

(450) Reuben D. High fiber cook book. Cancer Book House.

(451) Rey DK, Labuza TP. Characterization of the effect of solutes on the water-binding and gel strength properties of carrageenan. J Food Sci 1981 May-Jun; 46 (3): 786-9, 793.

(452) Reyes PS, Garcia E, Nelson PP, Gates JE, Spiller G, Briggs GM. Effects of dietary fibers on growth, blood parameters, coat and plasma cholesterol in guinea pigs (abstract). Fed Proc 1981 Mar 1; 40 (3 Pt II): 845.

(453) Rhee M, Pittz EP, Abraham R. Effect of combinations of Irideae carrageenan and cellulose on the absorption of some nutrients from the alimentary tract of rats. Ecotoxicol Environ Safety 1981 Mar; 5 (1): 1-14.

(454) Ristow KA, Gregory JF, Damron BL. The effect of dietary fiber on folic acid bioavailability (abstract). Fed Proc 1981 Mar 1; 40 (3 Pt II): 854.

(455) Rivellese A, Riccardi G, Giacco A, Pacioni D, Genovese S, Mattioli PL, Mancini M. A fibre-rich diet for the treatment of diabetes. In: Howard AN, McLean Baird I, eds. Recent advances in clinical nutrition: I. Proceedings of the first international symposium on clinical nutrition. London: John Libbey, 1981: 99-100.

(456) Robertson GL, Swinburne D. Changes in chlorophyll and pectin after storage and canning of kiwifruit. J Food Sci 1981 Sep-Oct; 46 (5): 1557-9, 1562. Correction. J Food Sci 1982 Mar-Apr; 47 (2): 693.

(457) Robertson I, Ford JA, McIntosh WB, Dunnigan MG. The role of cereals in the aetiology of nutritional rickets: the lesson of the Irish National Nutrition Survey 1943-8. Br J Nutr 1981 Jan; 45 (1): 17-22.

(458) Robertson JA, Eastwood MA. An examination of factors which may affect the water holding capacity of dietary fibre. Br J Nutr 1981 Jan; 45 (1): 83-8.

(459) Robertson JA, Eastwood MA. A method to measure the water-holding properties of dietary fibre using suction pressure. Br J Nutr 1981 Sep; 46 (2): 247-55.

(460) Robertson JA, Van Soest PJ. The detergent system of analysis and its application to could affect water-holding capacity of dietary fibre. J Sci Food Agric 1981 Aug; 32 (8): 819-25.

(461) Robertson JB, Van Soest PJ. The detergent system of analysis and its application to human foods. In: James WP, Theander O, eds. The analysis of dietary fiber in food. New York and Basel: Marcel Dekker Inc, 1981: 123-58. (Basic and clinical nutrition; vol 3.)

(462) Roche SW, Tobin M, Fielding JF. A palatability comparison between a granular and a tablet colloid bulk-forming agent. J Int Med Res 1981; 9 (5): 387-9.

(463) Roe B, Bruemmer JH. Changes in pectic substances and enzymes during ripening and storage of "Keitt" mangos. J Food Sci 1981 Jan-Feb; 46 (1): 186-9.

(464) Rogel AM, Vohra P. The effects of feeding various complex carbohydrates and simple sugars at increasing concentrations on growth of Tribolium larvae. Nutr Rep Int 1981 Oct; 24 (4): 847-53.

(465) Roland J-C, Vian B. Use of purified endopolygalacturonase for a topochemical study of elongating cell walls at the ultrastructural level. J Cell Sci 1981 Apr; 48: 333-43.

(466) Rosman MS. Glycosylated haemoglobin, blood glucose and serum cholesterol levels in diabetics treated with guar gum (letter). S Afr Med J 1981 May 16; 59 (21): 739-40.

(467) Ross JK, Leklem JE. The effect of dietary citrus pectin on the excretion of human fecal neutral and acid steroids and the activity of 7 α-dehydroxylase and β-glucuronidase. Am J Clin Nutr 1981 Oct; 34 (10): 2068-77.

(468) Rotenberg S. Some hematological parameters in heat-stressed rats receiving pectin in the diet. Acta Agric Scand 1981; 31 (1): 3-10.

(469) Roth NJ, Watts GH, Newman CW. Beta-glucanase as an aid in measuring neutral detergent fiber in barley kernels. Cereal Chem 1981 May-Jun; 58 (3): 245-6.

(470) Rotstein OD, Kay RM, Wayman M, Strasberg SM. Hypocholesterolemic effect of dietary fiber and lactulose (abstract). Arteriosclerosis 1981 Jan-Feb; 1 (1): 73-4.

(471) Rotstein OD, Kay RM, Wayman M, Strasberg SM. Prevention of cholesterol gallstones by lignin and lactulose in the hamster. Gastroenterology 1981 Dec; 81 (6): 1098-103.

(472) Rotstein OD, Kay RM, Wayman M, Siu KP, Strasberg SM. Effect of autohydrolyzed lignin and lactulose on gallbladder bile composition in hamsters. J Agric Food Chem 1981 May-Jun; 29 (3): 472-5.

(473) Rozen P, Hellerstein SM, Horwitz C. The low incidence of colorectal cancer in a 'high-risk' population: its correlation with dietary habits. Cancer 1981 Dec 15; 48 (12): 2692-5.

(474) Saito Y, Yoshida K, Yoshida N, Watanabe M. Digestibility of dietary fiber and its effect on mineral and thiamine balance in rats (abstract). XII International Congress of Nutrition. San Diego, California: 1981: 111.

(475) Salvioli G, Salati R, Pastorello M, Gibertini A. Cholesterol, bile acid and bile salt adsorption to bran in vitro. Pharmacol Res Commun 1981 Apr; 13 (4): 413-21.

(476) Salyers AA, Gherardini F, O'Brien M. Utilization of xylan by two species of human colonic Bacteroides. Appl Environ Microbiol 1981 Apr; 41 (4): 1065-8.

(477) Salyers AA, Arthur R, Kuritza A. Digestion of larch arabinogalactan by a strain of human colonic Bacteroides growing in continuous culture. J Agric Food Chem 1981 May-Jun; 29 (3): 475-80.

(478) Sandberg A-S, Andersson H, Hallgren B, Hasselblad K, Isaksson B, Hulten L. Experimental method for in vivo determination of dietary fibre and its effect on the absorption of nutrients in the small intestine. Br J Nutr 1981 Mar; 45 (2): 283-94.

(479) Sandberg A-S, Hallgren B, Hasselblad K. Analytical problems in the determination of dietary fibre. Naringsforskning 1981; 25 (4): 132-9.

(480) Sarett H. Safety of carrageenan used in foods (letter). Lancet 1981 Jan 17; 1 (8212): 151-2.

(481) Sartor G, Carlstrom S, Schersten B. Dietary supplementation of fibre (Lunelax) as a means to reduce postprandial glucose in diabetics. Acta Med Scand (Suppl) 1981: 656: 51-3.

(482) Sathe SK, Salunkhe DK. A research note. Isolation and partial characterization of an arabinogalactan from the great northern bean (Phaseolus vulgaris L.). J Food Sci 1981 Jul-Aug; 46 (4): 1276-7.

(483) Satoh H, Guth PH, Grossman MI. Gastric antral ulcers produced by indomethacin in the rat. II. Role of food (abstract). Gastroenterology 1981 May; 80 (5 Pt 2): 1272.

(484) Saunders DR, Wiggins HS. Conservation of mannitol, lactulose, and raffinose by the human colon. Am J Physiol 1981 Nov; 241 (5): G 397-402.

(485) Saunders DR, Wiggins HS. How do single doses of carbohydrates such as lactulose cause diarrhoea (abstract). Gastroenterology 1981 May; 80 (5 Pt 2): 1272.

(486) Saunders RM, Betschart AA. Dietary fiber in cereal foods: in vivo and in vitro studies (abstract). Cereal Foods World 1981 Sep; 26 (9): 492.

(487) Schwandt P, Richter WO, Weisweiler P. Soybean protein and serum cholesterol (letter). Atherosclerosis 1981 Nov-Dec; 40 (3-4): 371-2.

(488) Schwartz R, Wien EM, Wentworth RA. Use of nonabsorable markers for gastrointestinal contents in in vivo measurement of magnesium bioavailability. J Nutr 1981 Feb; 111 (2): 219-25.

(489) Schwartz SE, Levine RA, Rogus JB. Effect of chronic fiber ingestion on jejunal glucose and amino acid absorption in man (abstract). Gastroenterology 1981 May; 80 (5 Pt 2): 1278.

(490) Schweizer TF, Wursch P. Analysis of dietary fiber. In: James WP, Theander O, eds. The analysis of dietary fiber in food. New York and Basel: Marcel Dekker Inc., 1981: 203-16. (Basic and clinical nutrition; vol 3.)

(491) Segal I, Cooke SA, Hamilton DG, Ou Tim L. Polyps and colorectal cancer in South African Blacks. Gut 1981 Aug; 22 (8); 653-7.

(492) Segal I, Beck W, Van Zyl CJ. Diverticular disease in Johannesburg Blacks (abstract). S Afr Med J 1981 Aug 15; 60 (7): 293.

(493) Selvendran RR, Ring SG, Du Pont MS. Determination of the dietary fiber content of the EEC samples and a discussion of the various methods of analysis. In: James WP, Theander O, eds. The analysis of dietary fiber in food. New York and Basel: Marcel Dekker Inc, 1981: 95-121. (Basic and clinical nutrition; vol 3.)

(494) SerVaas C, Turgeon C, Birmingham F. Fiber and bran better health cookbook. New York: Bonanza Books, 1981.

(495) Shah NO, Pellett PL, Mahoney RR, Atallah MT. Effect of dietary fibre components and wheat bran on protein utilisation in rats (abstract). XII International Congress of Nutrition. San Diego, California: 1981: 55.

(496) Shah PJ. Unprocessed bran — a new approach to the treatment of idiopathic hypercalciuria. In: McLean Baird I, Ornstein MH, eds. Dietary fibre: progress towards the future. Proceedings of a symposium held at the Royal College of Physicians, London. Manchester, England: Kellogg Company of Great Britain Ltd, 1981: 47-51.

(497) Shim JL, McConnell JL. Modification of starch gels by xanthan gum (abstract). Cereal Foods World 1981 Sep; 26 (9): 495.

(498) Shogren MD, Pomeranz Y, Finney KF. Counteracting the deleterious effects of fiber in breadmaking. Cereal Chem 1981 Mar-Apr; 58 (2): 142-4.

(499) Sigleo S, Jackson MJ, Vahouny GV. Dietary fibers: altered intestinal morphology and nutrient transport (abstract). Fed Proc 1981 Mar 1; 40 (3 Pt II): 845.

(500) Simons LA, Gayst S, Balasubramaniam S. Effects of guar gum on lipid metabolism in hypercholesterolemic patients (abstract). XII International Congress of Nutrition. San Diego, California: 1981: 55.

(501) Simpson HC, Simpson RW, Lousley S, Carter RD, Geekie M, Hockaday TD, Mann JI. A high carbohydrate leguminous fibre diet improves all aspects of diabetic control. Lancet 1981 Jan 3; 1 (8210): 1-5.

(502) Simpson HC. High-carbohydrate, high-fibre diets for diabetics. Proc Nutr Soc 1981 May; 40 (2): 219-25.

(503) Simpson KM, Morris ER, Cook JD. The inhibitory effect of bran on iron absorption in man. Am J Clin Nutr 1981 Aug; 34 (8): 1469-78.

(504) Simpson RW, McDonald J, Wahlqvist M, Balazs N, Dunlop M. Effect of naturally occurring dietary fibre in Western foods on blood glucose. Aust NZ J Med 1981 Oct; 11 (5): 484-7.

(505) Simpson RW, McDonald J, Wahlqvist ML, Outch K. Acute effects of naturally occurring leguminous fibre on carbohydrate absorption (abstract). Proc Nutr Soc Aust 1981; 6: 163.

(506) Sinnett P, Whyte M. Part IV. Peasant agriculturalists. Papua New Quinea. In: Trowell HC, Burkitt DP, eds. Western diseases: their emergence and prevention. London: Edward Arnold, 1981: 171-87.

(507) Slavin JL, Sempos CT, Brauer PM, Marlett JA. Limits of predicting gastrointestinal transit time from other measures of bowel function. Am J Clin Nutr 1981 Oct; 34 (10): 2111-6.

(508) Slavin JL, Marlett JA. High performance liquid chromatography (HPLC) as a method for measuring the monosaccharides in neutral detergent fiber (NDF) (abstract). Fed Proc 1981 Mar 1; 40 (3 Pt II): 853.

(509) Slavin JL, Brauer PM, Marlett JA. Neutral detergent fiber, hemicellulose and cellulose digestibility in human subjects. J Nutr 1981 Feb; 111 (2): 287-97.

(510) Sly MR, Du Bryn DB, De Klerk WA. Some effects of fibre-and phytate-containing (cereal) diets in baboons. In: Howard AN, McLean Baird I, eds. Recent advances in clinical nutrition: I. Proceedings of the first international symposium on clinical nutrition. London: John Libbey, 1981: 102-3.

(511   Smith AN, Drummond E, Eastwood MA. The effect of coarse and fine Canadian Red Spring Wheat and French Soft Wheat bran on colonic motility in patients with diverticular disease. Am J Clin Nutr 1981 Nov; 34 (11): 2460-3.

(512) Smith AN, Shepherd J, Eastwood MA. Pressure changes after balloon distension of the colon wall in diverticular disease. Gut 1981 Oct; 22 (10): 841-4.

(513) Smith M, Liebman M, Ferreri LF, Thye FW, Driskell J, Stevens C. Effects of coarse wheat bran fiber and exercise on plasma lipids and lipoprotein cholesterol in males (abstract). Fed Proc 1981 Mar 1; 40 (3 Pt II): 904.

(514) Smith-Barbaro P, Hanson D, Reddy BS 1,2-Dimethylhydrazine-induced changes in hepatic, small intestinal, and colonic mucosal cytochromes P-450 and b5 of rats fed citrus pulp or wheat bran. Drug Metab Dispos 1981 Sep-Oct; 9 (5): 487-8.

(515) Smith-Barbaro P, Hanson D, Reddy BS. Carcinogen binding to various types of dietary fiber. JNCI 1981 Aug; 67 (2): 495-7.

(516) Smith-Barbaro PA, Hanson D, Reddy BS. Effect of bran and citrus pulp on hepatic, small intestinal and colonic HMG CoA reductase, cytochrome P450 and cytochrome b5 levels in rats. J Nutr 1981 May; 111 (5): 789-97.

(517) Snow P, O'Dea K. Factors affecting the rate of hydrolysis of starch in food. Am J Clin Nutr 1981 Dec; 34 (12): 2721-7.

(518) Sorenson AW, Street JC. The need for comprehensive diet studies to assess the relation of lipids to cancer. Cancer Res 1981 Sep; 41 (9 Pt 2): 3748-9.

(519) Souci SW, Fachmann W, Kraut H. Food composition and nutrition tables 1981-2. Stuttgart: Wissenschaftliche Verlagsgesellschaft mbH, 1981.

(520) Southgate DA. Use of the Southgate method for unavailable carbohydrates in the measurement of dietary fiber. In: James WP, Theander O, eds. The analysis of dietary fiber in food. New York and Basel: Marcel Dekker Inc, 1981: 1-19. (Basic and clinical nutrition; vol 3.)

(521) Southgate DA, White MA. Commentary on results obtained by the different laboratories using the Southgate method. In: James WP, Theander O, eds. The analysis of dietary fiber in food. New York and Basel: Marcel Dekker Inc, 1981: 37-50. (Basic and clinical nutrition; vol 3.)

(522) Southgate DA, Kritchevsky D. Terminology of dietary fiber. Prog Clin Biol Res 1981; 77: 219-22.

(523) Speth PA, Jansen JB, Lamers CB. Comparative study of different doses of acarbose, pectin, a combination of acarbose and pectin, and placebo in the dumping syndrome (abstract). Gut 1981 Oct; 22 (10). A863.

(524) Spiller GA, Freeman HJ. Recent advances in dietary fiber and colorectal diseases. Am J Clin Nutr 1981 Jun; 34 (6): 1145-52.

(525) Spiller GA. Effect of graded dietary levels of plant fibers on fecal output in pig-tailed monkeys. Nutr Rep Int 1981 Feb; 23 (2): 313-20.

(526) Srivastava U, Makhija SL, Nadeau M, Rakshit AK, Carbonneau N, Guennou L, Khare I. Proximate composition and mineral nutrient content of university meals. Nutr Rep Int 1981 Dec; 24 (6): 1139-51.

(527) Stace NH, Pomare EW, Peters S, Thomas L, Fisher A. Biliary lipids and dietary intakes (including dietary fiber) in four different female populations (abstract). Gastroenterology 1981 May; 80 (5 Pt 2): 1291.

(528) Stanway A. Taking the rough with the smooth. Revised ed. London: Pan, 1981.

(529) Stasse-Wolthuis M. Influence of dietary fibre on cholesterol metabolism and colonic function in healthy subjects. World Rev Nutr Diet 1981; 36: 100-40.

(530) Stein DT, Stone BT. Endoscopic removal of gastric phytobezoars (abstract). Gut 1981 Oct; 22 (10): A896.

(531)   Stephen AM. Faeces — how much fibre is left? Techniques of faecal fractionation. In: McLean Baird I, Ornstein MH, eds. Dietary fibre; progress towards the future. Proceedings of a symposium held at the Royal College of Physicians, London. Manchester, England: Kellogg Company of Great Britain Ltd, 1981: 14-20.

(532)   Stephen AM, Cummings JH. Effect of transit time on colonic nitrogen metabolism in man (abstract). Gastroenterology 1981 May; 80 (5 Pt 2): 1294.

(533)   Stephen AM, Cummings JH. The effect of wheat fibre on faecal pH in man (abstract). Gastroenterology 1981 May; 80 (5 Pt 2): 1294.

(534)   Stephen AM, Cummings JH. Degradation of dietary fibre in the human colon and its effect on the faecal microflora (abstract). XII International Congress of Nutrition. San Diego, California: 1981: 111.

(535)   Stephen AM, Cummings JH. Effect of changing transit time on colonic physiology in man (abstract). XII International Congress on Nutrition. San Diego, California: 1981: 112.

(536)   Stephen AM. Should we eat more fibre? J Hum Nutr 1981 Dec; 35 (6): 403-14.

(537)   Stokholm KH, Lauritsen KB, Larsen S. Reduced glycosuria during guar gum supplementation in non-insulin-dependent diabetics. A double-blind, randomised cross-over study. Dan Med Bull 1981; 28 (1): 41-2.

(538)   Story JA. The role of dietary fiber in lipid metabolism. Adv Lipid Res 1981; 18: 229-46.

(539)   Story JA, Kritchevsky D. Lignin and bile acid binding (letter). Lancet 1981 Aug 22; 2 (8243): 427.

(540)   Story JA, Baldino A, Czarnecki SK, Kritchevsky D. Modification of liver cholesterol accumulation by dietary fiber in rats. Nutr Rep Int 1981 Dec; 24 (6): 1213-9.

(541)   Strand LL, Ogawa JM, Bose E, Rumsey JW. Bimodal heat stability curves of fungal pectolytic enzymes and their implication for softening of canned apricots. J Food Sci 1981 Mar-Apr; 46 (2): 498-500, 505.

(542)   Sutton CD, Muir WM, Begin JJ. Effect of fiber on cholesterol metabolism in the Coturnix quail. Poult Sci 1981 Apr; 60 (4): 812-7.

(543)   Tabekha MM. Significance of dephytinization process of wheat bran for producing dietary fiber (abstract). XII International Congress of Nutrition. San Diego, California: 1981: 46.

(544)   Tadesse K. Is fibre metabolised? — An investigation of fibre breakdown in the colon. In: McLean Baird I, Ornstein MH, eds. Dietary fibre: progress towards the future. Proceedings of a symposium held at the Royal College of Physicians, London. Manchester, England: Kellogg Company of Great Britain Ltd, 1981: 12-3.

(545)   Takeda H, Tsujita J, Ebihara K, Kiriyama S. Decreased protein utilization in amaranth toxicity and its amelioration by the concurrent feeding of dietary fiber in rats. Nutr Rep Int 1981 Sep; 24 (3): 481-97.

(546)   Talbot JM. Role of dietary fiber in diverticular disease and colon cancer. Fed Proc 1981 Jul; 40 (9): 2337-42.

(547)   Tanaka Y, Okuda M, Sano T. Effects of chlorella feeding on experimental atherosclerosis in rabbits (abstract). XII International Congress of Nutrition. San Diego, California: 1981: 73.

(548)   Tangendjaja B, Buckle KA, Wootton M. Dephosphorylation of phytic acid in rice bran. J Food Sci 1981 Jul-Aug; 46 (4): 1021-4.

(549)   Tangprasertchai P, Stalnaker J, Salmon J, Wetzel DL. Fiber determination: nongravimetric alternative (abstract). Cereal Foods World 1981 Sep; 26 (9): 505.

(550)   Taranto MV, Kuo CM, Rhee KC. Possible role of the crude fiber of soy flour in texture formation during nonextrusion texturization processing. J Food Sci 1981 Sep-Oct; 46 (5): 1470-7.

(551)   Tasman-Jones C, Lindop R. Dietary fiber influences rat intestinal β-glucosidase and β-glucuronidase activities (abstract). XII International Congress of Nutrition. San Diego, California: 1981: 111.

(552)   Taverner MR, Hume ID, Farrell DJ. Availability to pigs of amino acids in cereal grains. 1. Endogenous levels of amino acids in ileal digesta and faeces of pigs given cereal diets. Br J Nutr 1981 Jul; 46 (1): 149-58.

(553) Taverner MR, Farrell DJ. Availability to pigs of amino acids in cereal grains. 4. Factors influencing the availability of amino acids and energy in grains. Br J Nutr 1981 Jul; 46 (1): 181-92.

(554) Taylor AJ, Brown JM, Downie LM. The effect of processing on the texture of canned mung bean (Phaseolus aureus) shoots. J Sci Food Agric 1981 Feb; 32 (2): 134-8.

(555) Teas J. The consumption of seaweed as a protective factor in the etiology of breast cancer. Med Hyphotheses 1981 May; 7 (5): 601-13.

(556) Tempero MA, West W, Zetterman RK. Failure of dietary cellulose fiber to prevent colon tumors in dimethylhydrazine (DMH)-treated rats on high cholesterol diets (abstract). Gastroenterology 1981 May; 80 (5 Pt 2): 1301.

(557) Theander O, Aman P. Analysis of dietary fibers and their main constituents. In: James WP, Theander O, eds. The analysis of dietary fiber in food. New York and Basel: Marcel Dekker Inc, 1981: 51-70. (Basic and clinical nutriton; vol 3.)

(558) Theander O. Review of the different analytical methods and remaining problems. In: James WP, Theander O, eds. The analysis of dietary fiber in food. New York and Basel: Marcel Dekker Inc, 1981: 263-76. (Basic and clinical nutrition; vol 3.)

(559) Thom D. The shapes and interactions of non-starch polysaccharides used in food systems (abstract). Cereal Foods World 1981 Sep; 26 (9): 503.

(560) Thompson SA, Weber CW. Effect of dietary fiber sources on tissue mineral levels in chicks. Poult Sci 1981 Apr; 60 (4): 840-5.

(561) Thomsen LL, Tasman-Jones C. Disaccharidase levels of the rat jejunum are altered by dietary fiber (abstract). XII International Congress of Nutrition. San Diego, California: 1981: 111.

(562) Thomson AW, Brent L, Sljivic V, Fowler EF. Carrageenan and the immune response (letter). Lancet 1981 Mar 21; 1 (8221): 671. Correction. 1981 Apr 11; 1 (8224): 852.

(563) Thornton JR. Are fibre supplements really necessary in diverticular disease of the colon (letter). Br Med J 1981 May 9; 282 (6275): 1546.

(564) Thornton JR. Gallstones — a disease of fibre deficiency or dietary excess? In: McLean Baird I, Ornstein MH, eds. Dietary fibre: progress towards the future. Proceedings of a symposium held at the Royal College of Physicians, London. Manchester, England: Kellogg Company of Great Britain Ltd, 1981: 65-70.

(565) Thornton JR, Emmett PM, Heaton KW. Effects of refined and unrefined carbo-hydrate diets on bile cholesterol saturation and bile acid metabolism (abstract). Gut 1981 Oct; 22 (10): A886.

(566) Thornton JR. High colonic pH promotes colorectal cancer. Lancet 1981 May 16; 1 (8229): 1081-3.

(567) Tolman RR. Absorption of peanuts (letter). N Engl J Med 1981 Feb 5; 304 (6): 359.

(568) Topping DL, Oakenfull DG. In vitro adsorption of bile acids by lignin — or by charcoal (letter). Lancet 1981 Jul 4; 2 (8236): 39.

(569) Tredger J, Sheard C, Marks V. Blood glucose and insulin levels in normal subjects following a meal with and without added sugar beet pulp. Diabete Metab 1981 Sep; 7 (3): 169-72.

(570) Trout DL, Bickard M, Bohn E, Ryan R, Emamali B, Cataland S. The nature and persistence of metabolic responses to xanthan gum in starved-refed rats (abstract). Fed Proc 1981 Mar 1; 40 (3 Pt II): 854.

(571) Trowell H, Godding EW. Fiber: new terminology or new concepts (letter). Am J Clin Nutr 1981 Jun; 34 (6): 1163-4.

(572) Trowell H, Burkitt D. Diseases of modern civilisation (letter). Br Med J 1981 Nov 7; 283 (6301): 1266.

(573) Trowell HC, Burkitt DP, eds. Western diseases: their emergence and prevention. London: Edward Arnold, 1981.

(574) Trowell H. Part I. Emergence of Western diseases in sub-Saharal Africans. Hypertension, obesity, diabetes mellitus and coronary heart disease. In: Trowell HC, Burkitt DP, eds. Western diseases: their emergence and prevention. London: Edward Arnold, 1981: 3-32.

(575) Trowell HC, Burkitt DP. Part VIII Summary. Contributors' reports. In: Trowell HC, Burkitt DP, eds. Western diseases: their emergence and prevention. London: Edward Arnold, 1981: 427-35.

(576) Trowell HC, Burkitt DP. Part VIII Summary. Treatment and prevention: a note on autoimmune disease in sub-Saharal Africans. In: Trowell HC, Burkitt DP, eds. Western diseases: their emergence and prevention. London: Edward Arnold, 1981: 436-43.

(577) Tsai AC, Peng B. Effects of locust bean gum on glucose tolerance, sugar digestion, and gastric motility in rats. J Nutr 1981 Dec; 111 (12): 2152-6.

(578) Tsu-Hsing Yang et al. An effective approach to the treatment of endemic blackfoot disease by the supplementation of rice bran oil to their ordinary diet (abstract). XII International Congress of Nutrition. San Diego, California: 1981: 29.

(579) Tucker DM, Sandstead HH, Logan GM Jr, Klevay LM, Mahalko J, Johnson LK, Inman L, Inglett GE. Dietary fiber and personality factors as determinants of stool output. Gastroenterology 1981 Nov; 81 (5): 879-83.

(580) Tuerena CE, Taylor AJ, Mitchell JR. A method for determining the methoxyl group distribution in low-methoxyl pectins — a preliminary report (abstract). J Sci Food Agric 1981 Aug; 32 (8): 847.

(581) Tweeten TN, Wetzel DL. Spectrometric pentosan determination as the hydrazone derivative of its reaction product in sealed tube headspace (abstract). Cereal Foods World 1981 Sep; 26 (9): 495-6.

(582) Ullrich IH, Lai H-Y, Vona L, Reid RL, Albrink MJ. Alterations of fecal steroid composition induced by changes in dietary fiber compositon. Am J Clin Nutr 1981 Oct; 34 (10): 2054-60.

(583) Ullrich IH, Albrink MJ. Dietary fiber protects against sucrose-induced hypertriglyceridemia (abstract). Arteriosclerosis 1981 Jan Feb, 1 (1). 79.

(584) Umadevi Sajjan S, Wankhede DB. Carbohydrate composition of winged bean (Psophocarpus tetragondobus). J Food Sci 1981 Mar-Apr; 46 (2): 601-2, 605.

(585) Umoh IB, Bassir O. Effects of traditional Nigerian peasant food preparatory methods on the mineral element composition (abstract). XII International Congress of Nutrition. San Diego, California: 1981: 44.

(586) Vadas L, Prihar HS, Pugashetti BK, Feingold DS. A gas chromatographic method for the quantitative determination of hexuronic acids in alginic acid. Anal Biochem 1981 Jul 1; 114 (2): 294-8.

(587) Vahouny GV, Cassidy MM, Lightfoot F, Grau L, Kritchevsky D. Ultrastructural modifications of intestinal and colonic mucosa induced by free or bound bile acids. Cancer Res 1981 Sep; 41 (9 Pt 2): 3764-5.

(588) Vahouny GV, Tombes R, Cassidy MM, Kritchevsky D, Gallo LL. Dietary fibers. VI: binding of fatty acids and monolein from mixed micelles containing bile salts and lecithin. Proc Soc Exp Biol Med 1981 Jan; 166 (1): 12-6.

(589) Van Itallie TB. Does fiber have a role in obesity management? In: McLean Baird I, Ornstein MH, eds. Dietary fibre: progress towards the future. Proceedings of a symposium held at the Royal College of Physicians, London. Manchester, England: Kellogg Company of Great Britain Ltd, 1981: 33-5.

(590) Van Itallie TB. Does fiber have a role in obesity management? In: McLean Baird I, Eastwood M, Mitchell K, Duggan J, Englyst H, Wordsworth H, Littlewood ER, Shah J, McLean Baird I, Tadesse K, Jenkins DJ, Burkitt D, Harrison JR, Black D, Cummings JH. Closing discussion. Final session. In: McLean Baird I, Ornstein MH, eds. Dietary fibre: progress towards the future. Proceedings of a symposium held at the Royal College of Physicians, London. Machester, England: Kellogg Company of Great Britain Ltd, 1981: 89-99.

(591) v.d. Trenck T, Sandermann H Jr. Incorporation of benzo (α)pyrene quinones into lignin. FEBS Lett 1981 Mar 9; 125 (1): 72-6.

(592) Vickery K. Are fibre supplements really necessary in diverticular disease of the colon (letter). Br Med J 1981 May 9; 282 (6275): 1546-7.

(593) Wailes A. Computer assessment of diet histories — fibre (abstract). Proc Nutr Soc Aust 1981; 5: 197.

(594) Walker AR. Part V. Migrants and mixed ethnic groups. South African Black, Indian and Coloured populations. In: Trowell HC, Burkitt DP, eds. Western diseases: their emergence and prevention. London: Edward Arnold, 1981: 285-318.

(595) Walkinshaw MD, Arnott S. Conformations and interactions of pectins. I. X-ray diffraction analyses of sodium pectate in neutral and acidified forms. J Mol Biol 1981 Dec 25; 153 (4): 1055-1073.

(596) Walkinshaw MD, Arnott S. Conformations and interactions of pectins. II. Models for junction zones in pectinic acid and calcium pectate gels. J Mol Biol 1981 Dec 25; 153 (4): 1075-85.

(597) Walter RH, Sherman RM. Apparent activation energy of viscous flow in pectin jellies. J Food Sci 1981 Jul-Aug; 46 (4): 1223-5.

(598) Wapnir RA, Lifshitz F. Weight gain and intestinal absorption of nutrients in rats: effect of antidiarrheal agents (astringents). Nutr Rep Int 1981 Mar; 23 (3): 557-64.

(599) Waszcznskyj N, Rao CS, Da Silva RS. Extraction of proteins from wheat bran: application of carbohydrases. Cereal Chem 1981 Jul-Aug; 58 (4): 264-6.

(600) Watkins DA. Are fibre supplements really necessary in diverticular disease of the colon (letter). Br Med J 1981 May 16; 282 (6276): 1631.

(601) Weisburger JH, Reddy BS. White or brown (letter). Nature 1981 Aug 20; 292 (5825): 666.

(602) West KM. Part III. Hunter-gatherers. North American Indians. In: Trowell HC, Burkitt DP, eds. Western diseases: their emergence and prevention. London: Edward Arnold, 1981: 129-37.

(603) White WB, Bird HR, Sunde ML, Prentice N, Burger WC, Marlett JA. The viscosity interaction of barley beta-glucan with Trichoderma viride cellulase in the chick intestine. Poult Sci 1981 May; 60 (5): 1043-8.

(604) WHO. Thickening agents. In: Evaluation of certain food additives. Geneva: WHO, 1981: 28-9. (Twenty-fifth report of the Joint FAO/WHO Expert Committee on Food Additives.)

(605) Wiemer K, Kies C. Lead and fiber interactions involving iron utilization in weanling mice. Nutr Rep Int 1981 Jul; 24 (1): 165-9.

(606) Wiemer K, Kies C, Fox HM. Fiber effects on iron utilization by human adolescents. Nutr Rep Int 1981 Oct; 24 (4): 659-66.

(607) Williams EH, Williams PH. Part IV. Peasant agriculturalists. Uganda West Nile District. In: Trowell HC, Burkitt DP, eds. Western diseases: their emergence and prevention. London: Edward Arnold, 1981: 188-93.

(608) Witmer JO, Purcell AE, Franz KB. Influence of dietary fiber and phytic acid on the biovailability of zinc from food (abstract). XII International Congress of Nutrition. San Diego, California: 1981: 46.

(609) Wood PJ. A new method for assay of barley β-(1$\rightarrow$3)-D-glucanohydrolase activity (abstract). Cereal Foods World 1981 Aug; 26 (9): 483.

(610) Wood PJ. Oat β-glucan — structure, location, properties (abstract). Cereal Foods World 1981 Sep; 26 (9): 497-8.

(611) Yamamoto S. Part VI. Far East. Japan. In: Trowell HC, Burkitt DP, eds. Western diseases: their emergence and prevention. London: Edward Arnold, 1981: 337-51.

(612) Yu MH, Miller LT. Influence of cooked wheat bran on bowel function and fecal excretion of nutrients. J Food Sci 1981 May-Jun; 46 (3): 720-3.

(613) Yudkin J. Book reviews. Let them eat bread! But which bread? Nature 1981 May 14; 291 (5811). 173-4.

(614) Yudkin J. Yudkin's answer (letter). Nature 1981 Aug 20; 292 (5825): 666.

(615) Zarling EJ, Moeller DD. Bezoar therapy. Complication using Adolph's meat tenderizer and alternatives from literature review. Arch Intern Med 1981 Nov; 141 (12): 1669-70.

(616) Zavoral JH, Fields D, Hanson M, Kuba K, Frantz I, Jacobs D. Familial type II hyper-cholesterolemia (FHC) families fed locust bean gum (LBG) food products (abstract). Arteriosclerosis 1981 Jan-Feb; 1 (1): 80.

(617) Ziegler RG, Blot WJ, Hoover, R, Blattner WA, Fraumeni JF Jr. Protocol for a study of nutritional factors and the low risk of colon cancer in southern retirement areas. Cancer Res 1981 Sep; 41 (9 Pt 2): 3724-6.

(618) Zimmet P, Whitehouse S. Part IV. Peasant agriculturalists. Pacific Islands of Nauru, Tuvalu and Western Samoa. In: Trowell HC, Burkitt DP, eds. Western diseases: their emergence and prevention. London: Edward Arnold, 1981: 204-24.

CHINESE

(619) Du SF, Wang H. Food fiber and diabetes. Sheng Li Ko Hsueh Chin Chan 1981 Mar; 12 (3): 234-8.

(620) Hou XC. On the requirements and dietary allowances of carbohydrates, fibers and trace elements. Sheng Li Ko Hsueh Chin Chan 1981 Feb; 12 (2): 152-6.

DANISH

(621) Arffmann S, Malchow-Moller A. Bulk laxatives. Ugeskr Laeger 1981 Apr 20; 143 (17): 1101-2.

(622) Rasmussen LP, Damsgaard EM, Iversen S. Granulated guar-gum (Slocose) for non-insulin dependent diabetic patients (English abstract). Ugeskr Laeger 1981 May 11; 143 (20): 1267-70.

DUTCH

(623) Lutjens A, Plooij M, Rustemeijer C, Verleur H. Effect of dietary fibre on the absorption of glucose in the intestine. Voeding 1981 Nov 15; 42 (11): 370-2.

(624) Pikaar NA. The importance of dietary fibre and the role of bread (English abstract). Voeding 1981 Apr 15; 42 (4): 114-7.

FRENCH

(625) Capron J-P, Zeitoun P, Julien D. A multicenter controlled trial of a combination of kaolin, sterculia gum, meprobamate, and magnesium salts, in the irritable bowel syndrome (English abtract). Gastroenterol Clin Biol 1981 Jan; 5 (1): 67-72.

(626) Cope R. Normalization of intestinal passage in patients with anal surgery. Action of a bran powder with polyenzymatic activity. Med Chir Dig 1981; 10 (4): 353-5.

(627) Cope R. Poly-Karaya and anal surgery. Med Chir Dig 1981; 10 (5): 463-4.

(628) Darnis F. Clinical study of a new medication in the treatment of functional colopathies. Med Chir Dig 1981; 10 (5): 461-2.

(629) Delmont J. The value of adding an antispasmodic musculotropic agent in the treatment of painful constipation in functional colopathies with bran. Med Chir Dig 1981; 10 (4): 365-70.

(630) Dietsch R, Bonneville B. Comparative study of Kaologeais and Smectite in the treatment of colopathies. Med Chir Dig 1981; 10 (6): 549-51.

(631) Dorf G, Licht H, Namias A, Paraf A. Action of Poly-Karaya in functional colopathies. Results of a multicentre study of 114 patients. Med Chir Dig 1981; 10 (6): 533-8.

(632) Melet JJ. The importance of nutrition among the risk factors in varicose veins (English abstract). Phlebologie 1981 Jul-Sep; 34 (3): 469-88.

(633) Meyer F, Le Quintrec Y. Relationship between dietary fibers and constipation (English abstract). Nouv Presse Med 1981 Jul 11-25; 10 (30): 2479-81.

GERMAN

(634) Forster H. Bulk in human nutrition — a critical review. Med Monatsschr Pharm 1981 Mar; 4 (3): 65-76.

(635) Matzkies F, Hubner M. Cholesterol and weight reduction with a new formula diet containing bran and guar as dietary fiber and a mixture of corn-, milk- and soya-protein (English abstract). Fortschr Med 1981 Feb 12; 99 (6): 195-9.

(636) Meier H, Kesting U, Poppe S. On the influence of native crude fibre on the digestibility of nitrogen and amino acids in pigs (English abstract). Arch Tierernaehr 1981 Mar; 31 (3): 187-93.

(637) Muller E, Rickenbach M. Nutrition and cancer — an overview (English abstract). Praxis 1981 Oct 20; 70 (43): 1903-12.
(638) Richter WO, Weisweiler P, Schwandt P. Therapy of hypercholesteremia with apple pectin. Dtsch Med Wochenschr 1981 May 8; 106 (19): 628.

ITALIAN
(639) Agazia B, Lorenzi S, Marchini P, Saporiti E. Possible therapeutic use of dietary fibre in uremic and dialytic hyperlipemia (English abstract). Minerva Nefrol 1981 Apr-Jun; 28 (2): 167-70.
(640) Alessandrini A, Fusco MA, Gatti E, Rossi PA. Dietary fibre and cholelithiasis. Results of a controlled study (abstract). Boll Soc Ital Biol Sper 1981; 57 (18 Pt II): 198.
(641) Arsenio L, Cavalli Sforza LT, Magnati G, Strata A. Clinical study of the use of a deproteinized guar flour in the treatment of obesity (English abstract). Acta Biomed Ateneo Parmene 1981. 52 (4): 149-57.
(642) Data PG, Cacchio M, Sergiacomo P, Di Tano G, Di Primio R, Battista P. Findings of the importance of dietetic fiber in the regulation of cholesterolemia (English abstract). Boll Soc Ital Biol Sper 1981 Jul 30; 57 (14): 1545-50.
(643) Losapio GM, Setti M, Nespoli M, Sculati O. Changes in the lipid pattern of atherosclerotic patients treated with a diet enriched with raw cereal fiber. Analysis of the results (English abstract). Minerva Dietol Gastroenterol 1981 Jan-Mar; 27 (1): 131-6.
(644) Magnoni V. Dietetic fiber in nutrition. Prophylactic and therapeutic activity and mechanism of action (English abstract). Minerva Med 1981 Feb 25; 72 (6): 287-96.

JAPANESE
(645) Kitano A, Kobayashi K, Oshiumi H, Ookawa K, Oka S, Tanaka Y, Kuwajuma S, Ono T. Studies of experimental ulcerative colitis induced by carrageenan in rabbits — especially long-term treatment with carrageenan and intestinal bacteria (English abstract). Nippon Shokakibyo Gakkai Zasshi 1981 Nov; 78 (11): 2104-11.
(646) Kuboyama N, Fujii A, Tamura T. Antitumor activities of bamboo leaf extracts (BLE) and its lignin (BLL) (English abstract). Nippon Yakurigaku Zasshi 1981 Jun, 77 (6). 579-96.

NORWEGIAN
(647) Uusitupa M, Karttunen P, Aro A. Effect of a small amount of guar gum mixed into a snack on blood glucose in healthy subjects and in insulin treated diabetics. Naringsforskning 1981; 25 (4): 125-7.

POLISH
(648) Bartnikowska E, Michajlik A. Use of pectins in the prevention and treatment of hyperlipidemia. Pol Tyg Lek 1981 Jan 5; 36 (1): 33-6.
(649) Bartnikowska E. Dietary fiber as a natural food component preventing the development of digestive tract diseases and arteriosclerosis. Pol Tyg Lek 1981 Jan 19; 36 (3): 109-11.
(650) Bulinski R, Kot A, Kotulas K, Szydlowska E. Nutritional and calorie value of dried fruit, vegetables and mushrooms (English abstract). Zywienie Czlowieka 1981; 8 (1): 57-62.
(651) Ludwicki J. Determination of the mercury content in wheat bran (English abstract). Rocz Panstw Hig 1981; 32 (4): 309-13.

RUSSIAN
(652) Levitan MKh, Dubinin AV, Beiul EA, Iurkov MIu, Shechovskaia AK. Treatment of colonic diverticulosis and irritable colon with wheat bran. Sov Med 1981; (8): 109-12.
(653) Rudenskaya MV, Lazarev PI, Ivanova TZ, Galperin YM. The phenomenon of formation of the dense fraction structures of enteral milieu in changes of its pH (English abstract). Sechenov Physiol J USSR 1981; 67 (2). 268-73.

SPANISH

(654) de la Vega, Holgado Silva C, Aznar Martin A, Vahi Serrano S, Aznar Reig A. Phytobezoar and diabetes mellitus. Rev Esp Enferm Apar Dig 1981 Mar; 59 (3): 379-84.
(656) Martinez Para MC, Torija Isasa ME, Fidanza AA. Estimation of alimentary fibre in
edible mushroom species: genus Agaricus (English abstract). An Bromatol 1981; 33
(1): 85-90.

SWEDISH

(656) Asp N-G, Anderson H. Dietary Fiber — theory and clinical aspects. Nord Med 1981
Feb; 96 (2): 51-4.
(657) Bergstrom G, Werner U. Bran and bulk preparations in the treatment of constipation in
geriatric patients. Lakartidningen 1981 Jul 17; 78 (25): 2438-9.

Englyst H: 65, 68, 163, 164, 228, 590
Erdman JW Jr: 165
Eshchar J: 166
Esterhuysen AJ: 76
Estes MK: 363
Evans JL: 176

Faber S: 422
Fachmann W: 519
Fairweather-Tait S: 167
Fang Pong S: 85
Faraji B: 168
Faridi HA: 428, 429
Farrell DJ: 20, 21, 51, 552, 553
Faturoti EO: 169, 170
Faubion JM: 171
Fehily AM: 95
Feingold DS: 586
Fernandez JA: 243
Fernandez R: 417
Ferreri LF: 513
Fetzer S: 267
Fidanza AA: 655
Fidanza F: 228
Fielden H: 231, 232
Fielding JF: 462
Fields D: 616
Finney KF: 498
Finney PL: 428, 429
Fioramonti J: 87
Fisher A: 527
Fisher N: 68, 590
Fleming CR: 448
Fleming S: 62
Fleming SE: 172, 334
Fletcher P: 432
Floch MH: 140, 173
Fogo M: 314
Foo LY: 174
Ford JA: 457
Forman LP: 175
Forster H: 634
Forsythe AB: 317, 319
Forsythe R: 156
Foster N: 178
Fotsis T: 4
Fowler EF: 562
Fowler J: 402, 403
Fox DB: 319
Fox DD: 317
Fox HM: 47, 229, 266, 267, 606
Foy WL Jr: 176
Francis B: 590

Frantz I: 616
Franz KB: 608
Frape DL: 177
Fraser GE: 178
Fraumeni JF Jr: 617
Fredlund PE: 54
Freeman HJ: 524
Friedland S: 284
Friedlander ML: 179
Frolich W: 180, 181
Fujii A: 646
Fulcher RG: 182
Furda I: 183, 228
Furmanska M: 287
Fusco MA: 640
Fussell ST: 184

Gallo LL: 588
Galperin YM: 653
Galton DJ: 135
Garcia E: 185, 452
Garcia L. JS: 445
Garcia-L SJ: 186
Garzon P: 445
Gassull MA: 232
Gates JE: 452
Gatti E: 640
Gayst S: 500
Gear JS: 187
Gee JM: 238
Geekie M: 501
Gelfand M: 179, 188
Gelroth JA: 428, 429, 430, 431
Genovese S: 455
Ghadirian P: 346
Gherardini F: 476
Giacco A: 455
Giaquinto CM: 386
Gibertini A: 475
Gibson RS: 13, 189
Gilat T: 438
Giri J: 190
Glauert HP: 191, 192
Glober GA: 193
Godara RB: 63, 194, 249
Godding EW: 37, 68, 571
Godfrey J: 109
Goel R: 195
Goering HK: 256
Goff DV: 231
Goldin BR: 4
Gomez Brenes R: 361
Gorbach SL: 4
Gordon C: 128
Gormley R: 196

Gould MR: 105, 106
Graff E: 438
Graham CH: 199
Graham DY: 363
Graham HD: 197
Graham S: 198
Graham SL: 199
Granger DN: 288, 289
Grau LE: 99, 587
Greenbaum DS: 200
Greenblatt DJ: 9
Greenfield MS: 113
Gregory JF III: 382, 383, 454
Griffith HM: 201
Griffiths DW: 202
Grisebach H: 321
Grobin W: 251
Grossman MI: 483
Gruden N: 354
Gueguen L: 40, 203
Guennou L: 526
Guild R: 204
Gumbmann MR: 62, 387
Gunnells CK: 385
Guoo JY: 103
Gupta ML: 283
Guth PH: 483

Hachida K: 378
Hadziyev D: 353
Hallgren B: 205, 478, 479
Hallmans G: 206, 391, 392
Hallmer H: 34
Hamilton DG: 491
Hamilton WD: 68
Hammett F: 306
Hanson D: 514, 515, 516
Hanson M: 616
Harbers LH: 207, 208
Harland BF: 209
Harmatz JS: 9
Harris CC: 134
Harrison JR: 590
Harrison SL: 210
Hartog M: 213, 326
Harwood JP: 209
Hasselblad K: 478, 479
Hautvast JG: 86
Haydar M: 353
Heading RC: 219
Heaton KW: 37, 68, 75, 211, 212, 213, 214, 326, 373, 565, 590
Heckman MM: 215
Hedlund B: 19
Hegewisch S: 279

        (1.12) Ileostomy
         48*, 427

        (1.13) Gallstones
         6, 72, 77*, 83*, 84*, 90*, 94, 109*, 120, 126, 131, 133, 134, 152*, 161*, 162,
         171, 179*, 198, 204*, 205*, 206, 216*, 219*, 234, 238*, 242, 256*, 264*,
         265*, 271*, 273, 275*, 277, 283, 313, 330*, 345, 351, 352, 389, 402*, 422,
         424*, 425*, 430*, 437*, 454, 473, 485*, 487*, 500, 502, 526*, 527, 563, 604

        (1.14) Phytobezoars
         13, 118, 119, 289, 483*, 576, 587, 593, 594, 608*, 609*

        (1.15) Miscellaneous gastrointestinal
         5, 6, 8, 13, 17, 21*, 43*, 57*, 62*, 83*, 163, 164*, 169, 176, 194*, 216*, 221*,
         222*, 224, 228, 236*, 241, 244*, 264, 265, 268*, 270*, 284*, 288, 294*, 319,
         324*, 325*, 333*, 345, 364, 370*, 374*, 416, 424, 425, 432*, 437*, 438*,
         439*, 443*, 444*, 448, 457*, 465*, 471, 482*, 514, 522, 523, 528, 555, 571*,
         580*, 597*, 608*, 609*

(2) *CARDIOVASCULAR*
        (2.1) Lipid metabolism, cholesterol, triglycerides
         3*, 4*, 5*, 6*, 7*, 17, 19*, 34, 37*, 39, 42, 44, 71, 72*, 75, 83*, 88, 89*, 94,
         95*, 108, 109, 120*, 125, 126, 133, 134, 136*, 140, 149, 152*, 169*, 176,
         179*, 195, 204*, 206, 211*, 217, 218*, 219*, 220*, 233*, 237, 238*, 242, 250,
         262*, 264*, 265*, 270*, 271, 274, 275*, 277, 278*, 282*, 292, 294, 300, 312,
         319*, 320*, 342, 346, 351, 352*, 361, 384, 389, 391*, 392*, 414, 415, 416*,
         418, 419*, 421*, 425*, 430*, 441*, 450*, 459*, 461, 471*, 473*, 476*, 478,
         484, 485, 486*, 489*, 490, 500, 514*, 519*, 526*, 527, 529*, 531*, 534, 535,
         554, 555*, 562*, 563, 564*, 565*, 580*, 587, 602*

        (2.2) Atherosclerosis, ischaemic heart disease
         7, 70*, 270*, 275*, 277, 279*, 301*, 351, 430*, 455, 456*, 470, 513, 527

        (2.3) Venous thrombosis, varicose veins, haemorrhoids
         156*, 328*, 345

        (2.4) Hypertension
         124, 156*

(3) *METABOLIC*
        (3.1) Diabetes mellitus, carbohydrate metabolism
         3*, 7*, 8, 9, 17, 19*, 24*, 39*, 41*, 44, 45*, 50, 64*, 75, 88, 89, 91, 112*,
         126*, 135*, 141, 149, 163, 164*, 165, 167*, 175*, 194*, 195, 199*, 208, 209,
         210, 211*, 214, 217, 223*, 228, 229, 230*, 231*, 232, 233*, 237, 240*, 243*,
         250, 259*, 262*, 274, 280, 281, 290*, 293*, 294*, 295*, 300, 304, 306*, 311*,
         312, 318*, 320*, 333*, 342, 346, 350, 352, 256*, 357*, 362*, 363*, 364, 371*,
         383, 384*, 388*, 394, 395, 397, 412, 416*, 431*, 439*, 443*, 450*, 455*,
         457*, 460, 461, 468*, 471*, 484, 492, 509*, 519*, 520, 522, 534, 535, 539*,
         540*, 546*, 547, 549*, 551, 555, 558*, 562*, 568, 576, 580*, 595*, 602*, 607*

        (3.2) Obesity
         3, 8*, 19*, 39, 45*, 178*, 211*, 274, 294, 296, 300, 309, 318*, 319*, 346, 455,
         546, 555

(4) *FIBRE AND FOOD*
        (4.1) Fibre: definition, terminology, composition, analysis
         11*, 25*, 35*, 36, 38, 47*, 49*, 52*, 53*, 56*, 73*, 92, 93, 96, 97, 98*, 99*,
         100*, 114*, 123*, 127*, 143*, 166*, 174, 183, 192*, 193*, 196*, 215, 235*,
         238, 244, 260*, 282, 307, 314, 321*, 322*, 329, 334, 336*, 337, 338*, 339*,
         340*, 341*, 344*, 354, 366*, 377, 387*, 390*, 400*, 413*, 428*, 477*, 495,
         496*, 497*, 498*, 499*, 507*, 512*, 514, 538*, 552, 561*, 570*, 573*, 577*,
         586*, 589*, 590*, 600*

(4.2)   Fibre in the diet and food, except cereals
2*, 16*, 35, 38, 49*, 53*, 59*, 63*, 74, 87*, 90*, 96, 106*, 115*, 116, 121*,
122, 127*, 131, 133, 142*, 143*, 144*, 181*, 183*, 186, 193*, 197, 202*,
207*, 231, 234, 235, 249, 260, 261, 266*, 279*, 282*, 287*, 301*, 302*, 303,
308*, 336*, 337*, 347, 366*, 367, 373*, 374, 398*, 400, 402*, 403, 405, 420,
426*, 428*, 445, 447, 451, 458*, 462, 469*, 475*, 488*, 495*, 496*, 498,
501*, 506, 507, 510*, 513, 515, 530, 532*, 536*, 537*, 541*, 542, 544, 560, 570*,
573*, 575, 577*, 588*, 600

(4.3)   Fibre in cereal and cereal foods
47, 56*, 96, 97, 98*, 99, 102*, 105, 115, 116*, 127, 128*, 143*, 180*, 235,
244, 305, 331*, 332, 334*, 337*, 348, 353*, 400, 452, 453, 498, 570*, 589*,
590*, 600

(4.4)   Modern dietary change
No paper relevant

(5) MISCELLANEOUS

(5.1)   Antitoxic action
85, 86*, 139*, 169*, 173*, 182, 256*, 257*, 263*, 432*, 556*, 598*

(5.2)   Ill-effects
13, 15*, 16*, 59, 106*, 130, 146, 160*, 239, 246*, 267, 284*, 285*, 292, 296,
315*, 367*, 374*, 377*, 417*, 443, 458*, 459, 464, 471, 475, 488*, 494*, 555,
556*, 571*, 587*, 592, 608*, 609*

(5.3)   Early views on whole foods and dietary fibre before 1940
No paper relevant

(5.4)   Experimental methods
81*, 306*, 436*, 518*

(5.5)   Other
1*, 2*, 10*, 11*, 21*, 38*, 51*, 52*, 60*, 61*, 63*, 70*, 72*, 73*, 77*, 78*,
82*, 84, 86*, 87*, 90*, 97*, 98*, 99*, 100*, 101*, 102*, 106*, 114*, 115*,
116*, 121*, 124, 128*, 129*, 152*, 157*, 161*, 169, 172*, 181*, 183*, 185*,
186*, 192*, 193*, 196*, 215*, 227*, 249, 266*, 270*, 279*, 284*, 285*, 287*,
293*, 300, 305, 307*, 318*, 322*, 330*, 336*, 338*, 339*, 340*, 341*, 344*,
352, 355, 376, 387*, 397, 398*, 399*, 400*, 403, 404*, 406, 407*, 411*, 417*,
428*, 434*, 435, 451*, 452, 453, 458*, 460*, 469*, 487*, 494*, 495, 497*,
499*, 501*, 503*, 507*, 514*, 515*, 538*, 561*, 610

(6) DIETARY FIBRE HYPOTHESES, GENERAL PRESENTATION

20, 27*, 28*, 65, 67, 68, 69, 247*, 272, 276, 381, 386, 440, 524, 527, 539*,
541, 543, 566, 572, 574, 605, 606

(7) BOOKS, SYMPOSIA, THESES

(7.1)   Books for the public
18*, 66*, 147*, 148*, 248*, 311*, 379*, 474*, 550*

(7.2)   Books for the scientist
168, 184*, 251*, 385*, 525*

(67) Burkitt DP. Dietary fiber: is it really helpful? Geriatrics 1982 Jan; 37 (1): 119-26.
(68) Burkitt DP. Western diseases and their emergence related to diet. S Afr Med J 1982 Jun 26; 61 (26): 1013-5.
(69) Burkitt D. Dietary fibre. World Med 1982 Dec 11; 18 (5): 10, 12.
(70) Burr ML, Sweetnam PM. Vegetarianism, dietary fiber, and mortality. Am J Clin Nutr 1982 Nov; 36 (5): 873-7.
(71) Burrows CF, Kronfeld DS, Banta CA, Merritt AM. Effects of fiber on digestibility and transit time in dogs. J Nutr 1982 Sep; 112 (9): 1726-32.
(72) Burton R, Manninen V. Influence of a psyllium-based fibre preparation on faecal and serum parameters. Acta Med Scand (Suppl) 1982; 688: 91-4.
(73) Cabib E, Roberts R, Bowers B. Synthesis of the yeast cell wall and its regulation. Annu Rev Biochem 1982; 51: 763-93.
(74) Calixto FS, Canellas J. Components of nutritional interest in carob pods (Ceratonia siliqua). J Sci Food Agric 1982 Dec; 33 (12): 1319-23.
(75) Calle A, Romeo SE, Cabrerizo L, Hernandez D, Bordiu E, Valle MA, Maranes JP, Charro AL. Dietary fibre and diabetes (abstract). Diabetologia 1982 Aug; 23 (2): 159.
(76) Calloway SP, Fonagy P. Fibre and duodenal ulcers (letter). Lancet 1982 Oct 16; 2 (8303): 878.
(77) Calvert GD, Yeates RA. Adsorption of bile salts by soya-bean flour, wheat bran, lucerne (Medicago sativa), sawdust and lignin; the effect of saponins and other plant constituents. Br J Nutr 1982 Jan; 47 (1): 45-52.
(78) Camire AL, Clydesdale FM. Interactions of soluble iron with wheat bran. J Food Sci 1982 Jul-Aug; 47 (4): 1296-7.
(79) Caprez A, Fairweather-Tait SJ. The effect of heat treatment and particle size of bran on mineral absorption in rats. Br J Nutr 1982 Nov; 48 (3): 467-75.
(80) Caprez A, Fairweather-Tait SJ. The effect of apple fibre on calcium, magnesium, iron, copper and zinc balance in the rat (abstract). Proc Nutr Soc 1982 Sep; 41 (3): 133A.
(81) Carryer PW, Brown ML, Malagelada J-R, Carlson GL, McCall JT. Quantification of the fate of dietary fiber in humans by a newly developed radiolabeled fiber marker. Gastroenterology 1982 Jun; 82 (6): 1389-94.
(82) Carter EG, Carpenter KJ. The bioavailability for humans of bound niacin from wheat bran. Am J Clin Nutr 1982 Nov; 36 (5): 855-61.
(83) Cassidy MM, Lightfoot FG, Vahouny GV. Morphological aspects of dietary fibers in the intestine. Adv Lipid Res 1982; 19: 203-29.
(84) Cassidy MM, Lightfoot FG, Vahouny GV. Dietary fiber, bile acids, and intestinal morphology. In: Vahouny GV, Kritchevsky D, eds. Dietary fiber in health and disease. New York: Plenum Press, 1982: 239-64.
(85) Catignani GL, Carter ME. Effects of dietary lignin on vitamin A stores in the rat (abstract). Fed Proc 1982 Mar 1; 41 (3): 386.
(86) Catignani GL, Carter ME. Antioxidant properties of lignin. J Food Sci 1982 Sep-Oct; 47 (5): 1745, 1748.
(87) Champion SA, Phillips GO, Williams PA. The effect of micro-crystalline cellulose on the organoleptic properties of ice cream. In: Phillips GO, Wedlock DJ, Williams PA, eds. Gums and stabilisers for the food industry. Interactions of hydrocolloids. Oxford: Pergamon Press, 1982: 361-6. (Prog Food Nutr Sci; vol 13.)
(88) Chang ML, Johnson MA. Effects of mucilaginous fibers on glucose tolerance and lipid metabolism in rats (abstract). Fed Proc 1982 Mar 1; 41 (3): 399.
(89) Chang ML. Effect of dietary pectin on esterification and excretion of exogenous cholesterol in rats. Nutr Rep Int 1982 Jul; 26 (1): 59-66.
(90) Chen ML, Chang SC, Guoo JY. Fiber contents of some Chinese vegetables and their in vitro binding capacity of bile acids. Nutr Rep Int 1982 Dec; 26 (6): 1053-9.
(91) Chen MS. The role of diet in the mechanism for decreased glucose tolerance of the aged (abstract). Diabetes 1982 May; 31 (Suppl 2): 82A.
(92) Chen W-J, Anderson JW. Analysis of fiber components (letter). Am J Clin Nutr 1982 Jan; 35 (1): 176.
(93) Chen W-J, Anderson JW. Plant fiber in selected cereals (letter). Am J Clin Nutr 1982 Feb; 35 (2): 408.

(94) Chen W-J, Anderson JW. Biliary bile acid and lipid metabolism of oat bran (abstract). Fed Proc 1982 Mar 1; 41 (3): 399.

(95) Cherry JA, Jones DE. Dietary cellulose, wheat bran, and fish meal in relation to hepatic lipids, serum lipids, and lipid excretion in laying hens. Poult Sci 1982 Sep; 61 (9): 1873-8.

(96) Cherry JP. Protein - polysaccharide interactions. In: Lineback DR, Inglett GE, eds. Food carbohydrates. Westport, Connecticut: AVI Publishing Company, 1982: 375-98.

(97) Christianson DD. Hydrocolloid interactions with starches. In: Lineback DR, Inglett GE, eds. Food carbohydrates. Westport, Connecticut: AVI Publishing Company, 1982: 399-419.

(98) Ciacco CF, D'Appolonia BL. Characterization of pentosans from different wheat flour classes and of their gelling capacity. Cereal Chem 1982 Mar-Apr; 59 (2): 96-100.

(99) Ciacco CF, D'Appolonia BL. Characterization and gelling capacity of water-soluble pentosans isolated from different mill streams. Cereal Chem 1982 May-Jun; 59 (3): 163-6.

(100) Clark AH, Richardson RK, Robinson G, Ross-Murphy SB, Weaver AC. Structure and mechanical properties of agar/BSA co-gels. In: Phillips GO, Wedlock DJ, Williams PA, eds. Gums and stabilisers for the food industry. Interactions of hydrocolloids. Oxford: Pergamon Press, 1982: 149-60. (Prog Food Nutr Sci; vol 13.)

(101) Coert A, Vonk Noordegraaf CA, Groen MB, van der Vies J. The dietary origin of urinary lignan HPMF. Experientia 1982 Aug 15; 38 (8): 904-5.

(102) Collins JL, Kalantari SM, Post AR. Peanut hull flour as dietary fiber in wheat bread. J Food Sci 1982 Nov-Dec; 47 (6): 1899-1902, 1920.

(103) Committee on diet, nutrition, and cancer. Assembly of Life Sciences National Research Council. Dietary fiber. In: Diet, nutrition and cancer. Washington, DC: National Academy Press, 1982.

(104) Connaughton J. McCarthy CF. Comparison of combination of isphagula/poloxamer 188 and placebo on gastrointestinal transit time. Ir Med J 1982 Mar; 75 (3): 93-4.

(105) Craddock D. Bread for health and bread for slimming. J R Coll Gen Pract 1982 Sep; 32 (242): 525, 528-9.

(106) Cruz R, Park YK. Production of fungal α-galactosidase and its application to the hydrolysis of galactooligosaccharides in soybean milk. J Food Sci 1982 Nov-Dec; 47 (6): 1973-5.

(107) Cummings JH. Polysaccharide fermentation in the human colon. In: Kasper H, Goebell H, eds. Colon and nutrition. Lancaster, England: MTP Press, 1982: 91-103.

(108) Cummings JH. Consequences of the metabolism of fiber in the human large intestine. In: Vahouny GV, Kritchevsky D, eds. Dietary fiber in health and disease. New York: Plenum Press, 1982: 9-22.

(109) Cummings JH, Branch WJ. Postulated mechanisms whereby fiber may protect against large bowel cancer. In: Vahouny GV, Kritchevsky D, eds. Dietary fiber in health and disease. New York: Plenum Press, 1982: 313-25.

(110) Cummings JH, Branch WJ, Bjerrum L, Paerregaard A, Helms P, Burton R. Colon cancer and large bowel function in Denmark and Finland. Nutr Cancer 1982; 4 (1): 61-6.

(111) Cummings JH. Health and the large intestine. In: Turner MR, ed. Nutrition and health. A perspective. The current status of research on diet-related diseases. Lancaster, England: MTP Press, 1982: 35-48.

(112) Daumerie C, Henquin J-C. Acute effects of guar gum on glucose tolerance and intestinal absorption of nutrients in rats. Diabete Metab 1982 Mar; 8 (1): 1-5.

(113) Davies NT. Effects of phytic acid on mineral availability. In: Vahouny GV, Kritchevsky D, eds. Dietary fiber in health and disease. New York: Plenum Press, 1982: 105-16.

(114) Dea IC. Polysaccharide conformation in solutions and gels. In: Lineback DR, Inglett GE, eds. Food carbohydrates. Westport, Connecticut: AVI Publishing Company, 1982: 420-57.

(115) De Fouw C, Zabik ME, Uebersax MA, Aguilera JM, Lusas E. Use of unheated and heat-treated navy bean hulls as a source of dietary fiber in spice-flavoured layer cakes. Cereal Chem 1982 May-Jun; 59 (3): 229-30.

(116) De Fouw C, Zabik ME, Uebersax MA, Aguilera JM, Lusas E. Effects of heat treatment and level of navy bean hulls in sugar-snap cookies. Cereal Chem 1982 Jul-Aug; 59 (4): 245-

(117) Delorme CB, Wojcik J. Interaction of dietary protein with cellulose in the adaptation to caloric dilution by weanling rats. J Nutr 1982 Jan; 112 (1): 21-8.

(118) Delpre G, Kadish U, Glantz I. New therapeutic approach and etiological considerations in postoperative phytobezoars (abstract). Scand J Gastroenterol 1982; 17 (Suppl 78): 245.

(119) DeLuca VA Jr. Phytobezoars — failure of the housekeeper. J Clin Gastroenterol 1982 Aug; 4 (4): 361-2.

(120) de Lumen BO, Lubin B, Chiu D, Reyes PS, Omaye ST. Bioavailability of vitamin E in rats fed diets containing pectin. Nutr Res 1982; 2 (1): 73-83.

(121) De Moor H, Rapaille A. Evaluation of starches and gums in pasteurised whipping cream. In: Phillips GO, Wedlock DJ, Williams PA, eds. Gums and stabilisers for the food industry. Interactions of hydrocolloids. Oxford: Pergamon Press, 1982: 199-207.

(122) Dierenfeld ES, Hintz HF, Robertson JB, Van Soest PJ, Oftedal OT. Utilization of bamboo by the giant panda. J Nutr 1982 Apr; 112 (4): 636-41.

(123) Dintzis FR. Dietary fiber analysis — concepts and problems. In: Lineback DR, Inglett GE, eds. Food carbohydrates. Westport, Connecticut: AVI Publishing Company, 1982: 312-32.

(124) Dodson PM, Shine B, Galton DJ, Landon J. Dietary fibre, sodium, hypertension and C-reactive protein (abstract). Proc Nutr Soc 1982 Jun; 41 (2): 51A.

(125) Dodson PM, Ferns G, Galton DJ, Taylor KG. High-density-lipoprotein subfractions: the effects of a high-fibre cereal, low-fat dietary regimen (abstract). Proc Nutr Soc 1982 Sep; 41 (3): 117A.

(126) Doi K, Matsuura M, Kawara A, Uenoyama R, Baba S. Effect of glucomannan (konjac fiber) on glucose and lipid metabolism in normal and diabetic subjects. In: Melish JS, Hanna J, Baba S, eds. Genetic environmental interaction in diabetes mellitus. Amsterdam: Excerpta Medica, 1982: 306-12.

(127) Dovell CJ, Harris ND. Development of a method to measure dietary fibre in oranges. J Sci Food Agric 1982 Feb; 33 (2): 185-93.

(128) Dreese PC, Hoseney RC. Baking properties of the bran fraction from brewer's spent grains. Cereal Chem 1982 Mar-Apr; 59 (2): 89-91.

(129) Duffus JH, Levi C, Manners DJ. Yeast cell-wall glucans. Adv Microb Physiol 1982; 23: 151-81.

(130) Dworkin BM, Deschner EE, Fath RB Jr, Winawer SJ. Degraded carrageenan as a model for acute right-sided colitis in mice|(abstract). Gastroenterology 1982 May; 82 (5 Pt 2): 1048.

(131) Eastwood MA, Brydon WG, Smith DM, Smith JH. A study of diet, serum lipids, and fecal constituents in spouses. Am J Clin Nutr 1982 Aug; 36 (2): 290-3.

(132) Eastwood MA, Watters DA, Smith AN. Diverticular disease — is it a motility disorder? Clin Gastroenterol 1982 Sep; 11 (3): 545-61.

(133) Eastwood MA, Baird JD, Brydon WG, Smith JH, Helliwell S, Pritchard JL. Dietary fiber and colon function in a population aged 18-80 years. In: Vahouny GV, Kritchevsky D, eds. Dietary fiber in health and disease. New York: Plenum Press, 1982: 23-33.

(134) Eastwood MA, Adamson I, Brydon WG. A comparison of the effect of yam, cassava and alfalfa based diets on cholesterol metabolism in the rat (abstract). Proc Nutr Soc 1982 Jun; 41 (2): 61A.

(135) Ebihara K, Kiriyama S. Comparative effects of water-soluble and water-insoluble dietary fibers on various parameters relating to glucose tolerance in rats. Nutr Rep Int 1982 Aug; 26 (2): 193-201.

(136) Eggum BO, Andersen JO, Rotenberg S. The effect of dietary fibre level and microbial activity in the digestive tract on fat metabolism in rats and pigs. Acta Agric Scand 1982; 32 (2): 145-50.

(137) Eggum BO, Thorbek G, Beames RM, Chwalibog A, Henckel S. Influence of diet and microbial activity in the digestive tract on digestibility, and nitrogen and energy metabolism in rats and pigs. Br J Nutr 1982 Jul; 49 (1): 161-75.

(138) Eggum BO, Juliano BO, Maningat CC. Protein and energy utilization of rice milling fractions by rats. Qual Plant Plant Foods Hum Nutr 1982; 31 (4): 371-6.

(139) Eggum BO, Beames RM, Wolstrup J. Excretion of nitrate and nitrite by the pig as influenced by dietary fibre levels and microbial activity in the digestive tract. Z Tierphysiol Tiernahr Futtermittelkd 1982 Oct; 48 (4): 195-200.

(140) Ehle FR, Robertson JB, Van Soest PJ. Influence of dietary fibers on fermentation in the human large intestine. J Nutr 1982 Jan; 112 (1): 158-66.

(141) El-Beheri Burgess BR. Rationale for changes in the dietary management of diabetes. Fat, carbohydrate, and fiber. J Am Diet Assoc 1982 Sep; 21 (3): 258-61.

(142) Ellis R, Morris ER, Hill AD, Smith JC Jr. Phytate: zinc molar ratio, mineral, and fiber content of three hospital diets. J Am Diet Assoc 1982 Jul; 81 (1): 26-9.

(143) Englyst H, Wiggins HS, Cummings JH. Determination of the non-starch polysaccharides in plant foods by gas-liquid chromatography of constituent sugars as alditol acetates. Analyst 1982 Mar; 107 (1272): 307-18.

(144) Englyst HN, Bingham SA, Wiggins HS, Southgate DA, Seppanen R, Helms P, Anderson V, Day KC, Choolun R, Collinson E, Cummings JH. Nonstarch polysaccharide consumption in four Scandinavian populations. Nutr Cancer 1982; 4 (1): 50-60.

(145) Espinoza J, Araya M, Krause S, Egana JI, Barrera G, Pacheco I, Brunser O. Fiber and fecal nutrient loss in environmental enteropathy (abstract). Fed Proc 1982 Mar 1; 41 (3): 712.

(146) Evans C. Facing up to the third F. World Med 1982 Nov 13; 18 (3): 57.

(147) Eyton A. The F-plan calorie and fibre chart. Harmondsworth, Middlesex: Penguin, 1982.

(148) Eyton A. The F-plan diet. Harmondsworth, Middlesex: Penguin, 1982.

(149) Fagerberg S-E. The effects of a bulk laxative (metamucil[R]) on fasting blood glucose, serum lipids and other variables in constipated patients with non-insulin dependent diabetes (abstract). Acta Endocrinol (Copenh) 1982; Suppl 247: 22.

(150) Fairweather-Tait SJ. The effect of different levels of wheat bran on iron absorption in rats from bread containing similar amounts of phytate. Br J Nutr 1982 Mar; 47 (2): 243-9.

(151) Fairweather-Tait SJ, Caprez A. A comparison between the effect of added sodium phytate and endogenous phytate in bran and oats on zinc absorption (abstract). Proc Nutr Soc 1982 Sep; 41 (3): 132A.

(152) Falk JD, Nagyvary JJ. Exploratory studies of lipid-pectin interactions. J Nutr 1982 Jan; 112 (1): 1052-6.

(153) Farah DA, Hall MJ, Mills PR, Russell RI. Effect of dietary fibre on zinc absorption (abstract). Gut 1982 Oct; 23 (10): A920.

(154) Farness PL, Schneeman BO. Effects of dietary cellulose, pectin and oat bran on the small intestine in the rat. J Nutr 1982 Jul; 112 (7): 1315-9.

(155) Fedail SS, Badi SE. The effects of sorghum and wheat brans on colonic functions of healthy Sudanese subjects (abstract). Scand J Gastroenterol 1982; 17 (Suppl 78): 503.

(156) Fehily AM, Milbank JE, Yarnell JW, Hayes TM, Kubiki AJ, Eastham RD. Dietary determinants of lipoproteins, total cholesterol, viscosity, fibrinogen, and blood pressure. Am J Clin Nutr 1982 Nov; 36 (5): 890-6.

(157) Fernandez R, Phillips SF. Components of fiber bind iron in vitro. Am J Clin Nutr 1982 Jan; 35 (1): 100-6.

(158) Fernandez R, Phillips SF. Components of fiber impair iron absorption in the dog. Am J Clin Nutr 1982 Jan; 35 (1): 107-12.

(159) Fielding JF. The necessity of concurrent high dietary fibre intake when testing for drug efficacy in the irritable bowel syndrome (abstract). Gastroenterology 1982 May; 82 (5 Pt 2): 1056.

(160) Fleming SE. Flatulence activity of the smooth-seeded field pea as indicated by hydrogen production in the rat. J Food Sci 1982 Jan-Feb; 47 (1): 12-5.

(161) Floren CH, Nilsson A. Binding of bile salts to fibre-enriched wheat bran. Hum Nutr: Clin Nutr 1982; 36C (5): 381-9.

(162) Floren C-H, Nilsson A. Adsorption of bile salts to fiber enriched wheat bran (abstract). Scand J Gastroenterol 1982; 17 (Suppl 78): 230.

(163) Florholmen J, Lenner RA, Jorde R, Burhol PG. The effect of metamucil on the postprandial blood glucose and plasma GIP in insulin-dependent diabetics (abstract). Acta Endocrinol (Copenh) 1982; Suppl 247: 23.

(164) Florholmen J, Arvidsson-Lenner R, Jorde R, Burhol PG. The effect of metamucil on postprandial blood glucose and plasma gastric inhibitory peptide in insulin-dependent diabetics. Acta Med Scand 1982; 212 (4): 237-9.

(165) Flourie B, Vidon N, Florent C, Bernier JJ. Effect of pectin on jejunal glucose absorption in man (abstract). Gut 1982 Oct; 23 (10): A911.

(166) Ford CW. A routine method for identification and quantitative determination by gas-liquid chromatography of galacturonic acid in pectic substances. J Sci Food Agri 1982 Apr; 33 (4): 318-24.

(167) Forman LP, Schneeman BO. Dietary pectin's effect on starch utilization in rats. J Nutr 1982 Mar; 112 (3): 528-33.

(168) Forum on nutritional aspects of bread and flour and the implications for public health and the food industry. Record of proceedings. Verbatim record of proceedings at the Forum on Nutritional Aspects of Bread and Flour which was held at the Royal Society on Wednesday, 10th February 1982. Based on DHSS report on health and social subjects no. 23. Medical mailing co, Freepost, The mailing house, London W13 9HL.

(169) Frape DL, Wayman BJ, Tuck MG, Jones E. The effects of gum arabic, wheat offal and various of its fractions on the metabolism of ^{14}C-labelled aflatoxin B_1 in the male weanling rat. Br J Nutr 1982 Jul; 48 (1): 97-110.

(170) Freeman HJ. Studies on the effects of single fiber sources in the dimethylhydrazine rodent model of human bowel neoplasia. In: Vahouny GV, Kritchevsky D, eds. Dietary fiber in health and disease. New York: Plenum Press, 1982: 287-97.

(171) Frenkiel P, Lee D, Marks J, Gilmore C, Bonorris G, Schoenfield L. Effect of diet on bile acid kinetics and secretion of biliary lipids in patients treated with urodeoxycholic acid (abstract). Gastroenterology 1982 May; 82 (5 Pt 2): 1061.

(172) Friend DR, Chang GW. Simple dye release assay for determining endopectinase activity. J Agric Food Chem 1982 Sep-Oct; 30 (5): 982-5.

(173) Fukuba H, Kanamori A. Effects of non-nutritional polysaccharides on the excretion of polychlorinated biphenyls. Nutr Rep Int 1982 Aug; 26 (2): 281-7.

(174) Fulcher RG, Wood PJ. Identification of cereal carbohydrates by fluorescence microscopy (abstract). Cereal Foods World 1982 Sep; 27 (9): 455.

(175) Gabbe SG, Cohen AW, Herman GO, Schwartz S. Effect of dietary fiber on the oral glucose tolerance test in pregnancy. Am J Obstet Gynecol 1982 Jul 1; 143 (5): 514-7.

(176) Gallaher D, Schneeman BO. Effect of dietary cellulose on the site of fat absorption (abstract). Fed Proç 1982 Mar 1; 41 (3): 399.

(177) Garcia-Lopez S, Wyatt CJ. Effect of fiber in corn tortillas and cooked beans on iron availability. J Agric Food Chem 1982 Jul-Aug; 30 (4): 724-7. Correction. 1982 Nov-Dec; 30 (6): 1262.

(178) Gawecki J, Jeszka J, Kubczak D. Effect of residue-rich food on postprandial energy output in rats. Acta Physiol Pol 1982 Sep-Dec; 33 (5-6): 441-6.

(179) Gibney MJ, Pathirana C, Smith L. Saponins and fibre. Lack of interactive effects on serum and liver cholesterol in rats and hamsters (letter). Atherosclerosis 1982 Dec; 45 (3): 365-7.

(180) Gill AA, Morgan AG, Smith DB. Total β-glucan content of some barley cultivars. J Inst Brewing 1982; 88 (5): 317-9.

(181) Glahn P-E. Hydrocolloid stabilization of protein suspensions at low pH. In: Phillips GO, Wedlock DJ, Williams PA, eds. Gums and stabilisers for the food industry. Interactions of hydrocolloids. Oxford: Pergamon Press, 1982: 171-7. (Prog Food Nutr Sci; vol 13.)

324

(182) Glauert HP, Bennink MR. Effect of diet on the metabolism of 1,2-dimethylhydrazine (DMH) in the rat (abstract). Fed Proc 1982 Mar 1; 41 (3): 356.

(183) Glicksman M. Food applications of gums. In: Lineback DR, Inglett GE, eds. Food carbohydrates. Westport, Connecticut: AVI Publishing Company, 1982: 270-95.

(184) Glicksman M. Food Hydrocolloids. Boca Raton, Florida: CRC Press, 1982.

(185) Glicksman M. The hydrocolloids industry in the '80s — problems and opportunities. In: Phillips GO, Wedlock DJ, Williams PA, eds. Gums and stabilisers for the food industry. Interactions of hydrocolloids. Oxford: Pergamon Press, 1982: 299-321. (Prog Food Nutr Sci; vol 13.)

(186) Goldin BR, Adlercreutz H, Gorbach SL, Warram JH, Dwyer JT, Swenson L, Woods MN. Estrogen excretion patterns and plasma levels in vegetarian and omnivorous women. N Engl J Med 1982 Dec 16; 307 (25): 1542-7.

(187) Golechha AC, Chadda VS, Chadda S, Sharma SK, Mishra SN. Role of isphagula husk in the management of irritable bowel syndrome (a randomized double-blind crossover study). J Assoc Physicians India 1982 Jun; 30 (6): 353-5.

(188) Graham DY, Moser SE, Estes MK. The effect of bran on bowel function in constipation. Am J Gastroenterol 1982 Sep; 77 (9): 599-603.

(189) Grammer JC, McGinnis J, Pubols MH. The effects of a pectic enzyme on the growth-depressing and rachitogenic properties of rye for chicks. Poult Sci 1982 Sep; 61 (9): 1891-6.

(190) Gruden N, Buben M. The effect of cellulose-zinc and/or lactose supplemented diet on ^{65}Zn absorption in rats. Nutr Rep Int 1982 Jul; 26 (1): 77-84.

(191) Guild R, Cerda J, Burgin C, Hogan M. The effect of pectin on the unstirred water layer in rabbit intestine (abstract). Gastroenterology 1982 May; 82 (5 Pt 2): 1076.

(192) Hales PW, Jefferies M, Pass G. Some physical properties of hydrocolloids in aqueous solution. In: Phillips GO, Wedlock DJ, Williams PA, eds. Gums and stabilisers for the food industry. Interactions of hydrocolloids. Oxford: Pergamon Press, 1982: 33-43. (Prog Food Nutr Sci; vol 13.)

(193) Hansen PM. Hydrocolloid-protein interactions: relationship to stabilization of fluid milk products. A review. In: Phillips GO, Wedlock DJ, Williams PA, eds. Gums and stabilisers for the food industry. Interactions of hydrocolloids. Oxford: Pergamon Press, 1982: 127-38. (Prog Food Nutr Sci; vol 13.)

(194) Hansen WE, Schulz G. The effect of dietary fiber on pancreatic amylase activity in vitro. Hepatogastroenterology 1982 Aug; 29 (4): 157-60.

(195) Harold M, Reeves R, Conley K. Effect of dietary fiber on insulin requirements and serum lipids in juvenile-onset diabetes mellitus (abstract). Diabetes 1982 May; 31 (Suppl 2): 157A.

(196) Harrop R, Phillips GO, Robb ID, Williams PA. Dispersion stability of micro-crystalline cellulose by polyelectrolytes. In: Phillips GO, Wedlock DJ, Williams PA, eds. Gums and stabilisers for the food industry. Interactions of hydrocolloids. Oxford: Pergamon Press, 1982: 331-40. (Prog Food Nutr Sci; vol 13.)

(197) Hasik J, Hryniewiecki L, Klincewicz H, Gadzinowska A. Feeding habits in patients with ulcerative colitis and colon diverticulitis. In: Kasper H, Goebell H, eds. Colon and nutrition. Lancaster, England: MTP Press, 1982: 153-7.

(198) Heaton KW. The colon and bile-acid metabolism. In: Kasper H, Goebell H, eds. Colon and nutrition. Lancaster, England: MTP Press, 1982: 117-24.

(199) Heaton KW, Manhire A, Henry CL, Hartog M. Does simple substitution of fiber-rich foods for refined foods aid in the treatment of diabetes mellitus? In: Vahouny GV, Kritchevsky D, eds. Dietary fiber in health and disease. New York: Plenum Press, 1982: 183-6.

(200) Heaton KW. Fibre and duodenal ulcers (letter). Lancet 1982 Oct 16; 2 (8303): 878.

(201) Hegde SN, Rolls BA, Coates ME. The effect of the gut microflora and dietary fibre on energy utilization by the chick. Br J Nutr 1982 Jul; 48 (1): 73-80.

(202) Helms, P, Jorgensen IM, Paerregaard A, Bjerrum L, Poulsen L, Mosbech J. Dietary patterns in Them and Copenhagen, Denmark. Nutr Cancer 1982; 4 (1): 34-40.

(203) Hill MJ. Influence of nutrition on the intestinal flora. In: Kasper H, Goebell H, eds. Colon and nutrition. Lancaster, England: MTP Press, 1982: 37-44.

(204) Hill MJ. Colonic bacterial activity: effect of fiber on substrate concentration and on enzyme action. In: Vahouny GV, Kritchevsky D, eds. Dietary fiber in health and disease. New York: Plenum Press, 1982: 35-43.

(205) Hill MJ. Bile acids and human colorectal cancer. In: Vahouny GV, Kritchevsky, D, eds. Dietary fiber in health and disease. New York: Plenum Press, 1982: 299-312.

(206) Hill MJ, Taylor AJ, Thompson MH, Wait R. Fecal steroids and urinary volatile phenols in four Scandinavian populations. Nutr Cancer 1982; 4 (1): 67-73.

(207) Hillman LC, Stace NH, Fisher A, Pomare EW. Dietary intakes and stool characteristics of patients with irritable bowel syndrome. Am J Clin Nutr 1982 Oct; 36 (4): 626-9.

(208) Hjollund E, Pedersen O, Richelsen B, Beck-Nielsen H, Schwartz Sorensen N. Increased insulin receptor binding (IRB) and insulin sensitivity (IS) in adipocytes from non-insulin dependent diabetics (NIDD) after a low-fat, high-starch, high-fiber diet (abstract). Acta Endocrinol (Copenh) 1982; Suppl 247:32.

(209) Hjollund E, Pedersen O, Richelsen B, Beck-Nielsen H, Sorensen NS. Increased insulin receptor binding and insulin sensitivity in adipocytes from type 2 (non-insulin dependent) diabetic patients after a low-fat, high-starch, high-fibre diet (abstract). Diabetologia 1982 Aug; 23 (2): 174.

(210) Hockaday TD. Beans in the management of diabetes. Proc Nutr Soc 1982 Jan; 41 (1): 81-2.

(211) Hoffman CR, Fineberg SE, Howey DC, Clark CM Jr, Pronsky Z. Short-term effects of a high-fiber, high-carbohydrate diet in very obese diabetic individuals. Diabetes Care 1982 Nov-Dec; 5 (6): 605-11.

(212) Hoverstad T, Bohmer T, Fausa O. Absorption of short-chain fatty acids from the human colon measured by the $^{14}CO_2$ breath test. Scand J Gastroenterol 1982; 17 (3): 373-8.

(213) Howe GR, Miller AB, Jain M, Cook G. Dietary factors in relation to the etiology of colorectal cancer. Cancer Detect Prev 1982; 5 (3): 331-4.

(214) Huttunen JK, Aro A, Pelkonen R, Puomio M, Siltanen I, Akerblom HK. Dietary therapy in diabetes mellitus. Description of a recommendation prepared by the Finnish Diabetes Association's Committee on Nutrition Therapy. Acta Med Scand 1982; 211 (6): 469-75.

(215) Hwang R. An approach to lignification in plants. Biochem Biophys Res Commun 1982 Mar 30; 105 (2): 509-14.

(216) Ikegami S, Tsuchihashi N, Nagayama S, Innami S. Effects of viscous indigestible polysaccharides on pancreatic exocrine and biliary secretion in rats. Nutr Rep Int 1982 Aug; 26 (2): 239-46.

(217) Illman RJ, Trimble RP, Snoswell AM, Topping DL. Daily variations in the concentrations of volatile fatty acids in the splanchnic blood vessels of rats fed diets high in pectin and bran. Nutr Rep Int 1982 Sep; 26 (3): 439-46.

(218) Imaizumi K, Tominaga A, Mawatari K, Sugano M. Effects of cellulose and guar gum on the secretion of mesenteric lymph chylomicrons in meal-fed rats. Nutr Rep Int 1982 Aug; 26 (2): 263-9.

(219) Indira M, Kurup PA. Effect of blackgram fibre on ethanol-induced hyperlipidemia in rats. Atherosclerosis 1982 Feb; 41 (2-3): 241-6.

(220) Irie N, Hara T, Goto Y. The effects of guar gum on postprandial chylomicronemia. Nutr Rep Int 1982 Aug; 26 (2): 207-14.

(221) Isaksson G, Lundquist I, Ihse I. In vitro inhibition of pancreatic enzyme activities by dietary fiber. Digestion 1982 May; 24 (1): 54-9.

(222) Isaksson G, Lundquist I, Ihse I. Effect of dietary fiber on pancreatic enzyme activity in vitro. The importance of viscosity, pH, ionic strength, adsorption, and time of incubation. Gastroenterology 1982 May; 82 (5 Pt 1): 918-24.

(223) Iwasaki Y, Aono M, Aoki N. Uchino H. Guar jelly for the treatment of diabetes mellitus in humans. Nutr Rep Int 1982 Aug; 26 (2): 203-6.

(224) Jacobs LR, Huber PW. Comparative effects of dietary oat bran, pectin and guar on rat colonic mucosal growth (abstract). Fed Proc 1982 Mar 1; 41 (3): 711.

(225) Jacobs LR. Comparative effects of dietary oat bran, pectin and guar on rat small intestinal mucosal growth and structure (abstract). Gastroenterology 1982 May; 82 (5 Pt 2): 1091.

(226) Jacobs LR, Lupton JR. Dietary wheat bran lowers colonic pH in rats. J Nutr 1982
Mar; 112 (3): 592-4.

(227) Jefferies M, Konadu EY, Pass G. Cation effects on the viscosity of gum ghatti. J Sci
Food Agric 1982 Nov; 33 (11): 1152-9.

(228) Jenkins DJ, Wolever TM, Taylor RH, Griffiths C, Krzeminska K, Lawrie JA, Bennett
CM, Goff DV, Sarson DL, Bloom SR. Slow release dietary carbohydrate improves
second meal tolerance. Am J Clin Nutr 1982 Jun; 35 (6): 1339-46.

(229) Jenkins DJ, Thorne MJ, Camelon K, Jenkins A, Rao AV, Taylor RH, Thompson LU,
Kalmusky J, Reichert R, Francis T. Effect of processing on digestibility and the blood
glucose response: a study of lentils. Am J Clin Nutr 1982 Dec; 36 (6): 1093-101.

(230) Jenkins DJ. Lente carbohydrate: a newer approach to the dietary management of
diabetes. Diabetes Care 1982 Nov-Dec; 5 (6): 634-41.

(231) Jenkins DJ, Ghafari H, Wolever TM, Taylor RH, Jenkins AL, Barker HM, Fielden H,
Bowling AC. Relationship between rate of digestion of foods and post-prandial
glycaemia. Diabetologia 1982 Jun; 22 (6): 450-5.

(232) Jenkins DJ, Taylor RH, Wolever TM. The diabetic diet, dietary carbohydrate and
differences in digestibility. Diabetologia 1982 Dec; 23 (6): 477-84.

(233) Jenkins DJ, Jepson EM. Leguminous seeds and their constituents in the treatment
of hyperlipidemia and diabetes. In: Noseda G, Fragiacomo C, Fumagalli R,
Paoletti R, eds. Lipoproteins and coronary atherosclerosis. Amsterdam: Elsevier
Biomedical Press, 1982: 247-56.

(234) Jensen OM, MacLennan R, Wahrendorf J. Diet, bowel function, fecal characteristics,
and large bowel cancer in Denmark and Finland. Nutr Cancer 1982; 4 (1): 5-19.

(235) Johansson C-G, Aman P, Asp N-G, Theander O. Enzymatic and neutral detergent
fibre methods for dietary fibre analysis comparison by recovery of dietary fibre.
Swed J Agric Res 1982; 12 (4): 157-61.

(236) Johnson DA, Sreebny LM. Effect of increasing the bulk content of the diet on the
rat parotid gland and saliva. J Dent Res 1982 May; 61 (5): 691-6.

(237) Johnson MA, Chang ML. Effects of molecular weight of carboxymethylcelluloses on
lipid metabolism and on the response to a glucose tolerance test in rats (abstract).
Fed Proc 1982 Mar 1; 41 (3): 399.

(238) Judd PA, Truswell AS. Comparison of the effects of high- and low-methoxyl pectins
on blood and faecal lipids in man. Br J Nutr 1982 Nov; 48 (3): 451-8.

(239) Judd PA. The effects of high intakes of barley on gastrointestinal function and
apparent digestibilities of dry matter, nitrogen and fat in human volunteers. J Plant
Foods 1982; 4 (2): 79-88.

(240) Kamath PS, Dilawari JB, Raghavan S, Batta RP, Mukewar S, Dash RJ. Plasma insulin
response to legumes and carbohydrate foods. Indian J Med Res 1982 Oct; 76: 583-90.

(241) Kanchana S, Shurpalekar KS. Influence of ragi (Eleusine coracana) husk on the growth
and body composition of albino rats. Nutr Rep Int 1982 Jan; 25 (1): 205-12.

(242) Kapur BM, Kumar K, Tandon RK. The association of refined carbohydrates with gallstones (abstract). Scand J Gastroenterol 1982; 17 (Suppl 78): 222.

(243) Kasper H, Schrezenmeir J. The effect of dietary fibre on D-xylose absorption. Hum
Nutr: Clin Nutr 1982; 36C (3): 243-50.

(244) Katz S, Williams KA. Effects of solvent extracts of rice bran and free-fatty acids upon
plaque and acid formation. J Dent Res 1982 Nov; 61 (11): 1269-73.

(245) Kaur AP, Bhat CM, Grewal RB. Effect of low fiber diet on physiological functioning
of gastro-intestinal tract and digestibility of nutrients. Philipp J Nutr 1982 Jul-Sep;
35 (3): 150-3.

(246) Kawaura A, Shibata M, Togei K, Otsuka H. Effect of dietary degraded carrageenan on
intestinal carcinogenesis in rats treated with 1,2-dimethylhydrazine dihydrochloride.
Tokushima J Exp Med 1982 Jun; 29 (1-2): 125-9.

(247) Kay RM. Dietary fiber. J Lipid Res 1982 Feb; 23 (2): 221-42.

(248) Keating L. Fibre and calorie counter. Emsworth, Hampshire: K Mason, 1982.

(249) Keeney PG. Hydrocolloid-lipid interactions. In: Phillips GO, Wedlock DJ, Williams PA,
eds. Gums and stabilisers for the food industry. Interactions of hydrocolloids. Oxford:
Pergamon Press, 1982: 181-9. (Prog Food Nutr Sci; vol 13.)

(250) Kelley MJ, Thomas JN, Liu VJ, Story JA. Effect of dietary fiber and meal pattern on modulation of HMG-CoA reductase (HMGR) activity (abstract). Fed Proc 1982 Mar 1; 41 (3): 398.

(251) Kellogg Company. Dietary fiber bibliography 1982 Jan; 1(2) and 1982 Sep; 1(3). Battle Creek, MI 49016: Kellog Company, 1982.

(252) Kelsay JL. Effects of fiber on mineral and vitamin bioavailability. In: Vahouny GV, Kritchevsky D, eds. Dietary fiber in health and disease. New York: Plenum Press, 1982: 91-103.

(253) Kendall PT, Holme DW. Studies on the digestibility of soya bean products, cereals, cereal and plant by-products in diets of dogs. J Sci Food Agric 1982 Sep; 33 (9): 813-22.

(254) Kendall PT, Holme DW, Smith PM. Methods of prediction of the digestible energy content of dog foods from gross energy value, proximate analysis and digestive nutrient content. J Sci Food Agric 1982 Sep; 33 (9): 823-31.

(255) Kerlin P, Phillips S. Transit of liquids and solids through the ileum of man (abstract). Gastroenterology 1982 May; 82 (5 Pt 2): 1099.

(256) Kimura T, Imamura H, Hasegawa K, Yoshida A. Mechanisms of toxicities of some detergents added to a diet and of the ameliorating effect of dietary fiber in the rat. J Nutr Sci Vitaminol (Tokyo) 1982 Oct; 28 (5): 483-9.

(257) Kimura T, Yoshida A. Toxicity of detergent feeding and effect of the concurrent feeding of dietary fiber in rats. Nutr Rep Int 1982 Aug; 26 (2): 271-9.

(258) King JC, Costa FM, Butte NF. Fecal mineral excretion of young men fed diets high in fiber components or phytate (abstract). Fed Proc 1982 Mar 1; 41 (3): 712.

(259) Kinmonth A-L, Angus RM, Jenkins PA, Smith MA, Baum JD. Whole foods and increased dietary fibre improve blood glucose control in diabetic children. Arch Dis Child 1982 Mar; 57 (3): 187-94.

(260) Kintner PK III, Van Buren JP. Carbohydrate interference and its correction in pectin analysis using the m-hydroxydiphenyl method. J Food Sci 1982 May-Jun; 47 (3): 756-9, 764.

(261) Kishi K, Inoue G, Yoshida A, Fuwa H, Koishi H, Koike G, Miyoshi T, Inoue T, Yoshida M, Omori A. Digestibility and energy availability of sea vegetables and fungi in man. Nutr Rep Int 1982 Aug; 26 (2): 183-92.

(262) Kishore N, Wahal PK, Sharma S, Sharma RK, Sharma BB. The effects of pectin on oral glucose tolerance and serum lipids. J Assoc Physicians India 1982 Dec; 30 (12): 885-7.

(263) Kiyozumi M, Mishima M, Noda S, Miyata K, Takahashi Y, Mizunaga F, Nakagawa M, Kojima S. Studies on poisonous metals. IX. Effects of dietary fibers on absorption of cadmium in rats. Chem Pharm Bull (Tokyo) 1982 Dec; 30 (12): 4494-9.

(264) Klapdor R, Hein C. Addition of fiber (wheat bran, bassorin) to the standard food does not influence biliary lipid composition in piglets. Res Exp Med (Berl) 1982; 180 (1): 21-4.

(265) Klurfeld DM, Tepper SA, Kritchevsky D. Distribution of exogenous radiolabeled cholesterol in rat intestine: effect of dietary fiber. Nutr Res 1982; 2 (1): 65-71.

(266) Knorr D. Functional properties of chitin and chitosan. J Food Sci 1982 Mar-Apr; 47 (2): 593-5.

(267) Kobayashi K, Kitano A, Kuwajima S, Yamamoto S. The role of intestinal bacteria in experimental ulcerative colitis induced by carrageenan (abstract). Scand J Gastro-enterol 1982; 17 (Suppl 78): 353.

(268) Komai M, Takehisa F, Kimura S. Effect of dietary fiber on intestinal epithelial cell kinetics of germ-free and conventional mice. Nutr Rep Int 1982 Aug; 26 (2): 255-61.

(269) Koopmans H, Rozen P, Kritchevsky D. Schmahl D, Kurtz W, Rosselin G. Discussion 10. In: Malt RA, Williamson RC, eds. Colonic carcinogenesis. Lancaster, England: MPT Press, 1982: 107-8.

(270) Kriek NP, Sly MR, de Bruyn DB, de Klerk WA, Renan MJ, Van Schalkwyk DJ, Van Rensburg SJ. Dietary wheaten bran in baboons: long-term effect on the morphology of the digestive tract and aorta, and on tissue mineral concentrations. Br J Exp Pathol 1982 Jun; 63|(3): 254-68.

(271) Kritchevsky D, Story JA. Dietary fiber and cancer. In: Vitale JJ, Broitman SA, eds. Advances in human clinical nutrition. The Hague, Netherlands: Martinus Nijhoff, 1982: 175-88.

(272) Kritchevsky D. Dietary fiber and disease. Bull NY Acad Med 1982 Apr; 58 (3): 230-41.

(273) Kritchevsky D. Can dietary change prevent disease? In: Kasper H, Goebell H, eds. Colon and nutrition. Lancaster, England: MTP Press, 1982: 269-78.

(274) Kritchevsky D. Fiber, obesity, and diabetes. In: Vahouny GV, Kritchevsky D, eds. Dietary fiber in health and disease. New York: Plenum Press, 1982: 133-7.

(275) Kritchevsky D. Fiber and lipids. In: Vahouny GV, Kritchevsky D, eds. Dietary fiber in health and disease. New York: Plenum Press, 1982: 187-92.

(276) Kritchevsky D. Dietary fiber in health and disease. In: Lineback DR, Inglett GE, eds. Food carbohydrates. Westport, Connecticut: AVI Publishing, 1982: 296-311.

(277) Kritchevsky D. Atherosclerosis and diet. In: Naito HK, ed. Nutrition and heart disease. Lancaster, England: MTP Press, 1982: 151-64.

(278) Kritchevsky D, Ryder E, Fishman A, Kaplan M, DeHoff JL. Influence of dietary fiber on food intake, feed efficiency and lipids in rats. Nutr Rep Int 1982 May; 25 (5): 783-7.

(279) Kromhout D, Bosschieter EB, de Lezenne Coulander C. Dietary fibre and ten-year mortality from coronary heart disease, cancer and all causes. The Zutphen study. Lancet 1982 Sep 4; 2 (8297): 518-22.

(280) Kuhl C, Molsted-Pedersen L, Hornnes PJ. Effect of guar on glucose control in pregnant insulin dependent diabetics (abstract). Acta Endocrinol (Copenh) 1982: Suppl 247: 40.

(281) Kuhl C, Molsted-Pedersen L, Hornnes PJ. Effect of guar gum on glycaemic control of pregnant insulin dependent diabetic patients (abstract). Diabetologia 1982 May; 22 (5): 389.

(282) Kurasawa S-I, Sugahara T, Hayashi J. Studies on dietary fibre of mushrooms and edible wild plants. Nutr Rep Int 1982 Aug; 26 (2): 167-73.

(283) Kurtz W, Thompson MH, Kovacs A, Schreve RH, Frommer D, Kirtchevsky D. Discussion 5. In: Malt RA, Williamson RC, eds. Colonic carcinogenesis. Lancaster, England: MTP Press, 1982: 57-8.

(284) Lamb DJ, Craig GT. Demineralization of human dental enamel by karaya gum solutions. Caries Res 1982; 16 (2): 118-22.

(285) Langeland T, Nyrud M. Contact urticaria to wheat bran bath: a case report. Acta Derm Venereol (Stockh) 1982; 62 (1): 82-3.

(286) Langman MJ. Nutritional and other epidemiological factors in the aetiology of inflammatory bowel disease. In: Kasper H, Goebell H, eds. Colon and nutrition. Lancaster, England: MTP Press, 1982: 173-9.

(287) Kaunay B, Pasquet E. Sucrose solutions with and without guar gum: rheological properties and relative sweetness intensity. In: Phillips GO, Wedlock DJ, Williams PA, eds. Gums and stabilisers for the food industry. Interactions of hydrocolloids. Oxford: Pergamon Press, 1982: 247-58. (Prog Food Nutr Sci; vol 13.)

(288) Lawaetz O, Bloom SR, Blackburn AM, Ralphs DN. Effect of pectin on gastric emptying and gut hormone release in the dumping syndrome (abstract). Scand J Gastroenterol 1982; 17 (Suppl 78): 18.

(289) Lawrence RE. A case of coconut bezoar and Meckel's diverticulum. Postgrad Med J 1982 Feb; 58 (676): 119-20.

(290) Leatherdale BA, Green DJ, Harding LK, Griffin D, Bailey CJ. Guar and gastric emptying in non-insulin dependent diabetes. Acta Diabetol Lat 1982 Oct-Dec; 19 (4): 339-43.

(291) Lee BH, Picard GA, Goulet G. Effects of processing methods on the nutritive value and digestibility of Oocystis alga in rats. Nutr Rep In 1982 Mar; 25 (3): 417-29.

(292) Lee HS, O'Donnell JA, Hurt HD, Hayes KC. Comparison of dietary fiber influence on cholesterolemia in cebus monkeys (abstract). Fed Proc 1982 Mar 1; 41 (3): 711.

(293) Lee SM. The effect of a high fibre diet on diabetic nephropathy in the db/db mouse. Diabetologia 1982 May; 22 (5): 349-53.

(294) Leeds AR. Modification of intestinal absorption by dietary fiber and fiber components. In: Vahouny GV, Kritchevsky D, eds. Dietary fiber in health and disease. New York: Plenum Press, 1982: 53-71.

(295) Leeds AR. Legumes and gastrointestinal function in relation to diets for diabetics. J Plant Foods 1982; 4 (1): 23-7.

(296) Leeds AR, Khumalo TD, Ndaba NG, Lincoln D. Haricot beans, transit time and stool weight. J Plant Foods 1982; 4 (1): 33-41.

(297) Lembcke B, Hasler K, Kramer P, Caspary WF, Creutzfeldt W. Plasma digoxin concentrations during administration of dietary fibre (guar gum) in man. Z Gastroenterol 1982 Mar; 20 (3): 164-7.

(298) Leshin HL, Jones RD, Karlin DA. The effect of dietary fiber supplements on breath hydrogen and methane excretion (abstract). Gastroenterology 1982 May; 82 (5 Pt 2): 1256.

(299) Levine RA, Schwartz SE, Singh A, Rogus JB, Track NS. Chronic pectin ingestion delays gastric emptying. In: Weinbeck M, ed. Motility of the digestive tract. New York: Raven Press, 1982: 379-85.

(300) Lindgarde F, Eriksson K-F, Lithell H, Saltin B. Coupling between dietary changes, reduced body weight, muscle fibre size and improved glucose tolerance in middle-aged men with impaired glucose tolerance. Acta Med Scand 1982; 212 (3): 99-106.

(301) Liu K, Stamler J, Trevisan M, Moss D. Dietary lipids, sugar, fiber, and mortality from coronary heart disease. Bivariate analysis of international data. Arteriosclerosis 1982 May-Jun; 2 (3): 221-7.

(302) Longe OG, Fetuga BL, Aken'ova ME. Changes in the composition and carbohydrate constituents of okra (Abelmoschus esculentus, Linn.) with age. Food Chem 1982 Jan; 8 (1): 27-32.

(303) Longe OG, Norton G, Lewis D. Comparative digestibility of carbohydrates of microbial products and their metabolisable energy values in chicks and rats. J Sci Food Agric 1982 Feb; 33 (2): 155-64.

(304) Lousley S, Jones DB, Slaughter P, Carter RD, Jelfs R, Barker K, Mann JI. Dietary fibre and poorly controlled diabetes (abstract). Diabetologia 1982 Nov; 23 (5): 470.

(305) Love M, Zenoble O. Substitution of microcrystalline cellulose and effect on the initial viscosity increase in white cake batters (abstract). Cereal Foods World 1982 Sep; 27 (9): 452.

(306) Low AG, Rainbird AL, Gurr MI. Animal models for studying the effect of fibre on gastrointestinal function. J Plant Foods 1982; 4 (1): 29-32.

(307) Luderitz T, Schatz G, Grisebach H. Enzymic synthesis of lignin precursors. Purification and properties of 4-coumarate: CoA ligase from cambial sap of spruce (Picea abies L.) Eur J Biochem 1982 Apr; 123 (3): 583-6.

(308) Lund ED, Smoot JM. Dietary fiber content of some tropical fruits and vegetables. J Agric Food Chem 1982 Nov-Dec; 30 (6): 1123-7.

(309) Makdani DD, Molnar IG. Satiety value of raw and cooked cellulose in the diets of rats (abstract). Fed Proc 1982 Mar 1; 41 (3): 400.

(310) Mallett AK. Effect of dietary pectin on the metabolic activity of the rat hindgut microflora. Chem Ind 1982; 24: 984-7.

(311) Mann J, The Oxford Dietetic Group. The diabetics' diet book. A new high-fibre eating programme. London, England: Martin Dunitz, 1982. (Positive health guide.)

(312) Manojlovic D, Micic J, Micic D, Popovic V, Lalic D, Djuric D. Influence of different carbohydrate and lipid content of food on glycaemia and serum lipoprotein levels in patients with impaired glucose tolerance (abstract). Diabetologia 1982 Aug; 23 (2): 185.

(313) Mansurov H. The effect of dietary fibre on the bile chemistry in obese patients with cholesterol gallstones (abstract). Scand J Gastroenterol 1982; 17 (Suppl 78): 139.

(314) Marlett JA, Neilson M, Chesters JG, Slavin JL. Analysis of fiber components (letter). Am J Clin Nutr 1982 Jan; 35 (1): 175-6.

(315) Marthinsen D, Fleming SE. Excretion of breath and flatus gases by humans consuming high-fiber diets. J Nutr 1982 Jun; 112 (6): 1133-43.

(316) Matek W, Riemann JF, Fruhmorgen P. Treatment of chronic constipation with swelling substances. In: Kasper H, Goebell H, eds. Colon and nutrition. Lancaster, England: MTP Press, 1982: 229.

(317) Math MV. Is bran useful in diverticular disease (letter). Br Med J 1982 May 8; 284 (6326): 1408-9.

(318) Matsuo T, Suzuoki Z. Feeding responses of riboflavin-deficient rats to energy dilution, cold exposure and glucoprivation. J Nutr 1982 Jun; 112 (6): 1052-6.

(319) Matzkies F, Budelski I, Webs B. Effect of fiber-containing dietary formula on metabolism. Fortschr Med 1982 May 20; 100 (19): 917-20.

(320) Mayne PD, McGill AR, Gormley TR, Tomkin GH, Julian TR, O'Moore RR. The effect of apple fibre on diabetic control and plasma lipids. Ir J Med Sci 1982 Feb; 151 (2): 36-41.

(321) Metraux JP. Thin-layer chromatography of neutral and acidic sugars from plant cell wall polysaccharides. J Chromatogr 1982 Mar 26; 237 (3): 525-7.

(322) Michel F, Doublier JL, Thibault JF. Investigations on high-methoxyl pectins by potentiometry and viscometry. In: Phillips GO, Wedlock DJ, Williams PA, eds. Gums and stabilisers for the food industry. Interactions of hydrocolloids. Oxford: Pergamon Press, 1982: 367-72. (Prog Food Nutr Sci; vol 13.)

(323) Miller B. Crohn's disease and nutrition: aetiological aspects. In: Kasper H, Goebell H, eds. Colon and nutrition. Lancaster, England: MTP Press, 1982: 251-6.

(324) Mizutani T, Mitsuoka T. Effect of konjac mannan on spontaneous liver tumorigenesis and fecal flora in C3H/He male mice. Cancer Lett 1982 Oct; 17 (1): 27-32.

(325) Mizutani T, Benno Y, Mitsuoka T. Effect of dietary fiber on tumorigenesis and longevity: with special reference to the fecal microflora. Nutr Rep Int 1982 Aug; 26 (2): 289-96.

(326) Mod RR, Ory RL, Morris NM, Normand FL. In vitro interaction of rice hemicellulose with trace minerals and their release by digestive enzymes. Cereal Chem 1982 Nov-Dec; 59 (6): 538-42.

(327) Mod RR, Ory RL, Morris NC, Normand FL. Effect of rice hemicelluloses on selected minerals in blood and feces of rats (abstract). Cereal Foods World 1982 Sep; 27 (9): 457.

(328) Moesgaard F, Nielsen ML, Hansen JB, Knudsen JT. High-fiber diet reduces bleeding and pain in patients with hemorrhoids. A double-blind trial of Vi-Siblin. Dis Colon Rectum 1982 Jul-Aug; 25 (5): 454-6.

(329) Mongeau R. Plant fiber in selected cereals (letter). Am J Clin Nutr 1982 Feb; 35 (2): 407-8.

(330) Mongeau R, Brassard R. Insoluble dietary fiber from breakfast cereals and brans: bile salt binding and water-holding capacity in relation to particle size. Cereal Chem 1982 Sep-Oct; 59 (5): 413-7.

(331) Mongeau R, Brassard R. Determination of neutral detergent fiber in breakfast cereals: pentose, hemicellulose, cellulose and lignin content. J Food Sci 1982 Mar-Apr; 47 (2): 550-5.

(332) Mongeau R, Brassard R. Comparison of the effects of two breakfast cereals on intestinal function in rats (abstract). Cereal Foods World 1982 Sep; 27 (9): 457.

(333) Monnier LH, Colette C, Aguirre L, Orsetti A, Combeaux D. Restored synergistic entero-hormonal response after addition of dietary fibre to patients with impaired glucose tolerance and reactive hypoglycaemia. Diabete Metab 1982 Sep; 8 (3): 217-22.

(334) Monte WC, Vaughan LA. An outline of 'fiber' analysis techniques. J Appl Nutr 1982; 34 (1): 46-62.

(335) Monte WC. The gastrointestinal clearance of ^{14}C polystyrene as influenced by addition of cellulose, bran and psyllium to the rat diet. J Appl Nutr 1982; 34 (2): 74-90.

(336) Morgan KC, Wright JL, Simpson FJ. Review of chemical constituents of the red alga Palmaria palmata (Dulse). Econ Bot 1980 Jan-Mar; 34 (1): 27-50.

(337) Mori B. Contents of dietary fiber in some Japanese foods and the amount ingested through Japanese meals. Nutr Rep Int 1982 Aug; 26 (2): 159-66.

(338) Morris ER, Taylor LJ. Oral perception of fluid viscosity. In: Phillips GO, Wedlock DJ, Williams PA, eds. Gums and stabilisers for the food industry. Interactions of hydrocolloids. Oxford: Pergamon Press, 1982: 285-96. (Prog Food Nutr Sci; vol 13.)

(339) Morris ER, Powell DA, Gidley MJ, Rees DA. Conformations and interactions of pectins. I. Polymorphism between gel and solid states of calcium polygalacturonate. J Mol Biol 1982 Mar 15; 155 (4): 507-16.

(340) Morris VJ, Belton PS. The influence of the cations sodium, potassium and calcium on the gelation of iota-carrageenan. In: Phillips GO, Wedlock DJ, Williams PA, eds. Gums and stabilisers for the food industry. Interactions of hydrocolloids. Oxford: Pergamon Press, 1982: 55-66. (Prog Food Nutr Sci; vol 13.)

(341) Morris VJ. Laser light scattering from unexcited and mechanically excited polysaccharide gels. In: Phillips GO, Wedlock DJ, Williams PA, eds. Gums and stabilisers for the food industry. Interactions of hydrocolloids. Oxford: Pergamon Press, 1982: 119-24. (Prog Food Nutr Sci; vol 13.)

(342) Munoz JM. Interactions of dietary fiber and nutrients. In: Vahouny GV, Kritchevsky D, eds. Dietary fiber in health and disease. New York: Plenum Press, 1982: 85-9.

(343) Murney RG Jr, Winship DH. The irritable colon syndrome. Clin Gastroenterol 1982 Sep; 11 (3): 563-92.

(344) McCleary BV, Neukom H. Effect of enzymic modification on the solution and interaction properties of galactomannans. In: Phillips GO, Wedlock DJ, Williams PA, eds. Gums and stabilisers for the food industry. Interactions of hydrocolloids. Oxford: Pergamon Press, 1982: 109-18. (Prog Food Nutr Sci; vol 13.)

(345) McCredie JA, Mangal SM, Babury MQ. High roughage diet and surgical diseases in Afghanistan. J R Coll Surg Edinb 1982 Jan; 27 (1): 38-41.

(346) McLean Ross AH, Eastwood MA, Brydon WG, McKay LF, Anderson DM, Anderson JR. Gum arabic metabolism in man (abstract). Proc Nutr Soc 1982 Jun; 41 (2): 64A.

(347) MacQuart-Moulin G, Durbec JP, Cornee J, Berthezene P. Nutritional risk factors in colorectal cancer. In: Kasper H, Goebell H, eds. Colon and nutrition. Lancaster, England: MTP Press, 1982: 231-3.

(348) McQuilkin Tarone C, Matthews RH. Proximate and mineral content of selected baked products. Cereal Foods World 1982 Jul; 27 (7): 308-13.

(349) McWhinnie DL, Mack AJ. The interaction of wheat bran and oral iron supplements in vivo. Hum Nutr: Clin Nutr 1982; 36C (4): 315-8.

(350) Nack SL, Albrink MJ, Ullrich IH, Goodwin C. The acute effect of dietary fiber on gastric emptying (abstract). Am J Clin Nutr 1982 Jun; 35 (6): xxvii.

(351) Naito HK. Nutritional modification for prevention and treatment of hyperlipidemia and hyperlipoproteinemia. In: Naito HK, ed. Nutrition and heart disease. Lancaster, England: MTP Press, 1982: 181-234.

(352) Nakamura H, Ishikawa T, Tada N, Kagami A, Kondo K. Miyazima E, Takeyama S. Effect of several kinds of dietary fibres on serum and lipoprotein lipids. Nutr Rep Int 1982 Aug; 26 (2): 215-21.

(353) Narasinga Rao BS, Prabhavathi T. Tannin content of foods commonly consumed in India and its influence on ionisable iron. J Sci Food Agric 1982 Jan; 33 (1): 89-96.

(354) Nayak BR, Pattabiraman TN. Studies on plant gums: characterisation of neem (Azadirachta indica) gum protease as a glycoprotein. J Sci Food Agric 1982 Mar; 33 (3): 263-8.

(355) Neale RJ. Binding of iron by fiber of wheat and maize (letter). Am J Clin Nutr 1982 Jun; 35 (6): 1500.

(356) Ney D, Hollingsworth DR, Cousins L. Decreased insulin requirement and improved control of diabetes in pregnant women given a high-carbohydrate, high-fiber, low-fat diet. Diabetes Care 1982 Sep-Oct; 5 (5): 529-33.

(357) Nguyen KN, Welsh JD, Manion CV, Ficken VJ. Effect of fiber on breath hydrogen response and symptoms after oral lactose in lactose malabsorbers. Am J Clin Nutr 1982 Jun; 35 (6): 1347-51.

(358) Nigro ND. A strategy for prevention of cancer of the large bowel. Dis Colon Rectum 1982 Nov-Dec; 25 (8): 755-8.

(359) Nomani MZ, Stansberry SC. Apparent digestibility of nitrogen and protein efficiency ratio as affected by dietary fiber fractions in rats on two feeding plans (abstract). Am J Clin Nutr 1982 Jun; 35 (6): xxv.

(360) Nomani MZ, Stansberry SC. Effect of dietary fiber fractions on the apparent digestibility of nitrogen and protein efficiency ratio in rats on two feeding plans. Nutr Rep Int 1982 Oct; 26 (4): 695-702.

(361) Normand FL, Ory RL, Mod RR, Saunders RM, Gumbmann MR. Effect of rice hemicellulose on rat fecal lipids (abstract). Fed Proc 1982 Mar 1; 41 (3): 471.

(362) Nutrition Sub-Committee of the British Diabetic Association's Medical Advisory Committee. Dietary recommendations for diabetics for the 1980s — a policy statement by the British Diabetic Association. Hum Nutr: Appl Nutr 1982 Oct; 36A (5): 378-94.

(363) Nygren C, Hallmans G. Effects of processed rye bran and raw rye bran on glucose metabolism in alloxan diabetic rats. J Nutr 1982 Jan; 112 (1): 17-20.

(364) Nygren C, Adolfsson R, Hallmans G, Sandman P-O, Stenling R, Winblad B. The effect of high bran bread on constipation and glucose tolerance in patients with senile dementia (abstract). Scand J Gastroenterol 1982; 17 (Suppl 78): 393.

(365) Nyman M, Asp N-G. Fermentation of dietary fibre components in the rat intestinal tract. Br J Nutr 1982 May; 47 (3): 357-66.

(366) O'Beirne B, Van Buren JP, Mattick LR. Two distinct pectin fractions from senescent Idared apples, extracted using nondegradative methods. J Food Sci 1982 Jan-Feb; 47 (1): 173-6.

(367) Odunfa SA. Carbohydrate changes in fermenting locust bean during iru preparation. J Plant Foods 1982; 4 (2): 105-10.

(368) Ohshima M, Yamada N, Ueda H. Some factors affecting plasma free amino acid concentrations in growing pigs fed a barley bran diet. Nutr Rep Int 1982 Jan; 25 (1): 1-6.

(369) Oku T, Konishi F, Hosoya N. Mechanism of inhibitory effect of unavailable carbohydrate on intestinal calcium absorption. J Nutr 1982 Mar; 112 (3): 410-5.

(370) Oku T, Konishi F, Hosoya N. Biochemical and morphological changes of gastrointestinal tract' by dietary fiber in rat. Nutr Rep Int 1982 Aug; 26 (2): 247-53.

(371) Oli JM, Ikeakor IP, Onwuameze IC. Blood glucose responses to common Nigerian foods. Trop Georg Med 1982; 34 (4): 317-22.

(372) Olness K, Tobin J Sr. Chronic constipation in children. Can it be managed by diet alone? Postgrad Med 1982 Oct; 72 (4): 149-54.

(373) Ologhobo AD, Fetuga BL. Carbohydrate constituents of some limabean (Phaseolus lunatus) varieties. Nutr Rep Int 1982 Dec; 26 (6): 981-8.

(374) Olson AC, Gray GM, Gumbmann MR, Wagner JR. Nutrient composition of and digestive response to whole and extracted dry beans. J Agric Food Chem 1982 Jan-Feb; 30 (1): 26-32.

(375) Omaye ST, Chow FI, Betschart AA. In vitro interaction of 1-^{14}C-ascorbic acid and 2-^{14}C-thiamin with dietary fiber. Cereal Chem 1982 Sep-Oct; 59 (5): 440-3.

(376) Omaye ST, Chow FI, Betschart AA. In vitro interactions between vitamins and sources of dietary fibers (abstract). Fed Proc 1982 Mar 1; 41 (3): 400.

(377) O'Neill C, Pan Q, Clarke G, Liu F, Hodges G, Ge M, Jordan P, Chang U, Newman R, Toulson E. Silica fragments from millet bran in mucosa surrounding oesophageal tumours in patients in Northern China. Lancet 1982 May 29; 1 (8283): 1202-6.

(378) Ornstein MH, Littlewood ER, McLean Baird I. Bran in diverticular disease — fact or fancy (abstract). Comment by WG Hardison. Gastroenterology 1982 Jan; 82 (1): 156.

(379) Ortiz EL. The fibre cook book. London, England: Jill Norman and Hobhouse, 1982.

(380) Osilesi O, Trout DL, Ryan RO. Influence of feeding conditions on slowing of gastric emptying by edible gums (abstract). Fed Proc 1982 Mar 1; 41 (3): 711.

(381) Owen DF, Cotton RH. Dietary fibers. Cereal Woods World 1982 Oct; 27 (10): 519-21.

(382) Painter NS. Diverticular disease of the colon. The first of the Western diseases shown to be due to a deficiency of dietary fibre. S Afr Med J 1982 Jun 26; 61 (26): 1016-20.

(383) Pedersen O, Hjollund E, Lindskov HO, Helms P, Ditzel J. Schwartz Sorensen N. Increased insulin binding to receptors on monocytes from insulin-dependent diabetics (IDDs) after a low-fat, high-starch, high-fiber diet (abstract). Acta Endocrinol (Copenh); Suppl 247: 51.

(384) Pedersen O, Hjollund E, Lindskov HO, Helms P, Sorensen NS, Ditzel J. Increased insulin receptor binding to monocytes from insulin-dependent diabetic patients after a low-fat, high-starch, high-fiber diet. Diabetes Care 1982 May-Jun; 5 (3): 284-91.

(385) Phillips GO, Wedlock DJ, Williams PA, eds. Gums and stabilisers for the food industry. Interactions of hydrocolloids. Oxford: Pergamon Press, 1982. (Prog Food Nutr Sci; vol 13.)

(386) Potter JD. Fibre in the prevention and management of chronic disease. Aust Fam Physician 1982 Apr; 11 (4): 292-3, 296-9.

(387) Powell DA, Morris ER, Gidley MJ, Rees DA. Conformations and interactions of pectins. II. Influence of residue sequence on chain association in calcium pectate gels. J Mol Biol 1982 Mar 15; 155 (4): 517-31.

(388) Poynard T, Slama G, Tchobroutsky G. Reduction of post-prandial insulin needs by pectin as assessed by the artificial pancreas in insulin-dependent diabetics. Diabete Metab 1982 Sep; 8 (3): 187-9.

(389) Premakumari K, Kurup PA. Lipid metabolism in rats fed rice and tapioca. Indian J Med Res 1982 Sep; 76: 448-93.

(390) Prentice N. Purification of beta-glucanase for beta-D-glucan assays. Cereal Chem 1982 May-Jun; 59 (3): 231-2.

(391) Prentice N, Qureshi AA, Burger WC, Elson CE. Response of hepatic cholesterol, fatty acid synthesis and activities of related enzymes to rolled barley and oats in chickens. Nutr Rep Int 1982 Oct; 26 (4): 597-604.

(392) Qureshi AA, Burger WC, Elson CE, Benevenga NJ. Effects of cereals and culture filtrate of Trichoderma viride on lipid metabolism of swine. Lipids 1982 Dec; 17 (12): 924-34.

(393) Raczynski G, Eggum BO, Chwalibog A. The effect of dietary composition on transit time in rats. Z Tierphysiol Tierernahr Futtermittelkd 1982; 47 (3): 160-7.

(394) Rainbird AL. Studies on the physiological action of dietary fibre in the gut of pigs (abstract). J Sci Food Agric 1982 Oct; 33 (10): 971-2.

(395) Rainbird AL, Low AG, Zebrowska T. Effect of guar gum on glucose absorption from isolated loops of jejunum in conscious growing pigs (abstract). Proc Nutr Soc 1982 Jun; 41 (2): 48A.

(396) Ranhotra GS, Gelroth JA, Novak FA, Bock MA, Winterringer GL. Digestibility of complex carbohydrates and protein in wheat breads. Cereal Chem 1982 Nov-Dec; 59 (6): 493-5.

(397) Rao PN, Gordon C, Davies D, Blacklock NJ. Are stone formers maladapted to refined carbohydrates? Br J Urol 1982 Dec; 54 (6): 575-7.

(398) Rao PN, Prendiville V, Buxton A, Moss DG, Blacklock NJ. Dietary management of urinary risk factors in renal stone formers. Br J Urol 1982 Dec; 54 (6): 578-83.

(399) Rao PU, Deosthale YG. Tannin content of pulses: varietal differences and effects of germination and cooking. J Sci Food Agric 1982 Oct; 33 (10): 1013-6.

(400) Rasper VF. Effect of preparative procedure on the evaluation of in vitro indigestible residue (dietary fiber). In: Lineback DR, Inglett GE, eds. Food carbohydrates. Westport, Connecticut: AVI Publishing Company, 1982: 333-55.

(401) Ray S, Pubols MH, Mcginnis J. The effect of a purified guar degrading enzyme on chick growth. Poult Sci 1982 Mar; 61 (3): 488-94.

(402) Reddy BS. Dietary fiber and colon carcinogenesis: a critical review. In: Vahouny GV, Kritchevsky D, eds. Dietary fiber in health and disease. New York: Plenum Press, 1982: 265-85.

(403) Reddy NR, Salunkhe DK, Sathe SK. Biochemistry of black gram (Phaseolus mungo L.): a review. CRC Crit Rev Food Sci Nutr 1982 Jan; 16 (1): 49-114.

(404) Rees DA, Williamson FB, Frangou SA, Morris ER. Fragmentation and modification of ι-carrageenan and characterisation of the polysaccharide order-disorder transition in solution. Eur J Biochem 1982 Feb; 122 (1): 71-9.

(405) Reichert RD, MacKenzie SL. Composition of peas (Pisum sativum) varying widely in protein content. J Agric Food Chem 1982 Mar-Apr; 30 (2): 312-7.

(406) Reinhold JG. Binding of iron by fiber of wheat and maize (letter). Am J Clin Nutr 1982 Jun; 35 (6): 1500-1.

(407) Reinhold JG, Garcia L. PM, Arias-Amado L, Garzon P. Dietary fiber-iron interactions: fiber-modified uptakes of iron by segments of rat intestine. In: Vahouny GV, Kritchevsky D, eds. Dietary fiber in health and disease. New York: Plenum Press, 1982: 117-32.

(408) Reissell P, Manninen V. Effect of administration of activated charcoal and fibre on absorption, excretion and steady state blood levels of digoxin and digitoxin. Evidence for intestinal secretion of the glycosides. Acta Med Scand (Suppl) 1982; 668: 88-90.

(409) Rendleman JA. Cereal complexes: binding of calcium by bran and components of bran. Cereal Chem 1982 Jul-Aug; 59 (4): 302-9.

(410) Rendleman JA, Grobe CA. Cereal complexes: binding of zinc by bran and components of bran. Cereal Chem 1982 Jul-Aug; 59 (4): 310-7.

(411) Ristow KA, Gregory JF III, Damron BL. Effects of dietary fiber on the bioavailability of folic acid monoglutamate. J Nutr 1982 Apr; 112 (4): 750-8.

(412) Rivellese A, Perrotti N, Genovese S, Santoro D, Giacco A, Riccardi G. The separate influence of dietary fibre and digestible carbohydrates on blood glucose control in diabetic patients (abstract). Diabetologia 1982 Aug; 23 (2): 195.

(413) Roberts RL, Cabib E. Serratia marcescens chitinase: one-step purification and use for the determination of chitin. Anal Biochem 1982; 127 (2): 402-12.

(414) Roediger WE, Rae DA. Trophic effect of short chain fatty acids on mucosal handling of ions by the defunctioned colon. Br J Surg 1982 Jan; 69 (1): 23-5.

(415) Roediger WE. Utilization of nutrients by isolated epithelial cells of the rat colon. Gastroenterology 1982 Aug; 83 (2): 424-9.

(416) Rogel AM, Vohra P. The effects of complex polysaccharides on growth, digestibility and blood parameters in pair-fed chicks. Nutr Res 1982; 2 (1): 39-49.

(417) Rosenberg S, Landay R, Klotz SD, Fireman P. Serum IgE antibodies to psyllium in individuals allergic to psyllium and English plantain. Ann Allergy 1982 May; 48 (5): 294-8.

(418) Rotenberg S, Eggum BO, Hegedus M, Jacobsen I. The effect of pectin and microbial activity in the digestive tract on faecal excretion of amino acids, fatty acids, thiamin, riboflavin, and niacin in young rats. Acta Agric Scand 1982; 32 (3): 309-19.

(419) Rotenberg S, Andersen JO. The effect of antibiotics on some lipid metabolism parameters in rats receiving corn starch, potato flour or pectin in the diet. Acta Agric Scand 1982; 32 (3): 321-40.

(420) Rozen P, Horwitz C, Gilat T. Can changes in dietary habits prevent colorectal cancer? In: Malt RA, Williamson RC, eds. Colonic carcinogenesis. Lancaster, England: MTP Press 1982: 101-5.

(421) Rozen P, Horwitz C, Gilat T. Dietary habits and colorectal cancer (abstract). Scand J Gastroenterol 1982; 17 (Suppl 78): 300.

(422) Rubinstein E, Andersen JR, Krag E. The effect of cereal fibers on bile lithogenicity in healthy, middle-aged, overweight women (abstract). Scand J Gastroenterol 1982; 17 (Suppl 78): 140.

(423) Rydning A, Berstad A, Aadland E, Odegaard B. Prophylactic effect of dietary fibre in duodenal ulcer disease. Lancet 1982 Oct 2; 2 (8301): 736-9.

(424) Sacquet E, Leprince C, Riottot M. Dietary fiber and cholesterol and bile acid metabolisms in axenic (germfree) and holoxenic (conventional) rats. I — Effect of wheat bran. Reprod Nutr Dev 1982; 22 (2): 291-305.

(425) Sacquet E, Leprince C, Riottot M. Dietary fiber and cholesterol and bile acid metabolisms in axenic (germfree) and holoxenic (conventional) rats. II — Effect of pectin. Reprod Nutr Dev 1982; 22 (3): 575-81.

(426) Salimath PV, Tharanathan RN. Carbohydrates of field bean (Dolichos lablab). Cereal Chem 1982 Sep-Oct; 59 (5): 430-5.

(427) Sandberg A-S, Hasselblad C, Hasselblad K, Hulten L. The effect of wheat bran on the absorption of minerals in the small intestine. Br J Nutr 1982 Sep; 48 (2): 185-91.
(428) Sanderson GR. The interactions of xanthan gum in food systems. In: Phillips GO, Wedlock DJ, Williams PA, eds. Gums and stabilisers for the food industry. Interactions of hydrocolloids. Oxford: Pergamon Press, 1982: 77-87. (Prog Food Nutr Sci; vol 13.)
(429) Sandstead HH. Copper bioavailability and requirements. Am J Clin Nutr 1982 Apr; 35 (4): 809-14.
(430) Santhakumari G, Bhaskaran Nair R, Varma RR. Effect of guar feeding on the lipid profiles of hypercholesterolaemic rats and rabbits. Planta Med 1982 Jan; 44 (1): 57-60.
(431) Sartor G, Carlstrom S, Schersten B. Dietary supplementation of fibre (Lunelax) as a means to reduce postprandial glucose in diabetics. Acta Med Scand 1982; Suppl 656: 51-3.
(432) Satoh H, Guth PH, Grossman MI. Role of food in gastrointestinal ulceration produced by indomethacin in the rat. Gastroenterology 1982 Jul; 83 (1 Pt 2): 210-5.
(433) Saunders RM. Digestibility of wheat bran in rats, chicks, calves and pigs (abstract). Cereal Foods World 1982 Sep; 27 (9): 459.
(434) Sayre RN, Saunders RM, Enochian RV, Schultz WG, Beagle EC. Review of rice bran stabilisation systems with emphasis on extrusion cooking. Cereal Foods World 1982 Jul; 27 (7): 317-22.
(435) Sayre RN, Fong RY, Randall JM, Schultz WG, Mossman AP, Nayyar D, Tribelhorn RE, Saunders RM. Stabilization of rice bran and recovery of edible oil (abstract). Cereal Foods World 1982 Sep; 27 (9): 454.
(436) Schemann M, Ehrlein H-J. The utility of cellulose meals for studies on gastrointestinal motility in dogs. Digestion 1982 Nov; 25 (3): 194-6.
(437) Schneeman BO. Pancreatic and digestive function. In: Vahouny GV, Kirtchevsky D, eds. Dietary fiber in health and disease. New York: Plenum Press, 1982: 73-83.
(438) Schneeman BO, Richter BD, Jacobs LR. Response to dietary wheat bran in the exocrine pancreas and intestine of rats. J Nutr 1982 Feb; 112 (2); 283-6
(439) Schrezenmeir J, Kasper H. The influence of dietary-fibre substances on the release of gastrointestinal hormones. In: Kasper H, Goebell H, eds. Colon and nutrition. Lancaster, England: MTP Press, 1982: 71-6.
(440) Schrijver M, Tytgat GN. Fibres, nutrition and the gut. Neth J Med 1982; 25 (2): 49-55.
(441) Schwandt P, Richter WO, Weisweiler P, Neureuther G. Cholestyramine plus pectin in treatment of patients with familial hypercholesterolemia. Atherosclerosis 1982 Sep; 44 (3): 379-83.
(442) Schwartz SE, Levine GD, Starr CM. Effects of dietary fiber on intestinal ion fluxes in rats. Am J Clin Nutr 1982 Dec; 36 (12): 1102-5.
(443) Schwartz SE, Levine RA, Singh A, Scheidecker JR, Track NS. Sustained pectin ingestion delays gastric emptying. Gastroenterology 1982 Oct; 83 (4): 812-7.
(444) Sculati O, Giampiccoli G, Gozzi B, Minissale V, Zambetti N, Iapichino G, Ipezzoli C, Giacomelli M, Lazzari P, Franzosi MG. Bran diet for an earlier resolution of post-operative ileus. J Int Med Res 1982; 10 (3): 194-7.
(445) Segal I, Walker AR. Diverticular disease in urban Africans in South Africa. Digestion 1982 May; 24 (1): 42-6.
(446) Segal I, Walker AR. Appendicitis in South African Blacks (letter). S Afr Med J 1982 Jan 30; 61 (5): 144.
(447) Segal I, Walker AR. Preliminary study of dietary factors in the aetiology of certain non-infective intestinal diseases (abstract). S Afr Med J 1982 Nov 20; 62 (22): 828.
(448) Shah N, Mahoney RR, Pellett PL. Effect of guar gum, pectin and lignin on protein utilization and proteolytic enzyme levels in growing rats (abstract). Fed Proc 1982 Mar 1; 41 (3): 399.
(449) Shah N, Atallah MT, Mahoney RR, Pellett PL. Effect of dietary fiber components on fecal nitrogen excretion and protein utilization in growing rats. J Nutr 1982 Apr; 112 (4): 658-66.
(450) Sharma RV, Sharma SC, Prasad Y. Effect of pectin on carbohydrate and fat metabolism. Indian J Med Res 1982 Nov; 76: 771-5.

(451) Sherman P. Hydrocolloid solutions and gels. Sensory evaluation of some textural characteristics and their dependence on rheological properties. In: Phillips GO, Wedlock DJ, Williams PA, eds. Gum and stabilisers for the food industry. Interactions of hydrocolloids. Oxford: Pergamon Press, 1982: 269-84. (Prog Food Nutr Sci; vol 13.)

(452) Sherwin LG, Melton SL. Effect of carboxymethylcellulose and soy protein isolates on development and breakdown of high fiber doughs during mixing (abstract). Cereal Foods World 1982 Sep; 27 (9): 470.

(453) Sherwin LG, Melton SL. Effect of carboxymethylcellulose and soy protein isolates on starch viscosity during heating of high fiber dough systems (abstract). Cereal Foods World 1982 Sep; 27 (9): 470.

(454) Shiau S-Y, Chang GW. Effects of dietary fiber on colonic mucin degradation and β-glucuronidase activity in rats (abstract). Fed Proc 1982 Mar 1; 41 (3): 400.

(455) Shima K, Tabata M, Tanaka A, Kumahara Y. Effect of dietary fiber (guar gum and konjac powder) on diabetic control. In: Melish JS, Hanna J, Baba S, eds. Genetic environmental interaction in diabetes mellitus. Amsterdam: Excerpta Medica, 1982: 313-8.

(456) Shima K, Ikegami H, Tanaka A, Ezaki A, Kumahara Y. Effect of dietary fiber, konjac mannan and guar gum, on absorption of sulfonylurea in man. Nutr Rep Int 1982 Aug; 26 (2): 297-302.

(457) Shimoyama R, Uehara S, Itagaki Y, Izumiyama S, Hirayama A. Effect of guar intake on plasma somatostatin-like immunoreactivity in diabetic patients. Hokkaido Igaku Zasshi 1982 Nov; 57 (6): 727-33.

(458) Silva HC, Braga GL. Effect of soaking and cooking on the oligosaccharide content of dry beans (Phaseolus vulgaris, L.). J Food Sci 1982 May-Jun; 47 (3): 924-5.

(459) Simons LA, Gayst S, Balasubramaniam S, Ruys J. Long-term treatment of hyper-cholesterolaemia with a new palatable formulation of guar gum. Atherosclerosis 1982 Oct; 45 (1): 101-8.

(460) Simpson HC, Mann JI, Chakrabarti R, Imeson JD, Stirling Y, Tozer M, Woolf L, Meade TW. Effect of high-fibre diet on haemostatic variables in diabetes. Br Med J 1982 May 29; 284 (6329): 1608.

(461) Simpson HC, Carter RD, Lousley S, Mann JI. Digestible carhobydrate — an inde-pendent effect of diabetic control in type 2 (non-insulin-dependent) diabetic patients? Diabetologia 1982 Sep; 23 (3): 235-9.

(462) Singh U, Kherdekar MS, Jambunathan R. Studies on desi and kabuli chickpea (Cicer arietinum L.) cultivars. The levels of amylase inhibitors, levels of oligosaccharides and in vitro starch digestibility. J Food Sci 1982 Mar-Apr; 47 (2): 510-2.

(463) Siragusa RJ, Cerda JJ. Methanol production from the degradation of pectin by human colonic bacteria (abstract). Am J Clin Nutr 1982 Apr; 35 (4): 822.

(464) Skovolsen P, Kirkegaard P, Poulsen SS. The effect of ileotransversotomy on carrageenan-induced colitis in guinea pigs (abstract). Scand J Gastroenterol 1982; 17 (Suppl 78): 353.

(465) Smalley JR, Klish WJ, Campbell MA, Brown MR. Use of psyllium in the management of chronic nonspecific diorrhea of childhood. J Pediatr Gastroenterol Nut 1982; 1 (3): 361-3.

(466) Smith AN. Effects of fibre on colonic function and motility. In: Kasper H, Goebell H, eds. Colon and nutrition. Lancaster, England: MTP Press, 1982: 181-7.

(467) Smith AN, Chalmers K, Wilson JM, Eastwood MA. Has the advent of fibre changed diverticular disease (abstract). Scand J Gastroenterol 1982; 17 (Suppl 78): 523.

(468) Smith CJ, Rosman MS, Levitt NS, Jackson WP. Guar biscuits in the diabetic diet. S Afr Med J 1982 Feb 6; 61 (6): 196-8.

(469) Smith J, Mitchell JR, Ledward DA. Effect of the inclusion of polysaccharides on soya extrusion. In: Phillips GO, Wedlock DJ, Williams PA, eds. Gums and stabilisers for the food industry. Interactions of hydrocolloids. Oxford: Pergamon Press, 1982: 139-47. (Prog Food Nutr Sci; vol 13.)

(470) Smith T. Chestnuts, fats, and fibre. Br Med J 1982 July 10; 285 (6335): 116-7.

(471) Smith U, Holm G. Effect of a modified guar gum preparation on glucose and lipid levels in diabetics and healthy volunteers. Atherosclerosis 1982 Oct; 45 (1): 1-10.

(472) Solomons NW. Biological availability of zinc in humans. Am J Clin Nutr 1982 May; 35 (5): 1048-75.

(473) Soni GL, George M, Singh R. Role of common Indian pulses as hypocholesterolemic agents. Indian J Nutr Diet 1982 Jun; 19 (6): 184-90.

(474) Sorenson J, Murray N. Increased fiber. Bishop's Corner, West Hartford, Connecticut: Witkower Press, 1982. (Menus for better health series.)

(475) Sosulski FW, Elkowicz L, Reichert RD. Oligosaccharides in eleven legumes and their air-classified protein and starch fractions. J Food Sci 1982 Mar-Apr; 47 (2): 498-502.

(476) Sosulski FW, Cadden AM. Composition and physiological properties of several sources of dietary fiber. J Food Sci 1982 Sep-Oct; 47 (5): 1472-7.

(477) Southgate DA. Definitions and terminology of dietary fiber. In: Vahouny GV, Kritchevsky D, eds. Dietary fiber in health and disease. New York: Plenum Press, 1982: 1-7.

(478) Southgate DA. Digestion and absorption of nutrients. In: Vahouny GV, Kritchevsky D, eds. Dietary fiber in health and disease. New York: Plenum Press, 1982: 45-52.

(479) Spiller GA. Nutritional factors in the aetiology and treatment of constipation. In: Kasper H, Goebell H, eds. Colon and nutrition. Lancaster, England: MTP Press, 1982: 189-92.

(480) Spiller GA. Colon cancer and dietary fiber: an overview. In: Vahouny GV, Kritchevsky D, eds. Dietary fiber in health and disease. New York: Plenum Press, 1982: 237-8.

(481) Spiller GA, Wong LG, Whittam JH, Scala J. Correlation of gastrointestinal transit time to fecal weight in adult humans at two levels of fiber intake. Nutr Rep Int 1982 Jan; 25 (1): 23-30.

(482) Stanley NF. The effect of carrageenan on peptic and tryptic digestion of casein. In: Phillips GO, Wedlock DJ, Williams PA, eds. Gums and stabilisers for the food industry. Interactions of hydrocolloids. Oxford: Pergamon Press, 1982: 161-70. (Prog Food Nutr Sci; vol 13.)

(483) Stein DT, Ballin R, Stone BG. Endoscopic removal of gastric phytobezoars. J Clin Gastroenterol 1982 Aug; 4 (4): 329-32.

(484) Story L, Anderson JW, Sieling B, Chen W. High-carbohydrate, high-fiber diets for lean insulin-treated diabetic men: long term effects (abstract). Diabetes 1982 May; 31 (Suppl 2): 58A.

(485) Story JA, Thomas JN. Modification of bile acid spectrum by dietary fiber. In: Vahouny GV, Kritchevsky D, eds., Dietary fiber in health and disease. New York: Plenum Press, 1982: 193-201.

(486) Story JA, Kelley MJ. Dietary fiber and lipoproteins. In: Vahouny GV, Kritchevsky D, eds. Dietary fiber in health and disease. New York: Plenum Press, 1982: 229-36.

(487) Story JA, White A, West LG. Adsorption of bile acids by components of alfalfa and wheat bran in vitro. J Food Sci 1982 Jul-Aug; 47 (4): 1276-9.

(488) Strobel S, Ferguson A, Anderson DM. Immunogenicity of foods and food additives — in vivo testing of gums arabic, karaya and tragacanth. Toxicol Lett 1982 Dec; 14 (3-4): 247-52.

(489) Sugano M, Fujisaki Y, Oku H, Ide T. 3-Hydroxy-3-methylglutaryl coenzyme A reductase activity in the small intestine of rats fed non-purified and semipurified diets. J Nutr 1982 Jan; 112 (1): 51-9.

(490) Swick A, Kies C, Fox HM. Blood serum lipid patterns of lacto-ovo-vegetarians and omnivore subjects fed vegetarian, lacto-vegetarian and omnivore diets supplemented with wheat bran (abstract). Fed Proc 1982 Mar 1; 41 (3): 774.

(491) Tadesse K. The effect of dietary fibre on gastric secretion and emptying in man (abstract). J Physiol (Lond) 1982; 332: 102P-3P.

(492) Takeda H, Tsujita J, Emoto T, Ebihara K, Kiriyama S. Nutritional significance of dietary fiber in counteracting the amaranth-toxicity in rats: a possible explanation of the mechanism. Nutr Rep Int 1982 Jan; 25 (1): 169-87.

(493) Tasman-Jones C, Owen RL, Jones AL. Semipurified dietary fiber and small-bowel morphology in rats. Dig Dis Sci 1982 Jun; 27 (6): 519-24.

(494) Taupin PJ, Anderson DM. Subchronic toxicity study in rats fed gum karaya. Food Chem Toxicol 1982 Oct; 20 (5): 513-7.

(495) Taylor AJ, Pritchard S. The potential of peapods as food thickeners. J Sci Food Agric 1982 Apr; 33 (4): 384-8.

(496) Testolin G, Bossi E, Vercesi P, Porrini M, Simonetti P, Ciappellano S. A rapid method for the analysis of alimentary fiber. Nutr Rep Int 1982 Jun; 25 (6): 859-65.

(497) Tharp BW. The effect of certain colloid/emulsifier blends and processing procedures on emulsion stability. In: Phillips GO, Wedlock DJ, Williams PA, eds. Gums and stabilisers for the food industry. Interactions of hydrocolloids. Oxford: Pergamon Press, 1982: 209-19. (Prog Food Nutr Sci; vol 13.)

(498) Theander O, Aman P. Studies on dietary fibre. A method for the analysis and chemical characterisation of total dietary fibre. J Sci Food Agric 1982 Apr; 33 (4): 340-4.

(499) Thom D, Dea IC, Morris ER, Powell DA. Interchain associations of alginate and pectins. In: Phillips GO, Wedlock DJ, Williams PA, eds. Gums and stabilisers for the food industry. Interactions of hydrocolloids. Oxford: Pergamon Press, 1982: 97-108. (Prog. Nutr Sci; vol 13.)

(500) Thomas JN, Kelley MJ, Petro MS, Story JA. Modification of cholesterol regression in rats by pectin and lignin (abstract). Fed Proc 1982 Mar 1; 41 (3): 398.

(501) Thomas WR. The practical application of microcrystalline cellulose in foods. In: Phillips GO, Wedlock DJ, Williams PA, eds. Gums and stabilisers for the food industry. Interactions of hydrocolloids. Oxford, Pegamon Press, 1982: 341-51. (Prog Food Nutr Sci; vol 13.)

(502) Thompson MH. The role of diet in relation to faecal bile acid concentration and large bowel cancer. In: Malt RA, Williamson RC, eds. Colonic carcinogenesis. Lancaster, England: MTP Press, 1982: 49-56.

(503) Thompson SA, Weber CW. Copper and zinc binding to dietary fiber sources: an ion exchange column method. J Food Sci 1982 Jan-Feb; 47 (1): 125-6, 133.

(504) Thomsen LL, Tasman-Jones C, Lee SP, Robertson AM. Dietary factors in the control of pH and volatile fatty acid production in the rat caecum. In: Kasper H, Goebell H, eds. Colon and nutrition. Lancaster, England: MTP Press, 1982: 47-51.

(505) Thomsen LL, Tasman-Jones C. Disaccharidase levels of the rat jejunum are altered by dietary fibre. Digestion 1982 Apr; 23 (4): 253-8.

(506) Thomson M, Logan RL, Sharman M, Lockerbie L, Riemersma RA, Oliver MF. Dietary survey in 40-year-old Edinburgh men. Hum Nutr: Appl Nutr 1982 Aug; 36A (4): 272-80.

(507) Toft K. Interactions between pectins and alginates. In: Phillips GO, Wedlock DJ, Williams PA, eds. Gums and stabilisers for the food industry. Interactions of hydro-colloids. Oxford: Pergamon Press, 1982: 89-96. (Prog Food Nutr Sci; vol 13.)

(508) Tovey FI, Jayaraj AP, Clark CG. Fibre and duodenal ulcers (letter). Lancet 1982 Oct 16; 2 (8303): 878.

(509) Track NS, Cannon MM, Flenniken A, Katamay S, Woods EF. Improved carbohydrate tolerance in fibre-fed rats: studies of the chronic effect. Can J Physiol Pharmacol 1982 Jun; 60 (6): 769-76.

(510) Treuherz J. Possible inter-relationship between zinc and dietary fibre in a group of lacto-ovo vegetarian adolescents. J Plant Foods 1982; 4 (2): 89-93.

(511) Trout DL, Ryan RO, Osilesi O. The amount and distribution of water and dry matter in the digestive tract of rats fed xanthan gum (abstract). Fed Proc 1982 Mar 1; 41 (3): 711.

(512) Trowell H. Indigestible residue or dietary fiber (letter). Am J Clin Nutr 1982 Jul; 36 (1): 194-5.

(513) Trowell J. Coronary disease (letter). Br Med J 1982 Sep 11; 285 (6343): 738.

(514) Tsuji K, Nakagawa Y, Iwao H, Okamatsu H, Yatake T, Tanaka S, Tanaka M. Influence of a microbial polysaccharide produced by Bacillus polymyxa no. 271 on cholesterol metabolism in rats. Nutr Rep Int 1982 Aug; 26 (2): 231-8.

(515)   Tucker GA, Robertson NG, Grierson D. Purification and changes in activities of tomato pectinesterase isoenzymes. J Sci Food Agri 1982 Apr; 33 (4): 396-400.

(516)   Turnlund JR. Bioavailability of selected minerals in cereal products. Cereal Foods World 1982 Apr; 27 (4): 152-7.

(517)   Uden P, Van Soest PJ. Comparative digestion of timothy (Phleum pratense) fibre by ruminants, equines and rabbits. Br J Nutr 1982 Mar; 47 (2): 267-72.

(518)   Uden P, Rounsaville TR, Wiggans GR, Van Soest PJ. The measurement of liquid and solid digesta retention in ruminants, equines and rabbits given timothy (Phleum pratense) hay. Br J Nutr 1982 Sep; 48 (2): 329-39.

(519)   Ullrich IH, Albrink MJ. Lack of effect of dietary fiber on serum lipids, glucose, and insulin in healthy young men fed high starch diets. Am J Clin Nutr 1982 Jul; 36 (1): 1-9.

(520)   Ullrich IH, Albrink MJ. Insulin-raising effect of dietary sucrose and its prevention by dietary fiber (abstract). Diabetes 1982 May; 31 (Suppl 2): 158A.

(521)   Ulman EA, Fisher H. Influence of simple versus complex carbohydrates on the arginine requirement of weanling rats (abstract). Fed Proc 1982 Mar 1; 41 (3): 540.

(522)   Uttenthal LO, Harris A, Yeats JC, Ghatei MA, Sagor GR, Polak JM, Bloom SR. Acarbose and guar have different effects on appetite and regulatory peptides in the rat (abstract). Diabetologia 1982 May; 22 (5): 397.

(523)   Uttenthal LO, Ghatei MA, Al-Mukhtar MY, Yeats JC, Sagor GR, Wright NA, Harris A, Polak JM, Bloom SR. Effect of acarbose and guar on gut regulatory peptides in the rat (abstract). Scand J Gastroenterol 1982; 17 (Suppl 78): 505.

(524)   Vahouny GV. Conclusions and recommendations of the symposium on 'Dietary fibers in health and disease,' Washington DC, 1981. Am J Clin Nutr 1982 Jan; 35 (1): 152-6.

(525)   Vahouny GV, Kritchevsky D, eds. Dietary fiber in health and disease. New York: Plenum Press, 1982.

(526)   Vahouny GV. Dietary fibers and intestinal absorption of lipids. In: Vahouny GV, Kritchevsky D, eds. Dietary fiber in health and disease. New York: Plenum Press, 1982: 203-27.

(527)   Vahouny GV. Dietary fiber, lipid metabolism, and atherosclerosis. Fed Proc 1982 Sep; 41 (11): 2801-6.

(528)   Valceschini G, Kies C, Fox HM. Protein status of humans fed moderate and low residue enteral formulas (abstract). Fed Proc 1982 Mar 1; 41 (3): 275.

(529)   Van Dokkum W, Wesstra A, Schippers FA. Physiological effects of fibre-rich types of bread. 1. The effect of dietary fibre from bread on the mineral balance of young men. Br J Nutr 1982 May; 47 (3): 451-60.

(530)   Van Dokkum W, De Vos RH, Cloughley FA, Hulshof KF, Dukel F, Wijsman JA. Food additives and food components in total diets in The Netherlands. Br J Nutr 1982 Sep; 48 (2): 223-31.

(531)   van Raaij JM, Katan MB, West CE, Hautvast JG. Influence of diets containing casein, soy isolate, and soy concentrate on serum cholesterol and lipoproteins in middle-aged volunteers. Am J Clin Nutr 1982 May; 35 (5): 925-34.

(532)   Van Staveren WA, Hautvast JG, Katan MB, Van Montfort MA, Van Oosten-Van Der Goes HG. Dietary fiber consumption in an adult Dutch population. J Am Diet Assoc 1982 Apr; 80 (4): 324-30.

(533)   Varel VH, Pond WG, Pekas JC, Yen JT. Influence of high-fiber diet on bacterial populations in gastrointestinal tracts of obese- and lean-genotype pigs. Appl Environ Microbiol 1982 Jul; 44 (1): 107-12.

(534)   Veeraraghavan K, Regunathan S, Srimathi V, Venugopala Rao A, Ramakrishnan S. Effect of dietary cane sugar and Bengal gram on blood lipids and insulin. Ind J Biochem Biophys 1982 Dec; 19 (6): 415-7.

(535)   Vessby B, Karlstrom B, Gustafsson I-B, Lithell H, Boberg M, Werner I. Comparison between the effects of two diabetic diets with different content of cereal fibre in type II diabetics. Acta Endocrinol (Copenh) 1982; Suppl 247: 61.

(536) Vidal-Valverde C, Blanco I, Rojas-Hidalgo E. Pectic substances in fresh, dried, dessicated and oleaginous Spanish fruits. J Agric Food Chem 1982 Sep-Oct; 30 (5): 832-5.

(537) Vidal-Valverde C, Herranz J, Blanco I, Rojas-Hidalgo E. Dietary fiber in Spanish fruits. J Food Sci 1982 Nov-Dec; 47 (6): 1840-5.

(538) Voragen AG, Schols HA, Pilnik W. HPLC analysis of anionic gums. In: Phillips GO, Wedlock DJ, Williams PA, eds. Gums and stabilisers for the food industry. Interactions of hydrocolloids. Oxford: Pergamon Press, 1982: 379-85. (Prog Food Nutr Sci: vol 13.)

(539) Vorster HH. The functional mechanism of dietary fibre — is chrome the answer? S Afr Med J 1982 Aug 14; 62 (8): 227-8.

(540) Wahren J, Juhlin-Dannfelt A, Bjorkman O, De Fronzo R, Felig P. Influence of fibre ingestion on carbohydrate utilization and absorption. Clin Physiol 1982 Aug; 2 (4): 315-21.

(541) Walker AF. Physiological effects of legumes in the human diet: a review. J Plant Foods 1982; 4 (1): 5-14.

(542) Walker AR, Segal I, Hathorn S. Dietary fibre and survival (letter). Lancet 1982 Oct; 2 (8305): 980.

(543) Walker AR, Burkitt DP. Plant fiber in the pediatric diet (letter). Pediatrics 1982 Jan; 69 (1): 130-1.

(544) Walker AR, Walker BF, Bhamjee D, Walker EJ, Ncongwane J, Segal I. Defaecation frequencies in Black, Indian, Coloured and White populations — what do they signify? S Afr Med J 1982 Aug 7; 62 (7): 195-9.

(545) Walker AR. The significance of non-infective bowel disease in urban black populations (abstract). Scand J Gastroenterol 1982; 17 (Suppl 78): 541.

(546) Ward GM, Simpson RW, Simpson HC, Naylor BA, Mann JI, Turner RC. Insulin receptor binding increased by high carbohydrate low fat diet in non-insulin-dependent diabetics. Eur J Clin Invest 1982 Apr; 12 (2): 93-6.

(547) Wedman B. Dietary prescription for high fiber diets (abstract). Diabetes 1982 May; 31 (Suppl 2): 109A.

(548) Weinreich J. Controlled studies with dietary fibre in the therapy of diverticular disease and irritable bowel syndrome. In: Kasper H, Geobell H, eds. Colon and nutrition. Lancaster, England: MTP Press, 1982: 239-49.

(549) Welsh JD, Manion CV, Griffiths WJ, Bird PC. Effect of psyllium hydrophilic mucilloid on oral glucose tolerance and breath hydrogen in postgastectomy patients. Dig Dis Sci 1982 Jan; 27 (1): 7-12.

(550) Westland P. The high-fibre cookbook. Recipes for good health. London: Martin Dunitz, 1982. (Positive health guide.)

(551) Williams CA, MacDonald I. Serum glucose and insulin responses in man, after varying the viscosity of starch (abstract). Proc Nutr Soc 1982 Jun; 41 (2): 47A.

(552) Williams PC, Starkey PM. A modification of the crude fiber test for application to flour. Cereal Chem 1982 Jul-Aug; 59 (4): 318.

(553) Williams VJ, Senior W. Effects of caecectomy on the digestibility of food and rate of passage of digesta in the rat. Austr J Biol Sci 1982: 35 (4): 373-9.

(554) Wilson JN, Wilson SP, Eaton RP. Effect of soluble fiber intake upon lipoprotein metabolism in genetic hyperlipemic rats (abstract). Am J Clin Nutr 1982 Apr; 35 (4): 862.

(555) Wirth A, Middelhoff G, Braeuning C, Schlierf G. Treatment of familial hypercholesterolemia with a combination of bezafibrate and guar. Atherosclerosis 1982 Dec; 45 (3): 291-7.

(556) Wise A, Mallett AK, Rowland IR. Dietary fibre, bacterial metabolism and toxicity of nitrate in the rat. Xenobiotica 1982 Feb; 12 (2): 111-8.

(557) Wojcik J, Delorme CB. The effect of dietary cellulose level on the utilization of amino acid-supplemented bread protein by weanling rats. Nutr Rep Int 1982 Apr; 25 (4): 709-20.

(558) Wolever TM, Jenkins DJ. The glycaemic index: implications of dietary fibre and the digestibility of different carbohydrate foods in the management of diabetes. J Plant Foods 1982; 4 (3): 127-38.

(559) Wong MA, Oace SM. Cecal microflora are required for pectin digestion and pectin induced vitamin B-12 deficiency symptoms in the rat (abstract). Fed Proc 1982 Mar 1; 41 (3): 711.

(560) World Health Organisation. Thickening agents. In: Evaluation of certain food additives and contaminants. Geneva: WHO, 1982: 28-30. (Twenty-sixth report of the Joint FAO/WHO Expert Committee on Food Additives.)

(561) Wyn-Jones E, Pereira MC, Morris ER. Ultrasonic relaxation studies in sols and gels. In: Phillips GO, Wedlock DJ, Williams PA, eds. Gums and stabilisers for the food industry. Interactions of hydrocolloids. Oxford: Pergamon Press, 1982: 21-31. (Prog Food Nutr Sci; vol 13.)

(562) Yoshida M, Izumi K, Nakata Y, Terada A, Furasawa M, Onodera C, Nakamura H. Fiber content in Japanese food and application of a high-fiber diet in the treatment of diabetes. In: Melish JS, Hanna J, Baba S, eds. Genetic environmental interaction in diabetes mellitus. Amsterdam: Excerpta Medica, 1982: 319-22.

(563) Zoppi G, Gobio-Casali L, Deganello A, Astolfi R, Saccomani F, Cecchettin M. Potential complications in the use of wheat bran for constipation in infancy. J Pediatr Gastroenterol Nutr 1982; 1 (1): 91-5.

BULGARIAN

(564) Apostolov I, Goranov I, Balabanski L, Krusteva A, Popova D. Serum lipid studies in hyperlipoproteinemia patients during diet therapy with pectin preparations (English abstract). Vutr Boles 1982; 21 (1): 51-4.

(565) Todorova S, Veleva N, Arnaudov I, Taneva T, Andreev D. Effect of dietetic fruit products prepared with sorbitol and pectin on the blood sugar and insulin levels in diabetic patients (English abstract). Vutr Boles 1982; 21 (5): 88-96.

CZECH

(566) Zamrazilova E. Dietary fiber. Cesk Gastroenterol Vyz 1982 Sep; 36 (6): 339-43.

DANISH

(567) Christensen MF. Do bulk preparations help in cases of recurrent abdominal pain in children (English abstract). Ugeskr Laeger 1982 Mar 8; 144 (10): 714-5.

(568) Pedersen O, Schwartz Sorensen N, Helms P, Winther E, Palmvig B. Diet for diabetics (English abstract). Ugeskr Laeger 1982 Oct 4; 144 (40): 2921-9.

(569) Rasmussen SN, Bondesen S, Edmund C, Frandsen I, Andersen I, Kempel K, Nielsen K. Treatment of irritable bowel with dietary fiber. A controlled clinical study (English abstract). Ugeskr Laeger 1982 Aug 16; 144 (33): 2415-7.

DUTCH

(570) Katan MB, van de Bovenkamp P. Analysis of total dietary fibre and pectin in Dutch foodstuffs (English abstract). Voeding 1982 May 15; 43 (5): 153-60.

(571) van Olffen GH, Tytgat GN. A belly full of bran. Ned Tijdschr Geneeskd 1982 Oct 30; 126 (44): 1993-5.

FINNISH

(572) Tarpila S. Dietary fiber and health. Duodecim 1982; 98 (2): 1738-47.

FRENCH

(573) Bezanger-Beauquesne L, Pinkas M. Trotin F. Uronic gums and mucilages (English abstract). Ann Pharm Fr 1982 Jul; 40 (2): 179-90.

(574) Chevrel B. Dietary fibres. Med Chir Dig 1982; 11 (2): 147-9.

(575) Curtois J-E. Request for authorization to use carboxymethyl-cellulose in various food products. Bull Acad Natl Med (Paris) 1982 Jun; 166 (6): 853-4.

(576) Grimaldi A, Engels J, Brassier D, Maisani E. Phytobezoar secondary to diabetic gastro-
       pathy (letter). Nouv Presse Med 1982 Jan 30; 11 (4): 282.
(577) Pradeau D, Bellenger P, Hamon M. Methods for identification of various industrial
       carbohydrate thickeners (English abstract). Ann Pharm Fr 1982; 40 (6): 555-66.

GERMAN
(578) Brandes J-W, Korst HA, Littmann K-P. Sugar-free diet as a long term treatment or
       intermittent treatment during remission in Crohn's disease — a prospective study
       (English abstract). Leber Magen Darm 1982 Nov; 12 (6): 225-8.
(579) Gruhn K, Hashish S, Richter G. Determination of the digestibility of the crude
       nutrients and the amino acids of two varieties of horse bean (Vicia faba L.) in colo-
       stomised laying hens (English abstract). Arch Tierernahr 1982 Sep; 32 (9): 651-8.
(580) Hansen WE. Effects of dietary fiber on the upper gastrointestinal tract (English
       abstract). Klin Wochenschr 1982 Dec 15; 60 (24): 1475-83.
(581) Harmuth-Hoene AE, Meier-Ploeger A, Leitzmann C. Effect of carob bean gum on
       absorption of minerals and trace elements in man (English abstract). Z Ernahrungswiss
       1982; 21 (3): 202-13.
(582) Jacorzynski B, Filutowicz H. Excretion of carbohydrates by rats fed legume seeds
       (English abstract). Nahrung 1982; 26 (10): 875-85.
(583) Kasper H. Fiber-rich and fiber-poor diets. Use in gastrointestinal diseases. MMW 1982
       Dec 10; 124 (49): 1108.
(584) Matek W, Fruhmorgen P, Reimann J F, Demling L. Treatment of chronic constipation
       with swelling substances (English abstract). Fortschr Med 1982 Jan 14; 100 (1-2):
       16-9.
(585) Meixner B, Hennig A. Screening of ergotropic agents with broilers using hydrocolloid-
       rich feed mixtures (English abstract). Z Versuchstierkd 1982; 24 (4): 219-24.
(586) Nuske J, Grimmecke HD, Reuter G. Polysaccharide structure of cell wall preparations
       from the food protein yeast Candida spec. H. (English abstract). Z Allg Mikrobiol
       1982; 22 (7): 477-86.
(587) Rabast U, Gotz ML. Negative effects of dietary bulk. Med Klin (Prax) 1982 Apr 9;
       77 (8): 42-9.
(588) Stransky M, Wild R, Schonhauser R, Blumenthal A. Nutrient and fiber content of
       infant food (English abstract). Helv Paediatr Acta 1982 Jun; 37 (3): 205-13.
(589) Thomann R, Piechaczek R. Gell chromatographic investigations of rye pentosans
       (English abstract). Nahrung 1982; 26 (10): 915-21.
(590) Thomann R, Scheinemann K. A favourable method for determination of soluble
       pentosans (English abstract). Nahrung 1982; 26 (6): 515-8.
(591) Zilly W, Kuhlmann J, Kasper H, Richter E. Effect of a fiber-rich diet on digoxin
       resorption (English abstract). Med Klin (Prax) 1982 Sep 10; 77 (19): 42-8.

HEBREW
(592) Rattan J. Should we be wary of a high-fiber diet (editorial). Harefuah 1982 Mar 1;
       102 (5): 212-3.

ITALIAN
(593) Bertoncini M, Nanni G, Sganga G, Pepoli R, Ticozzelli GF, Bergamini C. Mechanical
       ileus caused by phytobezoar of the small intestine after gastric surgical interventions.
       Observations on two cases (English abstract). Minerva Chir 1982 May 15; 37 (9):
       807-12.
(594) Falchi A, Androsoni GP, Arganini E, Gervino L, Palagi P, Rapisarda V. An unusual
       late complication of gastric resection. Intestinal occlusion caused by phytobezoars.
       Minerva Chir 1982 Nov 30; 37 (22): 2035-8.
(595) Nardi R, D'Anastasio C, Agostini D, Ferroni R, Pieromaldi S, Vecchi F, Zanichelli L.
       Effects of guar gum in non-diabetic obese women aged over 50 years (English abstract).
       Minerva Dietol Gastroenterol 1982 Oct-Dec; 28 (4): 341-6.
(596) Scevola F. The importance of intestinal pH in the appearance of colo-rectal tumours.
       Minerva Med 1982 Feb 25; 73 (7): 348-50.

JAPANESE
(597) Kitagawa K, Takashima T, Ida M, Truber E, Fuchs H. Imaging of the small intestine using an aqueous solution of methylcellulose (English abstract). Rinsho Hoshasen 1982 Sep; 27 (9): 963-7.
(598) Suzuki M, Aoyama H. Preventive effects of fiber against the toxicity of edible tar dyes in rats (English abstract). Nippon Eiseigaku Zasshi 1982 Oct; 37 (4): 714-21.

NORWEGIAN
(599) Skjerven O. Dietary fibers in the nursing homes of Troms. Tidsskr Nor Laegeforen 1982 Sep 30; 102 (27): 1395-6.

POLISH
(600) Gronowska-Senger A, Sobczak Z, Smaczny E. Dietary fibre determination in foods by the enzymatic method (English abstract). Rocz Panstw Zakl Hig 1982; 33 (3): 179-84.
(601) Los-Kuczera M, Piekarska J. Effect of dietary fibre on absorption of minerals. Zywienie Czlowieka 1982; 9 (3-4): 111-6.
(602) Zarnecka M. Pectins and disorders of lipid and carbohydrate metabolism. Zywienie Czlowieka i Metabolizm 1982; 9 (1-2): 23-32.

PORTUGUESE
(603) Coelho JV, Ribiero T de C, Paula Castro L. de. Effect of dietary fiber content in nutrition on various stool parameters in man (English abstract). Arg Gastroenterol 1982 Jan-Mar; 19 (1): 17-21.

RUSSIAN
(604) Dederer IM, Ustinov GG. Nutrition and biliary calculi. Vopr Pitan 1982 May-Jun; (3): 7-12.
(605) Mansurov KK. Dietary fiber and diseases of the digestive organs. Sov Med 1982; (7): 60 8.
(606) Rigo J. Role of food fibers in nutrition (English abstract). Vopr Pitan 1982 Jul-Aug; (4): 26-30.

SPANISH
(607) Garcia R, Graza S, de la Graza S, Espinosa-Campos J, Ovalle-Berumen F. High fiber diet prepared with regional foods as an aid in the control of patients with diabetes (English abstract). Rev Invest Clin 1982 Apr-Jun; 34 (2): 105-11.

SWEDISH
(608) Ahlman H. Total obstruction of oesophagus after intake of natural products. Lakartidningen 1982 Apr 14; 79 (15): 1479.
(609) Edstrom S, Pettersson G. Esophageal rupture after intake of natural products. Lakartidningen 1982 Apr 14; 79 (15): 1478-9.
(610) Tibbling L. Bulk laxatives — are the rules harder against the natural preparations than against the drugs. Lakartidningen 1982 Jul 14; 79 (28-9): 2621-2.

Ferns G: 125
Ferroni R: 595
Fetuga BL: 302, 373
Ficken VJ: 357
Fielden H: 231
Fielding JF: 159
Filutowicz H: 582
Fineberg SE: 211
Finney KF: 60
Fireman P: 417
Fisher A: 207
Fisher H: 521
Fishman A: 278
Fleming SE: 160, 315
Flenniken A: 509
Floren C-H: 161, 162
Florent C: 165
Florholmen J: 163, 164
Flourie B: 165
Fonagy P: 76
Fong RY: 435
Fontana D: 44
Ford CW: 166
Forman LP: 167
Fotsis T: 2
Fox HM: 490, 528
Francis T: 229
Frandsen I: 569
Frangou SA: 404
Franzosi MG: 444
Frape DL: 169
Freeman HJ: 170
Frenkiel P: 171
Friend DR: 172
Frommer D: 283
Fruhmorgen P: 316, 584
Fuchs H: 597
Fujisaki Y: 489
Fukuba H: 173
Fulcher RG: 174
Furasawa M: 562
Fuwa H: 261

Gabbe SG: 175
Gadzinowska A: 197
Gallaher D: 176
Galton DJ: 124, 125
Garcia R: 607
Garcia L. PM: 407
Garcia-Lopez S: 177
Gardner RS: 10, 11
Garza S: 607
Garzon P: 407
Gawecki J: 178
Gayst S: 459
Ge M: 377
Gee JM: 50

Gelroth JA: 396
Genovese S: 412
George M: 473
Gervino L: 594
Ghafari H: 231
Ghatei MA: 522, 523
Giacco A: 412
Giacomelli M: 444
Giampiccoli G: 444
Gibney MJ: 179
Gidley MJ: 339, 387
Gilat T: 420, 421
Gill AA: 180
Gilmore C: 171
Glahn P-E: 181
Glantz I: 118
Glauert HP: 182
Glicksman M: 183, 184, 185
Gobio-Casali L: 563
Goff DV: 228
Goldin BR: 2, 186
Golechha AC: 187
Goodwin C: 350
Goranov I: 37, 564
Gorbach SL: 2, 186
Gordon C: 397
Gormley TR: 320
Goto Y: 220
Gotz ML: 587
Goulet G: 291
Gozzi B: 444
Graham DY: 188
Grammer JC: 189
Gray GM: 374
Green DJ: 290
Gregory JF III: 411
Grewal RB: 245
Grierson D: 515
Griffin D: 290
Griffiths C: 228
Griffiths WJ: 549
Grimaldi A: 576
Grimmecke HD: 586
Grisebach H: 307
Grobe CA: 410
Groen MB: 101
Gronowska|Senger A: 600
Grossman MI: 432
Gruden N: 190
Gruhn K: 579
Gueguen L: 31, 32
Guild RT: 33, 191
Gumbmann MR: 361, 374
Guoo JY: 90
Gurr MI: 306
Gustafsson I-B: 535
Guth PH: 432

Hales PW: 192
Hall MJ: 153
Hallmans G: 45, 363, 364
Hamon M: 577
Hansen JB: 328
Hansen PM: 193
Hansen WE: 194, 580
Hara T: 220
Harding LK: 290
Harmuth-Hoene AE: 581
Harold M: 195
Harris A: 522, 523
Harris ND: 127
Harrop R: 196
Hartog M: 64, 199
Hasegawa K: 256
Hashish S: 579
Hasik J: 197
Hasler K: 297
Hasselblad C: 427
Hasselblad K: 427
Hathorn S: 542
Hautvast JG: 531, 532
Hayashi J: 282
Hayes KC: 292
Hayes TM: 156
Heaton KW: 64, 198, 199,
    200
Hegde SN: 201
Hegedus M: 418
Heikkinen R: 2
Hein C: 264
Helliwell S: 133
Helms P: 110, 144, 202, 383,
    384, 568
Henckel S: 137
Hennig A: 585
Henquin J-C: 112
Henry CL: 199
Herman GO: 175
Hernandez D: 75
Herranz J: 537
Hill AD: 142
Hill MJ: 203, 204, 205, 206
Hillman LC: 207
Hjollund E: 208, 209, 383,
    384
Hryniewiecki L: 197
Hintz HF: 122
Hobson BM: 16
Hockaday TD: 210
Hodges G: 377
Hoffman CR: 211
Hogan M: 191
Hollingsworth DR: 356
Holly RG: 39
Holm G: 471

Rotenberg S: 136, 418, 419
Rounsaville TR: 518
Rowland IR: 556
Rozen P: 269, 420, 421
Rubinstein E: 422
Russell RI: 153
Ruys J: 459
Ryan RO: 380, 511
Ryder E: 278
Rydning A: 423

Saccomani F: 563
Sacquet E: 424, 425
Sagor GR: 522, 523
Saito N: 3
Salimath PV: 426
Saltin B: 300
Salunkhe DK: 403
Sandberg A-S: 427
Sanderson GR: 428
Sandman P-O: 364
Sandstead HH: 46, 429
Santhakumari G: 430
Santoro D: 412
Sarson DL: 228
Sartor G: 24, 431
Sathe SK: 403
Satoh H: 432
Satterlee LD: 1
Saunders RM: 361, 433, 434,
    435
Savage DC: 41
Sayre RN: 434, 435
Scala J: 481
Scevola F: 596
Schatz G: 307
Scheidecker JR: 443
Scheinemann K: 590
Schemann M: 436
Schersten B: 24, 431
Schippers FA: 529
Schlierf G: 555
Schmahl D: 269
Schneeman BO: 154, 167,
    176, 437, 438
Schoenfield L: 171
Schols HA: 538
Schonhauser R: 588
Schreve RH: 283
Schrezenmeir J: 243, 439
Schrijver M: 440
Schultz WG: 434, 435
Schulz G: 194
Schwandt P: 441
Schwartz S: 175
Schwartz SE: 299, 442, 443
Schwartz Sorensen N: 208,

383, 384, 568
Sculati O: 444
Segal I: 445, 446, 447,
    542, 544
Senior W: 553
Seppanen R: 144
Sganga G: 593
Shah N: 448, 449
Sharma BB: 262
Sharma RK: 262
Sharma RV: 450
Sharma S: 262
Sharma SC: 450
Sharma SK: 187
Sharman M: 506
Sherman P: 451
Sherwin LG: 452, 453
Shiau S-Y: 454
Shibata M: 246
Shima K: 455, 456
Shimoyama R: 457
Shine B: 124
Shurpalekar KS: 241
Sieling B: 484
Siltanen I: 214
Silva HC: 458
Simonetti P: 496
Simons LA: 459
Simpson FJ: 336
Simpson HC: 460, 461, 546
Simpson RW: 546
Singh A: 299
Singh R: 473
Singh U: 462
Siragusa RJ: 463
Skjerven O: 599
Skovolsen P: 464
Slama G: 388
Slaughter P: 304
Slavin JL: 314
Sly MR: 270
Smaczny E: 600
Smalley JR: 465
Smith AN: 132, 466, 467
Smith CJ: 468
Smith DB: 180
Smith DM: 131
Smith J: 469
Smith JC Jr: 142
Smith JH: 131, 133
Smith L: 179
Smith MA: 259
Smith PM: 254
Smith T: 470
Smith U: 471
Smoot JM: 308
Snoswell AM: 217

Sobczak Z: 600
Solomons NW: 472
Soni GL: 473
Sorensen NS: 209
Sorenson J: 474
Sosulski FW: 475, 476
Southgate DA: 144, 477, 478
Spiller GA: 479, 480, 481
Sreebny LM: 236
Srimathi V: 534
Stace NH: 207
Stamler J: 301
Stanley NF: 482
Stansberry SC: 359, 360
Starkey PM: 552
Starr CM: 442
Staub H: 8
Stegner J: 9
Stein DT: 483
Stenling R: 364
Stirling Y: 460
Stone BG: 483
Story JA: 250, 271, 485,
    486, 487, 500
Story L: 484
Stransky M: 588
Street CA: 16
Street JC: 49
Strobel S: 488
Sugahara T: 282
Sugano M: 218, 489
Suzuki M: 598
Suzuoki Z: 318
Sweetnam PM: 70
Swenson L: 186
Swick A: 490

Tabata M: 455
Tada N: 352
Tadesse K: 491
Takahashi Y: 263
Takashima T: 597
Takeda H: 492
Takehisa F: 268
Takeyama S: 352
Taljedal I-B: 45
Tanaka A: 455, 456
Tanaka M: 514
Tanaka S: 514
Tandon RK: 242
Taneva T: 565
Tannock GW: 57
Tarpila S: 572
Tasman-Jones C: 493, 504,
    505
Taupin PJ: 494
Taylor AJ: 206, 495

Taylor KG: 125
Taylor LJ: 338
Taylor RH: 228, 229, 231,
    232
Tchobroutsky G: 388
Tepper SA: 265
Terada A: 562
Testolin G: 496
Tharanathan RN: 426
Tharp BW: 497
Theander O: 235, 498
Thibault JF: 322
Thom D: 499
Thomann R: 589, 590
Thomas JN: 250, 485, 500
Thomas WR: 501
Thompson LU: 229
Thompson MH: 206, 283,
    502
Thompson SA: 503
Thomsen LL: 504, 505
Thomson M: 506
Thorbek G: 137
Thorne MJ: 229
Tibbling L: 610
Ticozzelli GF: 593
Tobin J Sr: 372
Todorova S: 565
Toft K: 507
Togei K: 246
Tominaga A: 218
Tomkin GH: 320
Topping DL: 217
Toulson E: 377
Tovey FI: 508
Tozer M: 460
Track NS: 299, 443, 509
Treuherz J: 510
Trevisan M: 301
Tribelhorn RE: 435
Trimble RP: 217
Trotin F: 573
Trout DL: 380, 511
Trowell HC: 27, 28, 512
Trowell J: 513
Truber E: 597
Truswell AS: 238
Tsuchihashi N: 216
Tsuji K: 514
Tsujita J: 492
Tuck MG: 169
Tucker GA: 515
Turner RC: 546
Turnlund JR: 516
Tytgat GN: 440, 571

Uchino H: 223

Uden P: 517, 518
Uebersax MA: 115, 116
Ueda H: 368
Uehara S: 457
Uenoyama R: 126
Ullrich IH: 7, 350, 519, 520
Ulman EA: 521
Ustinov GG: 604
Utille J-P: 56
Uttenthal LO: 522, 523

Vahouny GV: 83, 84, 524,
    525, 526, 527
Valceschini G: 528
Valle MA: 75
Van Buren JP: 260, 366
van de Bovenkamp P: 570
van der Vies J: 101
Van Dokkum W: 529, 530
Van Montfort MA: 532
van Olffen GH: 571
Van Oosten-Van Der Goes
    HG: 532
van Raaij JM: 531
Van Rensburg SJ: 270
Van Schalkwyk DJ: 270
Van Soest PJ: 122, 140, 517,
    518
Van Staveren WA: 532
Varel VH: 533
Varma RR: 430
Vaughan LA: 334
Vecchi F: 595
Veeraraghavan K: 534
Veleva N: 565
Venugopala Rao A: 534
Vercesi P: 496
Vessby B: 535
Vidal-Valverde C: 536, 537
Vidon N: 165
Vohra P: 416
Vonk Noordegraaf CA: 101
Voragen AG: 538
Vorster HH: 539

Wadsworth J: 41
Wagner JR: 374
Wahal PK: 262
Wahren J: 540
Wahrendorf J: 234
Wait R: 206
Walker AF: 541
Walker AR: 445, 446, 447,
    542, 543, 544, 545
Walker BF: 544
Walker EJ: 544
Ward GM: 546

Warram JH: 186
Watters DA: 132
Wayman BJ: 169
Weaver AC: 100
Webs B: 319
Weber CW: 503
Weder JK: 43
Wedlock DJ: 10, 11, 385
Wedman B: 547
Weinreich J: 548
Weisweiler P: 441
Welsh JD: 357, 549
Welsh K: 44
Werner I: 535
Wesstra A: 529
West CE: 531
West LG: 487
Westin SI: 22
Westland P: 550
White A: 487
Whittam JH: 481
Wiggans GR: 518
Wiggins HS: 143, 144
Wijsman JA: 530
Wild R: 588
Williams CA: 551
Williams KA: 244
Williams PA: 97, 190, 389
Williams PC: 552
Williams VJ: 553
Williamson FB: 404
Wilson JM: 467
Wilson JN: 554
Wilson SP: 554
Winawer SJ: 130
Winblad B: 364
Winship DH: 343
Winterringer GL: 396
Winther E: 568
Wirth A: 555
Wise A: 556
Wojcik J: 117, 557
Wolever TM: 228, 231, 232,
    558
Wolstrup J: 30, 139
Wong LG: 481
Wong MA: 559
Wood PJ: 174
Woods EF: 509
Woods MN: 2, 186
Woolf L: 460
Wright JL: 336
Wright NA: 523
Wyatt CJ: 177
Wyn-Jones E: 561

Yamada N: 368

General Index

Diabetics, 29
  Mineral balance in, 77
  Obese, 49, 53
Dietary fibre
  Analysis, 83, 85
  Blood lipids, and, 23
  Collaborative trials, 87
  Components, 84
  Composition of foods (tables), 88, 89
  Definition, 83
  Diabetes, and, 47
  Digestibility, 4, 7, 61
  Food products, and, 83
  Fractionation methods, 85, 86
  Gallstones, and, 3
  Gravimetric methods, 85
  Intakes, 89, 90
  Large gut, and, 3
  Mineral absorption, and, 72
  Neutral detergent (NDF), 6
  Obesity, 61, 68
  Overweight, 68
  Water insoluble, 7
Dietary intake, 47
  Energy, 31, 40, 41
  Fat, 31, 41
  Protein, 4, 6
  Sugar, 41
Dietary simple sugars in diabetes, 55
Diets
  High carbohydrate, high fibre, 29, 31, 47, 48, 49,
    50, 52, 94
  High fibre, 48, 51
  Low carbohydrate, 47, 50
  Modified fat, 24
Digestibility
  Carbohydrate, 64
  Fibre, 4, 7, 61
  Protein, 64
Digestion of foods (*in vitro*), 54
Diverticular disease, 11, 95

Emotional stress, 5
Energy density of food, 61
Eubacteria, 8
Exercise, 5
Experimental carcinogenesis, 14

Faecal
  Acid steroids, 4, 5
  Amino acids, 4
  Bulk, 5
  Carbohydrate, 4
  Fat, 4, 31, 65
  Flora, 8
  Minerals, 4
  Nitrogen, 4, 65
  Weight, 3, 4, 8, 10, 11, 12
Fibre tablets, 68
Flatus, 9, 10
Flavones, 14
Food products, 83
Formate, 8

Fruits, 7, 11, 23, 24, 26, 76, 85
  Fibre content, 88
Fusobacteria, 8

Galacto-mannans, 8
  See guar gum
Gallstones, 23, 40
Gases, 7, 9
Gastric emptying, 52, 53, 64, 65
Glucose, blood, 47, 49, 50, 51, 52, 54, 65, 91, 93
Glucose kinetic studies, 52
beta-Glucuronidase, 8, 15
Glycaemic index, 54
beta-Glycans, 91
  Soluble, 25
Glycoproteins, 8
Grains, 7
  Fibre content, 89
Guar gum, 3, 6, 9, 15, 16, 27, 29, 31, 32, 47, 52, 53,
  55, 62, 64, 65, 91, 92, 93, 99
  Bread, 49, 93, 94, 95
  Crispbread, 49, 93
  Granola bar, 94, 95
  Granulated, 49, 53
  Pasta, 94
Gum acacia, 27
Gum karaya, 27
Gut hormones, 32, 52, 65

Haemorrhoids, 16, 95
Hemicellulose, 7, 44, 64
Hiatus hernia, 16
High fibre foods, 90
Hormones
  Gut, 32, 52, 65
  Insulin, 40
Hunger, 63
Hydrogen, 8
  Breath hydrogen, 9, 10, 51
3 Hydroxy-3 methyl glutaryl coenzyme A
  (HMGCoA) reductase, 40, 42
Hypercholesterolaemia, 24
Hyperglycaemia, 40
Hyperlipidaemia, 90
  See cholesterol
Hypertriglyceridaemia, 40

Ileostomy studies, 31, 64, 73
Indole, 8, 14
Inflammatory bowel disease, 13
Insulin, 40
  Insulin responses, 31, 52, 65, 91, 93
  Insulin sensitivity, 52
  Insulinogenic hormones, 52
Intestinal absorption
  Carbohydrate, 52
  Cholesterol, 31
  Fat, 31
Intestinal convective mixing, 53
Iron, 72, 73, 75, 78
Irritable bowel syndrome, 12, 95
Ischaemic heart disease (IHD), 23
Isothiocyanates, 14